Thinking with Metaphors in Medicine

While medical language is soaked in metaphor, and thinking with metaphor is central to diagnostic work, medicine – that is, medical culture, clinical practice and medical education – outwardly rejects metaphor for objective, literal scientific language. This thought-provoking book argues that this is a misstep, and critically considers what embracing the use of metaphors, similes and aphorisms might mean for shaping medical culture, and especially the doctor–patient relationship, in a healthy way.

Thinking with Metaphors in Medicine explores:

- how metaphors inhabit medicine – sometimes for the better and sometimes for the worse – and how these metaphors can be revealed, appreciated and understood;
- how diagnostic work utilizes thinking with metaphors;
- how patient–doctor communication can be better understood and enhanced as a metaphorical exchange;
- how the landscape of medicine is historically shaped by leading or didactic metaphors, such as 'the body as machine' and 'medicine as war', which may conflict with other values or perspectives on healthcare, for instance, person-centred care.

Outlining the kinds of metaphors that inhabit medicine and how they shape practices and identities of doctors, colleagues and patients, this book demonstrates how the landscape of medicine may be reshaped through metaphor shift. It is an important work for all those interested in the use of language in medicine, whether hailing from a humanities, social science or healthcare background.

Alan Bleakley is Emeritus Professor at the University of Plymouth's Peninsula Schools of Medicine and Dentistry, UK.

Routledge Advances in the Medical Humanities

New titles

Medicine, Health and the Arts
Approaches to the Medical
Humanities
Edited by Victoria Bates,
Alan Bleakley and Sam Goodman

Suffering Narratives of Older
Adults
A Phenomenological Approach to
Serious illness, Chronic Pain,
Recovery and Maternal Care
Mary Beth Morrissey

Medical Humanities and Medical
Education
How the Medical Humanities Can
Shape Better Doctors
Alan Bleakley

Learning Disability and Inclusion
Phobia
Past, Present and Future
C. F. Goodey

Collaborative Arts-based Research
for Social Justice
Victoria Foster

Person-centred Health Care
Balancing the Welfare of Clinicians
and Patients
Stephen Buetow

Digital Storytelling in Health and
Social Policy
Listening to Marginalized Voices
Nicole Matthews and
Naomi Sunderland

Bodies and Suffering
Emotions and Relations of Care
Ana Dragojlovic and Alex Broom

Thinking with Metaphors in
Medicine
The State of the Art
Alan Bleakley

Forthcoming titles

The Experience of
Institutionalisation
Social Exclusion, Stigma and Loss
of Identity
Jane Hubert

Thinking with Metaphors in Medicine

The State of the Art

Alan Bleakley

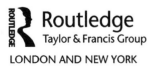

Routledge
Taylor & Francis Group

LONDON AND NEW YORK

First published 2017 by Routledge

2 Park Square, Milton Park, Abingdon, Oxfordshire OX14 4RN
52 Vanderbilt Avenue, New York, NY 10017

Routledge is an imprint of the Taylor & Francis Group, an informa business

First issued in paperback 2019

British Library Cataloguing in Publication Data
A catalogue record for this book is available from the British Library

Library of Congress Cataloging in Publication Data
Names: Bleakley, Alan (Alan Douglas), author.
Title: Thinking with metaphors in medicine : the state of the art /
Alan Bleakley.
Other titles: Routledge advances in the medical humanities.
Description: Abingdon, Oxon ; New York, NY : Routledge, 2017. |
Series: Routledge advances in the medical humanities | Includes
bibliographical references and index.
Identifiers: LCCN 2017005930| ISBN 9781138229440 (hbk) |
ISBN 9781315389448 (ebk)
Subjects: | MESH: Metaphor | Physician-Patient Relations | Language |
Interprofessional Relations | Education, Medical
Classification: LCC R727.3 | NLM W 62 | DDC 610.69/6–dc23
LC record available at https://lccn.loc.gov/2017005930

ISBN: 978-1-138-22944-0 (hbk)
ISBN: 978-0-367-22439-4 (pbk)

Typeset in Times New Roman
by Wearset Ltd, Boldon, Tyne and Wear

I would like to thank my loving family, especially my wife Sue, who puts up with my grumpy behaviour when I am writing; and when I am not writing.

Overheard in a hospital corridor:

'That's the surgeon who stitched me up.'

Overheard on the way into theatre from a senior gastrointestinal surgeon:

'That bloody medical student's late again – I'll have his guts for garters!'

Contents

Forewords

Introduction to forewords

Doctors and poets share the attribute of 'close noticing'. It is the basis of both creative writing and diagnostic acumen. Here is the poet Anthony Hecht: 'Each hanging waterdrop burns with a fierce/Bead of the sun's instilling'; and here, the surgeon Richard Selzer (who retired from surgery to write full time): 'in that place where he *knows* the duct to be, there is none. Only masses of scar curtained with blood vessels of unimagined fragility.' Hecht's waterdrop 'burns' (fiercely), while Selzer's scar is 'curtained' – both writers realize close noticing as poetic observation. Both waterdrop and blood vessels are pregnant with possibility. Hecht's observation treats the body of language, whereas Selzer's has a dual role – treating both the human body and the language that describes it, saving the latter from impoverishment (the given role of the poet, such as Hecht, in the world of lay observation).

I am honoured that two poets – both experts in close noticing – have contributed separate forewords to this book. One is a physician (Shane Neilson), the other an academic (Jeffery Donaldson). Their paths intertwine – Shane is, at the time of writing, a PhD candidate in English (researching and writing about pain) at McMaster University in Canada, where Jeffery is his supervisor. Jeffery has written a groundbreaking book on metaphor and science: *Missing Link: The Evolution of Metaphor and the Metaphor of Evolution* (2015). At one time, they had considered writing a joint contribution, but decided on separate forewords to this book. I am the beneficiary of their decisions, receiving a double bounty of curtained scars and fiercely burning waterdrops. They are generous in their observations of my work, and go well beyond mere commentary to offer original insights. They are experts in treating otherwise languishing language by shifting so skilfully into poetic registers that their close noticing in itself shines, sometimes with an unnerving dark glow, as well as shedding light on the surroundings. Their work enriches our lives, and their respective forewords substantially enrich this book.

Foreword 1

Shane Neilson: Carrying the day

Medical metaphors as disciplinary self-improvement instruments

As a poet who learned from other poets and their poetry before entering medical school, my belief in the power and primacy of metaphor was pre-established. If anything, medical school only reinforced my predisposition. From learning that a very sick patient could be said to 'circle the drain' before they might die in a controlled ICU setting, to the stultifyingly ubiquitous 'cancer=war' metaphor, I saw little reason to trade in a metaphor habit for a supposedly more objective means of conceptualizing clinical encounters since I'd have to reach for a metaphor anyway in order to explain what I'd just seen to the impatiently attending physician. Wanting the facts presented to them in as concise a fashion as possible, I might say 'Mr. Snide's circling the drain', and the senior doctor would immediately know how dire the situation was. No time factor about prognosis need be relayed, no fallible prediction of how long the patient might have before the physician need arrive at the bedside, no prolonged recitation of central line measurements. Language like 'The patient's condition is critical' or 'The patient is about to die' just can't convey the immediacy of the aforementioned drain metaphor. That kind of language is dead, a passively emergent code. (In the ICU, everyone is 'critical' and, in a sense, everyone might die. Nothing quite puts a needed spring in the step like a metaphor!) Metaphoric communication is rich, special, resonant: the human as near-effluent, the human essence about to be siphoned away. Or how about 'Mrs. Langille's crashing', as if the human is being hurled into a concrete embankment. Metaphors such as these have a practical function: they make doctors move, releasing them from a state of perpetual management of static emergency into the apprehension of the real thing.

When relating patient histories, my command of metaphor and narrative meant that I distinguished myself from other students inclined to skip to the application of rulers to skin lesions. I might not have been the student with the most encyclopaedic factual knowledge, I was comically far from the best proceduralist, and I chafed under authority, but I got through by listening, interpreting, and using metaphors. I owe metaphors for carrying me across the student threshold. Unlike many of my colleagues, I've *always* felt metaphors to be important, pervasive, and fundamentally *practical*. If a poem can't get by without them, then medicine can't, either.

As it happens, medicine doesn't get by without them. Medicine needs metaphor. Yet the twentieth- and twenty-first-century biomedical imperative elides metaphor in favour of statistical significance, in favour of research data that, no matter how strongly biomedicine seeks to obscure metaphor, will always be somehow structured by metaphor itself. Go ahead: explain statistical significance to me without throwing that statistical football long down the field towards the entity known as 'significance' … and what about 'face validity'? Not to mention the rather impressive system of metaphor research itself is predicated upon.

Medicine is not alone in neglecting the importance of metaphor. Even in the humanities, metaphor is thought of as old hat – a branch of rhetoric that, as a subject of academic study, has long been circling the drain. Literary studies left the literary long ago in favour of more fashionable things like race, gender, sexuality, class, and mad studies. Lately there's been a renaissance: the study of metaphor is making a comeback thanks to an ironic saviour. Ghettoized for too long as relevant only to arts and humanities practice, the analysis of metaphor has extended to the realm known as – I purposely put the term in scare quotes, for there is no pure concept without a metaphor lurking as impurity – 'Science'.

Implicit in the branches of various kinds of scientific inquiry, including medicine, are a host of metaphors used in systematic ways to broker how information is transformed into knowledge. Because the things we discover must enter into language in order to be known, and because language is inherently metaphorical, the renaissance is overdue. For if we are not aware of the metaphors we use, if we are not aware of how we know and how we come to know things, then we are ironically in the dark about our knowledge – its limits, the vistas we're not exploring, the self-satisfaction and complacency of a little going too long a way.

The specific domain of medicine is the quarry of Alan Bleakley's new book. A Professor Emeritus of Medical Education and Medical Humanities at Plymouth University Peninsula School of Medicine, Bleakley is an internationally renowned researcher, award-winning teacher, poet, and author of several acclaimed textbooks. He has written *Thinking with Metaphors in Medicine* not as a one-dimensional defence or exposé of metaphor in medical practice, education and research but, rather, as a contextualization of metaphor in a space uniquely suited to its study. He carries metaphor into unexpected places for the good of medical practice, research and education.

Metaphor, as Bleakley explains, is derived from the Greek *metapherein*, meaning 'to carry across'. Metaphors are meant to create understanding of things in relation to other things, for ideas to be carried across using other ideas. In other words, the metaphor creates a space for understanding that is somehow filled with likeness and unlikeness both – a liminal space in which seemingly contrary forces literally carry the day and create understanding, a message delivered where there was ignorance. As Bleakley demonstrates, medicine is a liminal field, both art and science, in the ideal circumstance not one component working against the other but both components working in collaboration to produce a host of metaphors that, depending on the situation, can be constructive, destructive, and often both at once.

Bleakley conducts a survey of Western literature, moving from Aristotle's poetics to the present day. He closely examines a burgeoning linguistics research undertaken in the past 20 years, punctuating these findings with a deep awareness of the classics (Bleakley is as comfortable discussing a medical humanities study as he is unpacking metaphors from the plays of Shakespeare). Enacted in every sentence are the stakes of his case: that metaphor is more than merely 'there', that metaphor works to create certain kinds of understanding and works against other kinds, and that to be aware of the implications of medical metaphors is to know how research and care might be better harnessed or improved. Bleakley shows how metaphor shouldn't be thrown out with the bathwater, à la Sontag, and instead should be interrogated and refined.

The effects of such a prescription might result in a course correction for Borg Biomedicine™, a powerful way to accumulate knowledge that's sailing too blind for safety and comfort. The unconscious metaphors we practice medicine by might become the metaphors we see by, metaphors that might constitute either headwinds to the goal or rocks threatening to sink the ship of medical progress (notwithstanding the fact that 'progress' itself is one of the dominant metaphors of medicine). A student on a hospital ward in Leeds might exclaim, 'Mr. Snide is circling the drain' and wonder about the connotations of juxtaposing 'the human' near 'sewage', spurring him to reach for a better metaphor. Prejudicial metaphors that reflect unconscious and conscious bias towards marginalized groups like the elderly, poor and racialized persons will appear on the radar of our disciplinary self-improvement. As Bleakley so beautifully writes, 'Metaphor is both a thing and a process; both that which is magnified and the magnifying lens.' May the art and science of medicine consider this book in order to get a better grasp of the thing known as metaphor and carry it across the field of inquiry like a magnifying lens.

Dr Shane Neilson is a Canadian prize-winning poet, writer, editor, critic and physician completing a PhD in English at McMaster University on pain. He lives in Guelph, Ontario with his family and has a medical practice in Erin, Ontario. Shane is poetry editor for Frog Hollow Press. His writing includes a collection of short stories (*Will* 2013) and a number of poetry collections, including *On Shaving Off His Face* (2015).

Foreword 2

Dr Jeffery Donaldson: The Patient Poem

It is a pleasure for me to twirl a baton at the front of Alan Bleakley's welcome parade, with its various floats, its marshalled demonstrations and dazzling manoeuvres. Its time has come. The planned route has gradually come clear to him, and onlookers are gathered in anticipation. Why, you can almost hear the different drummers around the bend. I speak metaphorically, of course, but I also mean what I say, and so does Bleakley.

Every living moment is shot through with relational tensions, the bodies and processes that science describes no less than the words we use to communicate them. Part of Bleakley's important work here is to open up our thinking, again metaphorically, to other ways in which our states of being might be explored and understood. He starts at the beginning, as one always must, with our general prejudice that metaphor is restricted to a certain language function and no more. You can say something as blatantly indicative as 'the patient is on the table' and feel that metaphor plays no part in its work. But relations abound. How do you know that 'patient' here is a noun and not an adjective? By context, you say: the word means 'to weave together'. What about the metaphoric leap that you have to make between the letters p-a-t-i-e-n-t and the physical body you have decided it captures in actual space? And how does the mere proximity to 'table' change your thoughts about the patient? It becomes a specimen, an object to be tinkered with or repaired. I need only say something like 'the patient is up his tree' (how do you picture him now?) for you to see how meanings and messages are transformed by relational tensions in the most innocent of expressions. And never mind any further point that you might wish to argue. Logic itself requires a series of leaps across minute gaps that are bridged by finer and finer component similarities that are ultimately inexhaustible. We have scarcely begun to understand how the diminutive A = B changes everything.

As the book unfolds, Bleakley's application of metaphor turns from product to process, from a listing of the metaphors we use to an exploration of relational energies, a practice of understanding. He offers a corrective to the constrained habit of thinking that to study metaphor is to study a mere list of deviant tropes. This was the largely structuralist approach of Lakoff and Johnson's powerful *Metaphors We Live By*, where we learned how our thought is constituted by metaphoric substitutions that determine and even distort our thinking. Bleakley walks us through all the implications for the practice of medicine and the behaviour of doctors, where the bias that MEDICINE IS WAR and THE BODY IS A MACHINE has dominated for decades. But he divides from this our need to engage more with the process of metaphoric thinking itself, both in how it informs doctor/patient relations and in the actual practice of medicine. Metaphors can be useful in communicating our states of health and illness, but Bleakley's deeper point is that the very state we seek to describe is metaphorical through and through. We are embodied metaphoric processes: 'Bodies … are not closed but open systems, working by "flows" and "interruptions,"' he writes (personal communication). The sooner we recognize this, the sooner we can harness all the powers of 'thinking more' that are the native right of every living body.

Metaphor is rarely mere substitution, but a play of identity and difference. I say 'my love is a gem' and quicker than thought your idea of love passes through your idea of a gem and becomes on the other side something that is neither your significant other alone nor a piece of hard glass. Something recognizable remains, but a change has occurred. The same goes for you and your body, as Bleakley shows: between the person you were yesterday and the one you may be tomorrow is a gap that is filled with relational energies, a space of play and risk. Inhabiting that gap, you become.

Our desire over the years to rein in metaphor aligns rather suggestively with our desire to rein in illness itself. Metaphors have outcomes and so do people. Parts fall into relation and things happen. We anxious egos have a very particular idea of what counts as a desirable outcome. Metaphors deviate from the status quo, transgress things as they are. They come to the rescue when thought calcifies, becomes too rigid or closed. But what if the status quo happens to be you and your health? You might resent and resist the intrusion. This is metaphor as catachresis, where the idea of error, deviance, and even abuse, predominates. Deviations from health require correctives, not encouragement. Doctors are summoned to control their increase, make them go away, restore us to our former selves. We hand them our bodies run amok, gone astray, deviated. We say, 'look what has happened'. We ask them to fix it, 'say it ain't so', eradicate the intruder. The war metaphors come rushing in. We, the patients, come bearing their standards. This puts doctors on the spot and is deeply counterintuitive so far as metaphoric thinking goes.

One of the outcomes of Bleakley's own metaphoric argument is that we need to engage more with the process of becoming that challenges our sense of what a promising outcome might be. Like metaphor, the processes that we call illness have always been with us and are a part of what makes life possible. When we see metaphor itself as a series of unruly substitutions that 'ain't so', we will constantly struggle to eradicate and contain its invasive ditherings. But if we treat metaphor as a process that pervades all physical and mental states – the hopeful as much as the menacing ones – our relation to it becomes part of a creative initiative, an active collaboration between what it is and who you are. Bleakley's coup (there's that war metaphor again) comes halfway through the book. The patient is a kind of poem: not something to impose meanings upon (as you learned to do in school?), but to be heard out, encouraged, let be. The patient poem (in both senses) is no longer a grumpy text mumbling at you incoherent complaints. It is a work in the making. Doctor and patient collaborate on a living 'body' that is still writing itself out.

Collaborate in the service of what? Good question. Every poem is a unity of relating parts, and so is every body. For a poem to hold together most effectively, certain additions might be unwelcome, because they don't seem to fit with what the entire expression seems to be getting at. Mention of a kitchen sink might not have struck Milton as a useful addition to the opening lines of *Paradise Lost*. As it unfolds, we see the poem itself telling us more and more about what it needs to be, and we negotiate with it, pushing back inventively while also observing its constraints. The unity of the whole is primary. Now let some new addition – a strange growth – multiply and take hold, point in an unfamiliar direction. You might feel that the unity had been spoiled. Or you might feel that it had simply changed and that the poem was now about something else altogether. At a certain point, you have to make a decision: try to undo the additions that have carried you off to strange places, or stop resisting and follow to see where they lead.

So with illness: in collaboration with your doctor, you might argue, for as long as the arguing makes sense, that 'this change is not who I am; let's see if we can get me feeling like my old self again'. But then perhaps you find that the change takes on a life of its own, as it were, becomes a part of who you are, so that there is no way of separating it from you ('surgery would be too risky at this stage'). In the mean time, your body is still becoming. You are still becoming.

Your task now is to make sure that you remain a whole expression of all you might possibly be, given your new reality, for as long as you possibly can.

In such relation, doctors might find themselves freed to pursue the kind of grace that I've always associated with a passage near the end of Henry Adams' *Education*:

> The clouds that gather round the setting sun do not always take a sober coloring from eyes that have kept watch on mortality; or, at least, the sobriety is sometimes scarcely sad. One walks with one's friends squarely up to the portal of life, and bids good-bye with a smile. One has done it so often!

Courage has no small part to play in the risks we take thinking and living metaphorically. But more of it, rather than less, is what the doctor orders. Which returns us to the idea of collaboration. A doctor and patient fall into relation. What will the outcome be? Part of my job might be to remind my fellow non-physicians that some of the new thinking has to come from outside the profession, and goes to what we expect of our doctors as much as what they expect of themselves.

Dr Jeffery Donaldson teaches American literature, poetry and creative writing in the English Department at McMaster University, Hamilton, Ontario, Canada and is passionate about creative pedagogy. He is an established poet (most recently *Slack Action* (Porcupine's Quill, 2013)), critic, and the author of an acclaimed book on metaphor: *Missing Link: the Evolution of Metaphor and the Metaphor of Evolution* (Montreal: McGill-Queens University Press, 2015).

Preface: forewarned

The future imperfect

The celebrated American novelist Don DeLillo's (2016) *Zero K* takes cryogenics as its platform for developing ideas about language and the human condition. DeLillo is a master of the dry and ominous metaphors that describe a world in which relationships are reduced to economic transactions – production and consumption of goods and services. In his masterwork *Underworld* (1997), a man in the throes of insight does not experience anything as trite as the pieces of a puzzle falling into place, or a lightbulb going on in his head; rather, his mouth fills with 'the foretaste of inner shiftings', while another character notes that the air has 'the feel of some auspicious design'. DeLillo's characters stray into the territory of the near future even as they inhabit the ground of the present. And isn't this what a metaphor does? It shifts us from familiar and tepid puddled ground to a hotter place of the future imperfect: 'by the time I reach 33 and complete my specialty surgical training, I will have been studying medicine for nearly 15 years. I am already feeling the burden of responsibility.'

In a world of personalized medicine, in which the genetic 'code' – long since 'cracked' – is now a personalized blueprint by which health and illness may be predicted and appropriate medical interventions planned, we are all living in the near future. De Lillo's novels typically deal with this habitat. *Zero K* imagines a world in which cryogenic suspension is available for the rich few as a choice to make before death – even well before death. This signifies a culture in which the burdens of inevitable illness as ageing encroaches are suspended – for the promise of awakening to a future time in which ageing may be permanently on hold, 'free of the flatlines of the past' (DeLillo 2016, p. 130).

In fact, the first cryopreservation was carried out in 1976, since when around 300 people have been cryopreserved in the USA and 2,500 have signed up for the procedure on their deaths (Brown 2016). To date, only 10 Britons have been 'frozen', including a recent high-profile case of a 14-year-old girl who tragically died from brain cancer. Her parents disagreed about whether she should be 'suspended', and a High Court judge ruled that her mother's opinion, in favour of the procedure, should hold sway. Cryogenics comfortably inhabits the world of metaphor, as does its ethical standing. While it is legal, cryogenic suspension (based in American facilities) is currently unregulated. Cryogenics remains in a suspended state.

What does a future hold in which the cryogenically suspended are released from their ice coffins, thawed and resparked, 'free of the flatlines of the past'? Well, claims one of DeLillo's characters, it will be a radically 'clear' future free of the messy business of metaphor that normally jump-starts our heart the moment we fall out of love with language: 'We will approximate the logic and beauty of pure mathematics in everyday speech. No similes, metaphors, analogies', a language that will 'not shrink' from new forms of 'objective truth'. This, however, merely restates the empiricist philosophical position that no cogent thinking can be done without cleansing language of metaphor and rhetoric, while this very statement itself works because of metaphor ('cleansing' language). DeLillo restates a fundamental contradiction in the logic of science (and, by implication, medicine) – that its practitioners wish to cleanse practice of metaphor, but cannot do this without employing metaphor: the genetic 'code', 'messenger' RNA, genetic 'engineering', cryogenic 'suspension', and so forth. In DeLillo's imagined world, the metaphors of 'codes' and 'engineering' would already seem archaic. First, they imply the building of bodies and cultures ('social engineering') rather than their morphing; second, such metaphors appear as gendered male; and third, they lack an aesthetic and ethical dimension.

In short, discourse is declared, oiled and enriched by metaphors, and the harder we work at eradicating them, the more we seem to draw upon metaphors. So let us bathe in them for a while to slough our thin skins of any residual resistance to metaphor.

Metaphor cleansing: the damned spot will not out

While I was working as a psychotherapist some time ago, a woman made a one-session appointment to talk about her teenage daughter's suspected eating disorder, which she found impossible to discuss face-to-face with her daughter. The opening remarks went something like this:

> I'm *worried sick* about Jane. She *eats like a horse* but is *thin as a rake* and always *on the go*. I'm sure she goes to the loo and makes herself *throw up*, but I just can't *pin her down* to talk – she's *tetchy* all the time, on a *short fuse*. I wondered if you might see her. She might *spill the beans* with you. I think that she's bulimic.

Here is a case of metaphor bulimia – nine in all.

The writer and commentator Susan Sontag famously riled against the abuse of metaphors by the medical profession, in particular where stigma is ascribed to patients' illnesses. For example, cancer is commonly described in terms of conflict and aggression, leaving some patients feeling as if they have failed because they did not fight hard enough. Sontag's (1978, p. 3) memorable opening to *Illness as Metaphor* reminds us that 'Everyone who is born holds dual citizenship, in the kingdom of the well and the kingdom of the sick'. She lets the reader know that she does not want to describe 'what it is really like to emigrate to the kingdom of the ill and live there', but rather, to analyse and contest 'the punitive or sentimental fantasies concocted about that situation'.

Using tuberculosis, cancer and in a second book AIDS (Sontag 1989), as her topics, Sontag argues that illness becomes subject to representation through negative or unhelpful metaphors that are equivalent to 'national stereotypes'. This argument was pushed to its limits. Illness, insists Sontag, is not a metaphor and should not be talked about as metaphor, let alone used as a negative or abusive metaphor. We should liberate ourselves from such 'seductive' metaphorical thinking, which offers a trap. Sontag herself suffered from breast cancer.

Yet Sontag could not help but rail against abuse of metaphors through metaphor-laden writing, reminding us that the best way to study the uses and abuses of metaphors seems to be through the lens of metaphor. Metaphors are an inevitable part of expression and communication – used both to illustrate and to persuade as rhetoric – but must be handled with care. In the opening chapter to *AIDS and Its Metaphors*, Sontag (1989) says that in rereading *Illness as Metaphor* 10 years on, 'I prefaced the polemic I wrote against metaphors of illness … with a brief, hectic flourish of metaphor, in mock exorcism of the seductiveness of metaphorical thinking.'

Sontag accepts that metaphor 'is the spawning ground of most kinds of understanding, including scientific understanding, and expressiveness'. The mock apology was in fact unnecessary. Critics have, perhaps, treated Sontag unfairly for apparently throwing the baby out with the bathwater in her refusal of metaphor in illness. But Sontag was critical only of the conscious or intentional *abuse* of metaphor (and not specifically of unaware misuse), such as martial or violence metaphors commonly used in cancer ('the war on cancer', 'aggressive therapies'), discussed at length in Chapter 4.

In this book, I examine uses and abuses of metaphors in medical contexts. Inevitably, this strays into the wider discourse of healthcare – for example, when discussing metaphors of clinical teamwork involving mixed professions. But I do not focus on the use of metaphors in, say, nursing or physiotherapy or pharmacy. My focus is on the medical profession and the ways that doctors use (and abuse) metaphors to make meanings, for diagnostic purposes, and to communicate with patients and colleagues in healthcare teams.

Acknowledgements

Thanks are due to a network of doctors who, over the years, have understood what I am trying to do in the world of medical education and have wholeheartedly supported my efforts, where others have soon tired of my left field interventions: Dr Robert Marshall, Dr David Levine, Dr Julie Thacker, Dr Ian Fussell, Dr Caroline Wellbery, Professor Allan Peterkin, Professor John Bligh, Dr Arno Kumagai, Professor Tony Pinching, Professor Tim Dornan, Dr Adrian Hobbs and Dr Adrian Flynn. Conversations with Rob Marshall about Homer and medicine have got me 'thinking otherwise' about metaphor.

I would also like to acknowledge the input of participants to the 2016 Dartington Hall symposium 'Thinking with Metaphors in Medicine: The State of the Art': Tess Jones, Arno Kumagai, Sue Bleakley, Stella Bolaki, Gianna Bouchard, Julie Bligh, Giskin Day, Bella Eacott, Martina Ann Kelly, Teo Manea, Mick Mangan, Robert Marshall, Martin O'Brien, Nicole Piemonte, Steve Reid, Caroline Wellbery, Tom Nutting and Victoria Bates. This symposium was partly supported by a generous grant from the Wellcome Trust. Without the support of the Wellcome Trust, the medical humanities would not have developed as an important inter-discipline in the UK. Arno Kumagai and Tess Jones in particular are the warmest of colleagues and have stretched my imagination in welcome ways.

Thanks are also due to Anita Wohlmann, who wrote to me about her important research that frames metaphors as 'pluripotent and empowering tools of the imagination, inviting ambiguity and complexity' at a time when I had become quite despondent about the ubiquity of metaphors that close down, rather than open up, thinking.

The project that culminated in the writing of this book was supported by a generous grant from the British Academy/Leverhulme Trust (SG150986 – Medical Metaphors: 'Food for Thought?').

1 The recovery of metaphor in medicine

Sticky brains

In the traditional curriculum model of undergraduate medical education – established by Abraham Flexner in North America over a century ago (Cooke *et al.* 2010; Bleakley *et al.* 2011) and still followed by most medical schools internationally – the first two years offer preclinical study of sciences. There is emphasis upon learning anatomy – traditionally through cadaver dissection – while the second phase of two or three years offers increasing levels of clinical experience.

The shift from classroom and anatomy laboratory to work-based learning in hospitals and clinics is abrupt, and one of the things that students learn is that medicine is a practice riddled with uncertainty and soaked in metaphor. This was almost certainly not spelt out in their preclinical learning and may come as a surprise, even a shock. Moreover, the landscapes of metaphors that medical students inhabit – characterizing the clinical medical culture – will not match those encountered in preclinical medical education, or the varied metaphorical landscapes inhabited by the patients they meet as they get their feet on the first rungs of the apprenticeship ladder.

Mara Buchbinder is an anthropologist working – at the time of writing – at the University of North Carolina, Chapel Hill in the field of social medicine. Studying at the University of California for her PhD, she looked at how clinicians, patients and their families made sense of chronic, unexplained pain in the context of a paediatric pain clinic (Buchbinder 2012, 2015). In particular, she focused upon what clinicians saw as 'difficult' or 'challenging' child patients suffering from intractable chronic pain, who were then classified as psychologically abnormal – a way, suggests Buchbinder, of rationalizing their lack of responsiveness to standard treatments. Such children were labelled as displaying 'pervasive developmental disorder' (PDD) – a pattern of 'perseverative thoughts' and 'quirky behaviour' including hyper-attentiveness, attention to detail and concrete thinking.

Paediatricians would, reductively, try to make sense of this observable behaviour through the use of metaphors that referred to unobservable brain functioning – in particular 'sticky neurons' and 'sticky brains'. The 'stickiness' refers to the perseverative behaviour of the children and adolescents observed by Buch-binder, and not, as one might first think, to a 'tacky' or 'gluey' neuronal sub-strate. The latter affords a dual meaning to the paediatricians' common view that these pain symptoms are all 'in the head' – on the one hand possibly psychoso-matic, and on the other possibly an unexplained neurological effect.

Buchbinder (2012, p. 102; 2015) sees the use of such metaphors as a discursive way of rationalizing the unknown, where the child is fixed as an abnormal type ('sticky' – for perseverative) that is ascribed to a hypostatized neurobiological configuration ('sticky neurons'/'sticky brains'). She then places metaphorical thinking at the centre of clinical, diagnostic reasoning, as 'the interactional pro-cesses through which clinical difficulties are managed, interpreted, and explained', where doctors are seen to be engaged in 'performative work of dia-gnosis and institutionalized misrecognition'. Here, she suggests, are medically constructed 'sticky encounters' between doctors, children as patients, and the parents of those children. The medical world, too, sticks to its 'explanation' of unexplained symptoms (either 'there is nothing physically wrong' or 'it is neuro-logical but we cannot pin it down'), while the patient and family stick to their view ('the child is suffering terribly – something must be wrong'). Buchbinder (2015) notes that the slice of the medical world that she observed is shaped by the wider medical culture's didactic metaphor of 'the body as machine'. Doctors are puzzled if they cannot find what has broken down in the machine of the body, which can ordinarily be oiled, made more efficient, and where parts can be repaired or replaced.

In an area of clinical and psychobiological uncertainty, a combination of per-formative and mental 'stickiness' again offers an appropriate 'scatter' or 'blanket' metaphor for challenging behaviour (perversely sticking to details), a psychological or psychosomatic condition (it may be 'all in the mind') and an assumed underlying neural substrate. Medical students on clinical placements in this paediatric clinic quickly learned, too, how a metaphorical language could describe a territory of the unknown to make sense of this alien world. Metaphor offers an heuristic, perhaps even a comfort blanket, in the absence of clear dia-gnosis and abundant uncertainty. As scientists, medical students are encouraged to assume that observed symptomatic behaviour has a functional neurobiological underpinning; yet, unless a range of brain imaging tests are applied, the precise brain mechanism can only be described metaphorically – again, in terms of 'stickiness'. Simultaneously, the research team processed stories from these chil-dren, their parents, and paediatric psychiatry and psychology professionals that appeal to a literary sensibility. These stories have common threads, or stick together, suggesting a syndrome, and continuing to weave the comfort blanket for clinicians and their students. Science becomes an art, as clinical observation is translated into narrative and supposed functional brain mechanisms are framed as metaphors.

As Lynne Greenberg (2009) suggests, medicine 'is not a science of black-and-white facts but rather an art, capable of endless possibilities and as open ended as literary interpretation'. Greenberg is right to challenge medicine's claim to be a science, but the opposition of science with art is unhelpful. Medicine is both a science and an art – better, as Kathryn Montgomery (Hunter 1993; Montgomery 2006) suggests, medicine is a 'science using' practice that requires both scientific knowledge and clinical practice artistry, ethical acumen and humanity.

Following Aristotle, Montgomery describes medicine as *phronesis* – theory put to practical use in activity or, better, as performance (http://performingmedi-cine.com/category/performance/). Where medicine is honed in expertise, such as doctors working for many years within a specialty, then practice develops as 'connoisseurship' (Bleakley 2015). This is an educated sensibility for close noticing and appreciation (diagnostic acumen) and sensitivity towards patients in the recommendation and management of treatments; and – most importantly – in working with patients to develop meanings for their illnesses, largely through appropriate metaphorical framing.

As Danielle Ofri (undated; http://danielleofri.com/poetry-in-medicine/) notes, 'interpreting metaphors is a critical clinical skill in diagnosis; patients' symp-toms often present in metaphorical manners and we doctors need to know how to interpret our patients' metaphors'. Such sensitivity and metaphorical framing should, of course, be extended further to healthcare colleagues with whom doctors work in teams around patients. Both sensibility and sensitivity in clinical praxis require appreciation and understanding of analogy (metaphor and resem-blance) – defined fully below.

Metaphors in science

Those who work in the arts and humanities are familiar with the extent to which metaphor pervades their work. When the question is asked in Shakespeare's *Cymbeline* (1: 1) 'What's his name and birth?' and the answer comes 'I cannot delve him to the root', we know exactly what this means and we do not take it literally. The language, however, considerably enhances the exchange. Where the painter Lucian Freud captures skin tone in a portrait through skilled and imaginative application of oil paint on canvas, the painting is necessarily a meta-phor for the heightened presence of the person who is captured on canvas. The skin is super-real, more skin-like than skin itself. Something has gone up a gear. Depth of character is captured in the expression.

We often imagine that such metaphorical activity does not occur in science, stereotyped as bracketing out the metaphorical and foregrounding the literal and factual. Certainly, medical students from science backgrounds would be sur-prised to see their vocation described as 'soaked' in metaphor. Indeed, unless this is explicitly pointed out to them and appears of use in their learning and practice, they will simply park this information as 'interesting but of little use' as they carry on with the task at hand. For them, medicine is about problem-solving through fact and reason – and not about problem stating (Reddy 1993) or 'sense-making' (Kolko 2010) through metaphor.

But science is a metaphor-using activity too (van Rijn-van Tongeren 1997; Temmerman 2000). When we talk of 'messenger' ribonucleic acid (RNA), this is a metaphoric way of expressing that genetic information is conveyed from DNA to the ribosome, where such information (as nucleotide combinations) specifies the amino acid sequence that will generate specific proteins. 'Messenger' is not a particularly vibrant or sexy metaphor, but at a level beyond the genetic code, it is key to medicine and surgery, where much of the tension around communicating with patients is in breaking bad news.

'Don't shoot the messenger' may be the metaphor ringing at the back of a doctor's mind as she breaks bad news to an aggressive and emotionally unhinged family member who assumed his or her loved one would emerge from difficult surgery with ease. This metaphor can be traced to Sophocles' *Antigone* (*c*.441 BC) where 'no one loves the messenger who brings bad news', and is repeated famously in Shakespeare's *Antony and Cleopatra* (*c*.1606), where, upon learning that Antony has married Octavia, Cleopatra goes into a rage, physically striking and heaping her venom on the messenger, threatening to gouge out his eyes, scalp him and worse:

> Horrible villain! or I'll spurn thine eyes
> Like balls before me; I'll unhair thy head:
>
> (*She hales him up and down*) (drags him across the stage)
>
> Thou shalt be whipp'd with wire, and stew'd in brine,
> Smarting in lingering pickle.

To which the alarmed messenger responds: 'I that do bring the news made not the match.'

'Messenger' RNA may, then, not pack much of a punch, where 'don't shoot the messenger' in Shakespeare certainly does. Returning to science, when we describe a hadron 'collider' that smashes atoms and analyses the results, 'collider' is a literal description just edging towards the metaphorical. But when we talk of the results of such collisions in terms of 'exotic' hadrons and the greater understanding of 'black holes', then we are in metaphorical territory, although this is grounded in substance – the metaphor is embodied (albeit 'substances' are now subatomic particles).

Getting to grips with 'metaphor' as both cause and effect of complexity

'I buttered the bread' is a plain and literal description of something I just did (A = A). 'You know which side your bread is buttered' is more complex. This is an idiom – used since the sixteenth century to mean knowing where your best interests lie. An idiom is a non-literal way of expressing something that is already familiar to users of a language. 'Between a rock and a hard place' is another example of an idiom. A metaphor, however, is a non-literal use of language that is possible to understand even when you have never heard it before, such as 'drowning in paperwork'. Here, A = B. 'Paperwork' isn't a pond, a river or a raging ocean. Yet, 'drowning' (A) can be imaginatively connected to 'paperwork' (B). The first (A) is understood in a different, usually deeper, way through relationship to, and by means of, the second (B). (I am borrowing the elegant 'A = B' formula from Jeffery Donaldson (2015), detailed below.)

A metaphor is, then, a link between two previously unconnected things, usually acting as a catalyst for a deeper understanding. I say 'usually' because metaphors can also be negative and mislead – but more on this later. The beauty of a metaphor is that it is not only the link itself (a linguistic product of cognition) but also the means by which we appreciate, value and understand this link (embodied and social cognition). Metaphor is both a thing and a process; both that which is magnified and the magnifying lens, or that which is refracted and the medium for refraction.

For Jeffery Donaldson (2015), metaphor is fundamental not only to consciousness, but also to the evolutionary process that has made consciousness possible. Metaphor, as connection, is the intangible current in life that makes the imagination tangible, or brings meaning to experience through paradox. If two things are linked literally (A = A), then we will appreciate this as mechanical and linear – the car skids lightly into the tree and the front light is smashed. What, however, if several elements are interrelating within a system that is not linear but contains uncertainty, ambiguity and paradox? The weather suddenly turns foul, a freak rainstorm impeding vision so badly that the driver panics, hitting the brakes a fraction too hard, but luckily the car just gently skids off the road and skims a tree, with damage only to a front light. The weather and the human body are such complex systems.

As the incident unfolds, the emotions of surprise, fear and relief that the driver goes through are an emergent property of several, interacting, 'open' complex systems – including the weather and the human body (but not necessarily the car, which is a mechanical, 'closed', engineered system – complicated but not complex). They are also complex because the interaction between elements in the system is multiple and to some extent unpredictable. Metaphor is our primary linguistic medium for grasping the qualities, idiosyncrasies and expressions of dynamic, adaptive, complex systems. And, of course, metaphor as process is itself an expressive complex system.

Such systems stay close to chaos but do not fall into chaos. They are constantly adapting during perturbations and may develop further complexity as 'activity systems' or 'networks' (Bleakley 2015). A network develops through translations across its components that give greater meaning or capacity. Evolution is biology's biggest network process. Rainforests, deserts, weather systems and human social groups are large, in-process network outcomes, or evolving complex systems. Within such open, complex, adaptive systems appear 'state spaces' – these are all possible states of the dynamic system. For example, a person can be relatively ill or well with somatic or psychological symptoms. State spaces are generally relatively stable, while dynamic (the body's main dynamism is entropy – enervated flesh will eventually run down into death), because within the system certain 'attractors' appear that offer stability through process.

Mind the gap

Attractors in the body are organ systems: the central and autonomic nervous systems, the enteric nervous system mesh that controls digestion and gastrointestinal functions, the vascular system, and so forth. Communications occur between attractors, while the relative stability and influence of attractors within the overall complex system and across all possible state spaces differ. Thus, there are 'gaps' between attractors and there are attractors themselves, just as there are gaps between nerve axons (synapses) and gaps between paired words ('drowning' and 'paperwork'). The synapse or gap can be described as a metaphor. Metaphor also describes the means by which the gap is jumped, as one meaning develops into another more complex and imaginative meaning, and the means by which this leap (of faith) – or A = B – is achieved, appreciated, imagined and understood. This, again, casts metaphor as both the 'missing link' in life and the experience of that life's missing link, as Donaldson (2015) suggests.

For Donaldson, the creation of the Cosmos at the 'Big Bang' (now there is a strange metaphor – coined by the astronomer Fred Hoyle in 1949 – as there was nobody present to judge its size or its noise level and quality) is the 'gap' that we can only fill with the notion of 'metaphor', and metaphor is our best way of appreciating that gap. Metaphor is the best word we have to describe how meanings are changed when one thing is put in relation to another; but also, metaphor production is, again, the process by which, and the lens through which, we appreciate the imaginative transformations that occur when non-literal relations are expressed.

In Shakespeare's *Romeo and Juliet*, the Capulets and the Montagues are enemies. Juliet is a Capulet and Romeo a Montague. A fight breaks out between the rival houses in which Tybalt (a Capulet) stabs Mercutio (neither a Montague nor a Capulet) under Romeo's arm (Romeo is trying to stop the fight). Mercutio says that he is hurt but, showing manly courage in front of his peers, says it is only a 'scratch', while asking his Page to fetch a surgeon. Romeo says: 'Courage, man. The hurt cannot be much'. Mercutio replies:

> No, 'tis not so deep as a well nor so wide as a church door, but 'tis enough, 'twill serve. Ask for me tomorrow, and you shall find me a grave man. I am peppered, I warrant, for this world.

The description of the wound appears to be hyperbolic, but, as it does indeed turn out to be fatal, serves as a metaphor. 'Peppered', too, is a metaphor. Just as 'peppered with requests' means overwhelmed or showered, so Mercutio says that he is overwhelmed, or dying. Shakespeare's imaginative metaphors shift ordinary and literal description: 'I've been stabbed and I am dying' into an extra-ordinary and emotionally draining experience.

Yet, metaphors can keel over and die, or become so jaded and overused that they no longer have impact. The pharmaceutical 'blister' pack is a child of the 1960s and is forever associated with the introduction of the oral contraceptive pill. I can clearly remember when 'blister' pack first circulated in everyday speech as a strange mixture of the pathologized (the blister that is raised to protect a hurt, such as a burn) and the sanitized (the transparent blister, the protective foil). Pressing blister packs simulated little births as the pill popped out, yet this very pill protected against possible future births. Yet, 'blister' pack is already a dead (overused) metaphor, displaced by 'smart' packaging (also called 'active' and 'intelligent' packaging), popularized only in the last decade. 'Intelligent' packag-ing, for example for food, contains internal or external indicators to provide information about the contents, such as the freshness of the food; or packages may contain sachets or pads that soak up moisture to prevent mould developing.

Metaphors, too, can be malignant – stigmatizing, as Susan Sontag suggests and as I have already noted, or closing down thinking, as Shane Neilson (2015) suggests. This book spends a good deal of time exploring what many believe to be two dead metaphors in medical discourse – the body as machine and medi-cine as war – as malignant, both stigmatizing and closing off thinking, within both medical and lay culture. Such metaphors produce insensibility or dulling that resists and frustrates the creation of imaginative metaphors more suited to a healthcare that refuses to objectify the patient, and sees medical intervention in terms of collaboration rather than confrontation.

Paul Ricoeur (2003) reminds us of two linguistic contexts: semantics (the meanings of words, etymology) and semiotics (the use of words). It is in the use of words that metaphor gains power, through, as Jeffery Donaldson (2015) reminds us, putting one word in *relation* to another (again – mind the gap). Metaphor is concerned with this range of relationships: a vehicle or source with a tenor or target where A does not equal A, but B. 'I've had enough' is perhaps a good enough description, but 'that is the final straw' (also the straw that broke the camel's back) is far more potent. The imagination is immediately called into action: everything is in the balance, and then just one more straw causes the scales to tip. The literal 'enough is enough' is A=A. The imaginative 'the final straw' is A=B. There were no literal straws involved when I finally snapped and lost my temper in the face of my (ex) boss's persistent and unfair demands. Words in metaphors are in strange and productive relationships, where meanings move across a gap and gain imaginative depth and surprise: 'flogging a dead horse' and 'the elephant in the room' still surprise because they are so visually arresting, echoing the camel's back breaking under the weight of an extra straw.

Donaldson (2015) finds a place for 'everyday' metaphors that some claim as dead. While the brain works through synaptic connections between neurons that form large networks with massive connective possibilities, in fact, transmission and reception of neural impulses or 'messages' occur through interneurons, the workhorses of the brain's cortex, which are relays between sensory and motor neurons. Interneurons make up most of the brain's neuronal mass. Whereas sensory neurons take in stimuli and motor neurons cause action on such stimuli, in-between is a massive amount of processing and meaning making, or 'thinking more', as Donaldson puts it. This is metaphoric work for sticky neurons – which probably work best as non-stick connectors, easily cleaned after use.

Between seeing a friend at a distance, catching his or her eye, and greeting and exchanging conversation, is a heap of meaning making, memory stimulation, emotional colouring, planning and co-ordination of possibilities. This is the work of the extensive system of interneurons acting as a processual complex, adaptive system. The system's shifting from 'thinking' (reflex) to 'thinking more' (planning, adapting, imagining, emoting) may be fuelled by analogy, or oiled by metaphor, but is far from machine-like. Further, this interneuronal networking is a social phenomenon, organized as an extended cognition in concert with others' brains – don't talk about 'kicking the bucket' at a funeral; never 'spill the beans' to a stranger; and don't say 'how time flies' when visiting a friend in prison. Then why do doctors talk about 'fighting cancer' to terminally ill cancer patients who have already 'lost' the fight and are in palliative care (Semino *et al.* 2015)?

Is medicine really 'soaked' or 'saturated' in – or even 'spiked', or 'spiced', with – metaphor?

Metaphor accounts for around 10 per cent of everyday speech, according to James Geary (2011, pp. 5–6), as roughly 1 metaphorical word or phrase for every 10–12 in a written sentence; but this is really a meaningless statistic, because metaphor is aligned with the quality and not the frequency of the word. And the contemplated written word differs from spontaneous utterances. If we think of what hits home in an utterance, then metaphor may account for much of the impact of speech. Indeed, the subtitle of Geary's book *I Is an Other* (*The Secret Life of Metaphor and How It Shapes the Way We See the World*) tells us that metaphor has a life to be exposed, and this tacit lifeform organizes perception, thinking, feeling and, most importantly, imagination.

Still, to claim that medicine is 'soaked' or 'saturated' in metaphor may seem a step too far – and is there any empirical evidence for this? Maier and Shibles (2011, p. 1) certainly agree with this assertion, mobilizing metaphors themselves for rhetorical 'explanation', where 'The meanings of medicine are generated by a constant stream of metaphors.' 'Stream' does indeed suggest a continuous soaking in metaphor that is not static.

Let us return to Susan Sontag's (1978, 1989) well-known studies on historically contingent metaphors of tuberculosis, cancer and AIDS that explore the abuses of metaphors through how they situate cancer and AIDS patients. Cancer patients must be fighters, and AIDS patients are suffering from a modern plague of their own making, and can then be freely judged. Ulrike Kistner (1998) describes how Sontag would bleach out ubiquitous and pervasive use of metaphors from medicine altogether where they are seen as disturbing or harmful, an unnecessary extra burden for patients to bear.

If Sontag is right, and metaphors in medicine are both ubiquitous and pervasive, then both 'soaked' and 'saturated' may be apt metaphors. A soaking occurs in a sudden rainstorm and not just in long-term immersion. 'Drenched' in metaphor may serve just as well. Metaphors may appear like rainstorms – as sudden downpours in specific contexts. If a patient's safety is at stake, for example in a tricky surgical operation, metaphors such as 'close shave', 'near miss', 'sailing close to the wind' and 'I am about to blow my top' may emerge in surgical team talk. Under the opposite set of conditions, with a straightforward procedure, this may also draw use of metaphor such as 'a piece of cake', 'a walk in the park' or a 'doddle'. But these are conversational metaphors and not specific to surgery or medicine. What of culture-specific medical metaphors?

Françoise Salager-Meyer (1990) studied the occurrence of metaphors in 90 medical texts across three languages – English, Spanish and French (30 texts in each language from 15 medical specialties, totalling 130,000 words). The appearance of metaphor was consistent across texts – 1.2 per cent in Medical English, 1.2 per cent in Medical Spanish and 1.1 per cent in Medical French – way below Geary's guess at incidence in everyday communication. This is a small amount of each text, and it may then seem that here is empirical evidence that metaphor is peripheral, where medicine appears to be dominated by non-metaphorical or literal (technical) language use. But this would be a false reading.

The author herself says that 'the words which bear a metaphorical status usually refer to concepts which are crucial to an optimum understanding of the text' (Salager-Meyer 1990, p. 148). In other words, again, *quality* of language is more important than frequency or quantity of occurrence of words. There are several other problems that arise from this empirical work.

First, this research does not take into account the role of didactic or leading metaphors (such as 'medicine as war' and 'the body as machine') – detailed in Chapter 4 – that historically shape medical culture and its texts (and that may be negative or counterproductive). These may be thought of as 'meta-metaphors': background, historically contingent effects insidiously shaping front-line metaphors. Further, such metaphors may have become so ingrained in the culture as to no longer surprise and then are called 'dead' metaphors, as explained previously.

Second, the research does not, again, account for the qualitative effect of metaphors. While a frequency count from a corpus analysis tells us the raw number of metaphors in a body of statements, which is then compared with the raw number of non-metaphorical uses of language, in some ways such data are meaningless, because the quality and influence of differing types of language in context are then not taken into account. Rhetorical language, for example, is primarily about impact, whereas descriptive, technical language is about information or supplement. The latter may provide a great deal of ineffectual wadding, while the kernel of a speech act may be the metaphor, and it is this part that may provide the impact of talk or text.

Third, this linguistic corpus analysis research looks at metaphors in medical textbooks but not in clinical practice, medical research, medical education, medical management and patient encounters. Context matters again. Medical texts account for a relatively small part of medical culture and practice. For example, the frequency of metaphor use in patient encounters, particularly in general practice and psychiatry, would surely be higher than the use of metaphors in a textbook context. Patients, as laypersons, would follow the general rule established by Lakoff and Johnson's (1980) work – explored in more depth later – that 'most of our everyday language is metaphorical' (Salager-Meyer 1990, p. 146).

This directly contradicts even Geary's assertion that metaphor accounts for only around 10 per cent of everyday speech. Of course, it all depends on what you mean by 'metaphor', as we shall see. Further, any social interaction – especially in highly rule-bound contexts such as medicine and healthcare – is only partly language-based. Mostly, it is non-verbal performance that is highly scripted and staged, based on a set of cultural metaphors as recurring tropes, such as management of personal space (proxemics) and hierarchies (power distribution).

Fourth, this corpus linguistics text-based research misses a whole slice of medical culture and practice that involves the 'dark' metaphors of medical slang (discussed in more depth later) (BBC News Channel 2003; Fox *et al.* 2003), likely to be more common in accident and emergency and intensive care than in other specialties, although there is no empirical evidence for this assertion. Fifth, this research does not embrace key areas of metaphor use in medicine, such as sense-based (often 'food' descriptions) resemblances, common in diagnostic work in radiology, dermatology and pathology, the 'visual' specialties (discussed in depth in Chapters 5 and 6). And sixth, this research does not embrace the use of aphorisms or maxims in medicine (see Appendix 3; Levine and Bleakley 2012).

What Salager-Meyer's work does tell us is that medical metaphors are more likely to appear in descriptions of technical structures (anatomy) than of processes (physiology). This is because the Greek or Latin origins of terms for processes have been maintained much more strongly than terms for structures. The latter then attract colloquial metaphorical descriptions such as the 'wall' of the intestine, a mitral 'valve', a coronary 'tree', the 'lining' of the stomach, the ear 'drum', the bones of the inner ear as 'stirrup', 'anvil' and 'hammer' – although there are some classical derivations offering strong and memorable images, such as 'lid' of the eye as cover or cap, 'cancer' as a crab or lobster, and 'pylorus' as gatekeeper. Functions, on the other hand, retain Greek and Latin roots, such as 'haematopoiesis' (the forming of new blood cells) and 'haemorrhage' (bleeding, often violently).

Further, medical language resists the narrative quality of literary writing; it is largely descriptive and functional, drawing from standard 'English for Medical Purposes' (EMP) (described in more detail later). Medical language explicitly favours the indicative (certainty and fact – 'this is') rather than the subjunctive mood (entertaining uncertainty or ambiguity – 'this may be'), and makes use of descriptive qualifying adjectives and concept-expressing nouns rather than action words such as process-expressing verbs.

The most frequently encountered morphological (form) metaphors in Salager-Meyer's analyses (across English, Spanish and French examples) are:

- architectural, such as 'tunnel' syndrome, aortic 'arch'
- geomorphical (earth-based), such as visual 'field', urinary 'stream'
- phytomorphical (plant-based), such as 'cauliflower' ear, nerve 'roots' (very common in medicine, drawing on 'tree', 'branch', 'trunk', 'root', 'stem')
- anatomical, such as femoral 'neck', foreign 'bodies'
- zoomorphical (animal-based), such as 'butterfly' rash, 'horseshoe' nuclei.

Amongst the most frequently encountered physiological (function) metaphors are:

- 'migratory' pain
- mechanical 'ventilation'.

As noted, Salager-Meyer's work described above is an example of corpus linguistics (Appendix 2 describes a protocol and method for such research). Here, a body of work (corpus) is analysed for its linguistic content and effects. For her Master's dissertation, Carolina Huang (described in Finatto 2010) carried out a linguistic corpus study on a Brazilian medical journal dealing with articles on AIDS between 1984 and 2002, to map out metaphor use. This expansive work offers a counterpoint to Sontag's reductive account of metaphors of AIDS. The key metaphor that emerged was 'personification' of AIDS – the disease or illness talked about as if it were an autonomous person rather than the manifestation of a viral infection in a person and in a population. AIDS was also seen to be in a 'race' with the medical establishment and drug companies fast-tracking research to find a cure.

Overall, 90 patterns of metaphor were identified in the corpus (2,578 contexts in which AIDS appeared as a metaphor), divided into seven main groups, guided by a framework provided by Lakoff and Johnson (1980):

1   personification (of course, the virus is realized in human experience, but turning the virus into human form affords a way in which it can be given a face and faced up to)
2   personification with an extra attribute such as 'strength'
3   time (as in a 'race against time')
4   process
5   container (what 'reserves' do you have?)
6   orientation (AIDS has a direction)
7   war (the 'fight' against AIDS).

Pamela Faber and Carlos Márquez Linares (Faber and Linares 2004) are members of the LexiCon Research group at the University of Granada (http://lexicon.ugr.es). Part of this research portfolio is linguistic corpus analysis of medical texts including use of metaphor. The authors note that the constructional meaning of concepts is extended by the use of metaphor. A complex linguistic expression such as metaphor usage goes beyond the sum of the meanings of its lexical and grammatical components to include its construal – the capacity to conceptualize the same situation in different ways. This is central to complex diagnoses in medicine.

Faber and Linares (2004, p. 2) carried out a corpus analysis of oncology texts from both English and Spanish sources (medical textbooks, encyclopaedias, CD ROM publications) of approximately 32 million words. First, they note 'the pervasiveness of metaphor in scientific communication'. From the corpus analysis, the authors describe several functions for metaphor usage in such texts, extending beyond oncology's master or didactic metaphor of 'medicine as war':

1   Metaphors extend conceptualization to personification
    Here, the dominant metaphors are to turn cells and genes into autonomous human forms that have existence – they may be 'immortal' or can 'commit suicide'. They morph when they are 'starved'. Existence includes personification of cells or genes that act as agents, such as disease agent and treatment agent. This can move out of the individual to the social, such as 'reporter' genes and 'gatekeeper' genes. Inter-domain mapping means that genes can also be 'emotional', such as cells being more or less 'fussy'; and cells have agency, whereby they can 'migrate', 'crawl', 'scout' and 'wander'.

2   Introduction of novel terms and phrases
    At the lexical level, metaphors are introduced that see cancer in new ways. Medicine maps the structures of the world onto our bodies (imitating the 'arms' and 'legs' of a chair, for example):

    • Medical metaphors are related to everyday objects – such as DNA 'ladders' and 'dumbbell' DNA.
    • Body parts are described as building structures: cell 'walls', DNA 'library'.

    Metaphors describe bodies as landscapes:

    • The body is often described in agricultural terms, with the doctor cast as farmer: bone marrow 'harvests' and 'transplants'; 'implants', 'grafts' and tumours 'seeding'; 'sickle cells' and 'radiation seeds'. There is a long history of medical anatomy borrowing terms from botany (roots, stems, branches).
    • The body is described in topographical terms, such as vascular 'lakes' and 'vascular 'waterfalls'; there are ocular ciliary 'valleys' and metastatic 'cascades'.

3   Metaphors introduce propositional meanings
    This suggests something to be considered, adopted or done, such as a diagnosis implying treatment regime. The focus is on the meaning of the activity. Where 2 above focuses on nouns (object concepts represented by nominal forms), propositional meanings focus on verbs. The metaphor

offers an extension of a verb's basic meaning. For example, something is 'implicated': there is evidence related to a certain body part or organ, and this suggests a disease.

4   Pragmatic context
Metaphors activate a particular kind of insight into how others behave or what signs may mean (again facilitating diagnostic acumen). The most common metaphorical conceptualization here is the 'crime story' or a 'mystery'. Kathryn Montgomery (Hunter 1993) famously describes medicine as 'sleuthing' – referring to diagnostic process as the close noticing and processing of cues and clues by experts in a specialty. Thus, for example, 'clue', 'mystery', 'sleuthing', 'footprint', 'suspect', 'interrogation', and of course 'evidence' (medicine is supposed to be an 'evidence-based' practice) are common metaphors.

While doctors learn a body of domain knowledge in scientific terms, and this becomes more specialized as they progress as experts, the conceptual apparatus by which the domain knowledge is exercised in clinical practice, developed in medical research, and progressed through innovation in patient care is transfer from the scientific conceptual domain to a metaphorical parallel. Cells do not 'attack' other cells – this is a metaphorical construct. Diagnosis is not a detective story – this is also a metaphorical construct. Yet, 'scaffolding' practice – through invoking metaphorical frames to deepen the literal frames that medical science provides – creates a more generous and adventurous practice in which innovation is possible. (I will have more to say on 'scaffolding' in the context of medical education in Chapter 8). As Faber and Linares (2004, p. 9) note, 'metaphor in scientific texts' (by which they specifically mean the oncology texts that form the corpus for their analysis) 'is a much more complex and pervasive phenomenon than is generally believed'.

Bearing in mind again that a corpus analysis of medical textbooks, extending to current CD ROM media, addresses a relatively small proportion of medicine's activities, nevertheless, corpus analysis research does offer a rich harvest. There is considerable overlap between these corpus analysis studies, as one might expect. With further studies, a meta-review could be carried out to ascertain a landscape of metaphors currently in use in medicine across several languages.

Perhaps to describe medicine as 'soaked' or 'saturated' in metaphor is also too 'watery', avoiding other element metaphor groups of fire, earth and air (Bachelard 1977, 1988, 1989, 1992, 1994, 2002; Stroud and Sardello 2015). Earlier, I noted agricultural metaphors in medicine and surgery such as 'harvesting' (organs), 'grafting' (bone) and 'transplanting' (skin). We also need metaphors that capture the heat and ferment of medical practice. So, metaphors other than 'soaked' and 'saturated' could be considered, such as medicine being 'spiked' or 'spiced' with metaphor. This, however, suggests sudden or abrupt metaphor episodes and misses the fact that medical culture is historically shaped by didactic or leading metaphors (again, 'medicine as 'war', 'the body as a machine' and also 'illness as a journey') that culturally shape patients' responses to medical episodes and produce identity constructions for both patients and doctors. 'Spiced' with metaphor may unnecessarily return us to analogy as ornamentation. Metaphors, then, come – sometimes overtly and often subtly – to structure both clinicians' and patients' responses to the disease or illness. Metaphors also come to constitute scientific knowledge (such as pharmaceutical research), forms of therapy and population issues such as public perceptions.

In short, medical metaphors are not for ornamentation but transcend such stylistic concerns, providing a framework for theorizing and shaping practice interventions in clinical settings. As introduced above, Susan Sontag (1989) argued that metaphors of cancer and AIDS could bring stigma and an unnecessary extra burden for the patient. But Sontag's argument that metaphor should be avoided in medicine misses the points raised by researchers such as Huang: first, that metaphor is so pervasive in medicine that the point is not to eradicate, but to understand the influence of, metaphor, and to shift didactic metaphors; and second, that the study of metaphors can offer potential ways of understanding how treatments may be better managed.

Such mappings of metaphors, suggests Finatto (2010, p. 655), afford a 'geography' of medicine. Following the groundbreaking work of Rita Temmerman (2000) in calling for a new and radical sociocognitive approach to how science works and how scientists think, going beyond the prejudices and resistances concerning rhetoric and metaphor to embrace these areas as central to scientific work, Finatto calls for the close and systematic study of medical texts through corpus linguistics and associated approaches. Elena Semino and colleagues at the University of Lancaster have initiated a very important empirical study, using both quantitative corpus linguistics and qualitative survey, looking at the use of metaphors in end-of-life (palliative) care (The Metaphor in End-of-Life Care Study). They interrogate the dominance of 'violence' metaphors in cancer discourse, where 'journey' metaphors offer an alternative tone (Demmen *et al.* 2015; Semino *et al.* 2015; Demjen *et al.* 2016; Potts and Semino 2017).

They also warn against quick judgement of the supposedly inappropriate use of 'violence' metaphors by healthcare practitioners, noting that patients may use such metaphors more frequently than practitioners, according to context. However, it is not clear whether patients use such metaphors within a false consciousness – without reflection or forethought, but habitually, and possibly as a response to the widespread use of the war metaphor beyond their own immediate medical concerns.

As noted earlier, the study of metaphor in medicine must go beyond written texts to spoken practices as performance, in particular conversations between doctors and patients. This must embrace non-verbal as well as verbal metaphors, such as gesture, proximity, expression and habitual style, and impression and impression management (Goffman 1959). One study in the philosophy of medicine, described next, is particularly interested in the doctor–patient relationship as a metaphorical expression in its own right. Goffman, noted above, would see such relationships as heavily rule bound, involving managing impressions on both sides – or as dramaturgical, with humans as actors. There is public (frontstage) behaviour where cultures mix (doctors and the lay public), and private (backstage) behaviour such as the use of unsavoury slang within medical culture. Doctors and patients have roles and scripts and engage in some improvisation. Central to those scripts is a core set of metaphors.

A 'metaphorical method'

Barbara Maier and Warren Shibles (2011) place thinking with metaphor at the centre of their rationale for a philosophy of medicine. They suggest that medical practice is shaped by language and that much of the everyday language used in medicine – 'caring', 'cause', 'help', 'patient' and even 'death' – is used casually, without critical awareness. Importantly, they claim that medical culture is indeed soaked in metaphor. They set out an approach to the philosophy of medicine shaped by thinking with metaphors, which they call a 'Metaphorical Method'. This is a radical version of 'thinking otherwise' or against the grain of convention. The fact that medicine strains to reject metaphorical thinking is seen as a symptom of its 'discussion illiteracy' or inability to adopt critically reflexive thinking about its key terms and practices (particularly the doctor–patient relationship). For Maier and Shibles, everything is a metaphor until proven otherwise, for every statement, even a scientific 'fact', is rhetorical. It is rhetorical because it is social, or the statement achieves its status and meaning according to social context and is, as it were, constantly arguing its case.

Discussion illiteracy has bedmates in 'emotion illiteracy' and 'ethics illiteracy'. The vacuum created by slack philosophical thinking in medicine is filled by simplistic managerialist approaches and by the instrumental ethics approach of principlism, which ignore messy, context-based human judgement. The authors' claim is not just academic posturing – Barbara Maier is an experienced clinician – but offers a significant challenge to medical education to recognize the importance of metaphor in medicine. The 'Metaphorical Method' – a new way of thinking about medicine, where 'Philosophy of medicine is metaphors about medicine' (Maier and Shibles 2011, p. 1) – should be core content in undergraduate medicine and surgery curricula.

So, again, what is a 'Metaphorical Method'? It is a questioning of every taken-for-granted idea and practice in medicine as a critical investigation of its standing and legitimacy. This is not a nihilistic approach but a comparative one. The illustrative examples given below will illuminate the method. First, as noted, one must assume that every statement made in medicine is rhetorical or acts to persuade, from a simple piece of information (perhaps offered within a context of a clear power differential), to a messy differential diagnosis, to a research paper. The authors suggest, again, that even scientific language used in medicine is rhetorical and draws heavily on metaphor, especially 'big metaphors' such as 'evidence-based practice' and 'the medical model'. These meta-metaphors cannot be taken at face value but require critical scrutiny, and are often used as smokescreen for 'truth' and 'fact'. Indeed, the 'medical model', suggest Maier and Shibles, is a metaphor taken literally.

   If a metaphor is defined as relating previously unrelated things, then medicine fundamentally follows metaphor, for 'illness' generally follows from 'health'. Where the generalized or population-based statistic meets the individual patient, medicine is necessarily a 'guesstimate', an 'as if' – again the employment of metaphor. The authors then put forward a surprising method in which they consider the analytic methods used in medicine as not countermetaphorical, but actually in themselves differing kinds of metaphor. Here are some typical metaphorical strategies used by doctors, drawing on Maier and Shibles' headings but where I provide the illustrative examples:

1   *Juxtaposition*: two words placed together create a new meaning, such as 'your tumour has spread'. 'Cancer' is derived from the Greek *karkinos* and Latin *carcinos* ('crab') – the crab has scuttled sideways, but what does this mean for the patient? 'Spread' is indeterminate. 'Metastatic' remains a shield behind which the doctor can hide.
2   *Analogy, simile or comparison*: the 'spread' of the cancer, explains the oncologist, is like an invading army. But the patient is not thinking in militaristic metaphors and does not experience this 'invasion'. How will she make sense of the 'spread'? Is it more like the spread of butter on toast, or the spread of a rumour?
3   *Symbolism*: the oncologist says to the patient that there is a 'beacon of hope' through a newly developed drug. We can put you in a randomized controlled trial (RCT), but we won't know which leg of the trial you are on. 'Random', 'controlled', 'trial', 'leg'? The patient is confused – 'I don't want a beacon of hope, I want certainty.'
4   *Reversal*: not only do many drugs have undesirable side effects (anti-inflammatory medicines may cover up symptoms but do not offer cure and can perforate your stomach), but also psychological interventions can have paradoxical effects, such as palliative care shortening life.

One area where Maier and Sibles are particularly strong is using their 'metaphoric method' to analyse differing kinds of doctor (or healthcare worker) (H)–patient (P) relationships. For example (the illustrative examples are mine):

1   $H = P$. The patient is on an equal footing with the doctor. For example, the patient is an expert in his or her own illness; but, and this is where Maier and Shibles' model of metaphor is very helpful, the doctor can also become a patient. 'Doctoring' and 'patient' roles now become metaphors as illness becomes the focal point.
2   H v. P. The doctor or patient or both adopt confrontational positions towards one another, disagreeing about treatments or management of illness. There may be a personality clash.
3   *Not H and not P*. A religious or legal decision trumps the position of either doctor or patient, or both. The metaphors of 'medicine' and 'care' shift as the dominant values change.

4   *H or P*. There is not necessarily a confrontation (*H* v. *P*), but either the doctor's paternalism or the patient's autonomy holds sway.

5   *H and P*. A dialogical relationship ensues, and decision-making is shared.

6   *H not P*. The patient is in a coma, at end of life, on the operating table, undergoing an investigation or procedure, in which the tenor never allows the vehicle to emerge. (See the following Chapter 2 for an explanation of 'tenor' and 'vehicle' in metaphor production.)

7   *P not H*. The patient decides not to turn up for an appointment, or refuses treatment by not complying with a prescription. The vehicle has slipped free of the tenor. (Again, see Chapter 2.)

8   *H does not equal P*. No metaphorical relationship can emerge between tenor and vehicle (again, see Chapter 2) due to unbridged differences arising from prejudice grounded in, for example, gender or ethnicity.

9   *H? P*. The doctor and/or the patient are both unstable and unpredictable due to mental illness or other health issues such as addictions and dependencies. Or, an unresolved sexual attraction or sinister obsession has emerged.

In framing medical work in terms of metaphor, Maier and Shibles are not asking us to adopt positions, but to 'think otherwise' about current scenarios, or to think critically using metaphor as the medium.

Conclusion

Medicine, then – a sci-art praxis – is soaked in, or spiked with, or grounded in, or air-dried in, or flaming with, embodied metaphors expressed through language and in performance, including speech acts. Metaphor in medicine manifests in various ways and serves a variety of functions. Attitudes towards metaphor in medicine differ – some see metaphors (particularly resemblances) as historical curiosities to be archived, which at best serve as mnemonics (Almendraia 2014) (see Chapters 5 and 6), while others see rich and complex purposes in the use of metaphors, such as diagnostic and pedagogical aids (Andrade-Filho and Pena 2001), or ways of communicating with patients without resorting to alienating technical language (Frieden and Dolev 2005). Maier and Shibles, as we saw above, see medicine as a flow of context-dependent metaphors to be reflexively interrupted and understood, and as a way of mapping medicine's geographies or habitats.

With the exception of the work of (to some extent) Samuel Vaisrub (1977) and (to a far greater extent) Geraldine van Rijn-van Tongeren (1997) – discussed in the following Chapter 2 – the use of analogies (metaphors and resemblances or similes) in medicine has not been systematically mapped and analysed. There are islands of literature that go beyond mere description of metaphors in medicine to explanation of their origins and usage – for example, shaping medical culture and practice, and generating theory – such as Salager-Meyer and Finatto, described above. Other key literature includes Thagard 1997; Andrade-Filho and Pena 2001; Bleakley 2004, 2006, 2015; Bleakley *et al.* 2003a, 2003b; Frieden and Dolev 2005; Pena and Andrade-Filho 2010; and Lakhtakia 2014.

There is an important body of literature looking at previously unexamined didactic metaphors in medicine, such as 'illness as a journey' (Galewski 2015; Semino *et al.* 2015), and the historical origins of the 'the body as machine' metaphor (Lynn undated; Osherson and AmaraSingham 1981; Ott 1995; Gleyse 2013). A significant critical literature addresses the metaphor of 'medicine as war' (or 'illness as violence'), which poses identity dilemmas such as 'Doctors at war, doctors washing feet', or doctor as heroic warrior and as humble servant in one and the same body (Miller 2014); suggests strategies such as 'The war is over – let us learn to work together' (Vogt and Mach 2015); or insists on a change of leading metaphor such as 'Stop using military metaphors for disease' (Wiggins 2012) and to replace them with pacific 'ecological' metaphors (Annas 1995, 1996). For challenges to martial and violence metaphors, see, for example, Sontag 1978; Burnside 1983; Hodgkin 1985; Sontag 1989; Warren 1991; Docherty 2001; Mitchell *et al.* 2003; Leaf 2004; Penson *et al.* 2004; Reisfield and Wilson 2004; Bell 2012; Slobod and Fuks 2012; Lane *et al.* 2013; Cooper 2014; George and Whitehouse 2014; McCartney 2014; Demmen *et al.* 2015; Galewski 2015; Semino *et al.* 2015; Potts and Semino 2017. At the time of writing, this literature has not been systematically reviewed.

The journalist Charles Krauthammer (1986) turns our current discussion on its head by reminding us that medical metaphors are borrowed in politics for rhetorical purposes, particularly 'medicine as war', whereby the political right in particular describes left wing uprisings as 'cancers' that must be 'cut out'. We see the same rhetoric at work against terrorist organizations in the current era, in which 'surgical strikes' at the 'heart' of such organizations raise hope of their excision.

Replacing once lively, but now unhelpful, tired, dead or even malignant, metaphors extends also to economic/'market' metaphors (healthcare as a business and service, patients as customers) (Mustacchi and Krevans 2001; Hudak *et al.* 2003). This embraces issues such as medicine's ethically sensitive relationship with the pharmaceutical industry. Mather (2005) explores how the doctor–industry relationship has been characterized by the contrasting metaphors of the 'pipeline' and the 'porcupine'. The pharmaceutical industry sees its connection to medicine in terms of a pipeline, the one feeding the other to their mutual benefit, largely ignoring the well-documented ethical conundrums this relationship raises. Doctors, in turn, see their relationship to 'Big Pharma' as one of 'dancing with the porcupine'.

I look at this literature on dominant metaphors more closely in Chapter 4, showing, for example, that historically contingent, leading martial metaphors are highly resistant to change and adapt to new medical cultures – for example, 'targets' are absorbed into 'personalized medicine', and the 'war on terror' is adapted to refresh the longstanding 'war on cancer' (Meisenberg and Meisenberg 2015) and 'war on Alzheimer's' (George and Whitehouse 2014) – despite longstanding criticism and call for such change. An array of emergent pacific metaphors has been suggested that may come to supplant martial metaphors. It may be that a single, dominant pacific metaphor (meta-narrative) does not supplant metaphors of war, but rather, a range of context-specific metaphors (small stories) become commonly used. Certainly, it is vital that metaphors used by doctors and healthcare professionals do not add to the suffering of patients, who may subscribe to different metaphors to best understand, tolerate or communicate their symptoms (Semino *et al.* 2015).

While there is a large body of work on the meanings and values of representations of medicine in fiction, film or television, there is no linguistic corpus analysis study of this 'mirror' literature of medicine. Anita Wohlmann (2015) at Johannes Gutenberg-Universität, Mainz, Germany is researching the use of metaphors in North American medical and fictional writing. She argues that such metaphors offer 'epistemic and experiential meeting places between medical and scientific information and individual lifeworlds' (www.grk.lifesciences-lifewriting.uni-mainz.de/research-projects/dr-anita-wohlmann-medical-metaphors/).

Wohlmann notes that the study of metaphor use in science received a boost after Lakoff and Johnson's work showing the ubiquity of metaphor, whereby metaphors in science were now read for their transformative potential rather than as displacement or ornamentation. Drawing on the work of Couser (2005) and Kirklin (2001, 2007), she also notes that 'the use of metaphors in relation to illness can involve harmful mystification of diseases or ethical problems with regard to truth telling'. However, Wohlmann has great faith in the transformative, invigorating and nourishing aspects of metaphor, which she describes as 'plurisignifying potential'. She is engaged in an important research project that does not isolate metaphors from the narratives in which they appear, but rather, reads metaphors as seeds for mini-narratives through which the larger narrative may be re-examined.

During correspondence with Anita Wohlmann, she was kind enough to send this summary of her current work, advertising the potentially rich process connections between medical and literary framings of the female body:

My research project is situated at the intersection of the humanities and medicine and focuses on metaphors in their capacities as potent epistemological and experiential devices. Metaphors, like narratives, are relevant in science and health contexts as they help explain complex and abstract information. At the same time, metaphors enable individuals to voice disruptive, personal experiences that are difficult to describe otherwise, for example through a coherent narrative. While narrative has been successfully implemented within interdisciplinary approaches, such as Medical Humanities and Narrative Medicine, research on metaphors has emphasized the problematic side of metaphors: Metaphors can be stigmatizing, essentializing or dehumanizing when the meaning of the source domain is substituted with that of the target (e.g., body as machine). Little attention has been paid so far to the fact that metaphors can also be pluripotent and empowering tools of the imagination, inviting ambiguity and complexity. Metaphors have the power to defamiliarize, contest and reimagine reductionist or allegedly set connotations. This research project asks: How can the plurisignifying potential of metaphors be activated and conceptualized so that limiting and harmful metaphors become liberating and productive?

The object of investigation is a corpus of fictional narratives by female American authors from 1850–1950, in which the writers negotiate, challenge and reimagine problematic metaphors of the female body. These metaphors were also used by doctors and scientists, who tried to explain the nature of womanhood. The analysis will exemplify how these metaphors of the female body, such as woman-as-flower or the body-as-a-closed-energy-system, can become spaces of individual agency and rhetorical resistance when their plurisignifying potential is activated. Thus, the project highlights how the definitions of the female body are in a state of flux and are constantly being negotiated and renegotiated between medical experts and female writers.

(Wohlmann 2016, personal correspondence, reproduced with permission)

Metaphors that no longer rise to the occasion ('dead' metaphors), or are actively harmful ('malignant metaphors'), may shape entire cultures, such as heroic medicine, the politically far right, or evangelical movements. But Wohlmann's work suggests to me that the same metaphors, when approached from perspectives, for example, of feminisms, liberation politics, social justice movements and pedagogies of the oppressed, are transformed, and can treat symptoms in the suffering body of metaphor itself.

Metaphor, too, can act as a softener where necessary. In the context of palliative care, Hutchings (1998, p. 283) suggests that the use of metaphor 'allows us to share a truth without the glare of reality', allowing healthcare practitioners to use 'veils that shield the dying from the glare of their prognosis'. Understanding metaphor use is important for doctors, in order to appreciate 'the inexplicable and unspeakable, the pain and isolation felt as a result of an illness experience'.

Metaphors can, then, be antidotes, shields (veiling the truth of a prognosis, for example), mirrors (metaphors as a medium for reflection), and levers (getting underneath something to reveal a hidden reality). Shielding, mirroring and providing leverage are differing forms of cognition reflecting 'thinking with metaphors', where metaphors are only 'explained' (rather, explored and appreciated) through further metaphors. For some, metaphor use is infrequent in medicine and still treated as a curiosity; for others, medicine is a performative activity in which language use drawing on metaphor is central. In the following chapter, I will trace how views on the importance of metaphor in medicine have changed historically, boosted especially by the work of George Lakoff and Mark Johnson (1980), who, fusing cognitive psychology, semantics (the meanings of language in social contexts) and semiotics (the study of the meaning of signs), prised metaphor studies away from a purely linguistic interest to study how metaphors shape concepts and thinking. More, Lakoff and Johnson's work shifts focus from the individual language user to social and cultural activities, or embodied and distributed cognition.

Imagine that metaphors are life forms living symbiotically with humans in overlapping habitats: culture, language, emotion and cognition. Metaphors appear especially as the aesthetics of performativity (or, life as poetry, rich in imagination and invention). Let us return to the 'sticky neurons' and 'sticky brains' metaphors used by the paediatricians studied – in their natural work habitats – by the anthropologist Mara Buchbinder (2015), described earlier. Buchbinder reasoned that these metaphors were used not just to approximate experience, but as political tools in the service of medicine – mobilized to label (and then control) awkward children (and the parents, who, in some cases, mirrored the children's symptoms) with pesky and unmanageable symptoms of overly perseverative thoughts, emotions and behaviours. By pragmatic clinicians, the descriptor 'sticky' was used, paradoxically, as a literal metaphor. You can practically touch the imagined, gluey neuronal clusters that gather on the inside, as stubbornness, fixity and overattention to detail manifest on the outer (perhaps more Velcro-like than gluey). This complex itself is glued by persistent and inexplicable felt pain.

The metaphor that life is 'sticky', like a piece of gum, was used to effect by Jean Paul Sartre to describe a key aspect of the existential experience of nausea (Shibles 1971, p. 6). Stickiness and glueyness are symptomatic of life itself, lived as a 'sickness unto death', as Kierkegaard described life's trajectory. We are urged now into perseverative behaviour as a virtue – a 'stickiness unto death': 'stick with it', 'stick to our guns', bearing with the 'sticky moments'. To come 'unstuck' is to fail. Experiencing and surviving 'sticky situations' builds resilience. The 'stickiness' metaphor circulates and infects like a virus, and metaphor is the medium through which life is refracted, for better or worse. So, why do we not note and tend our metaphors with greater diligence? Why has medicine in particular resisted metaphor, despite the latter's sticky tenacity? Why is the 'metaphorical method' (Shibles 1971) not taught to medical students as a meta-discursive strategy through which they can articulate how their medical- and specialty-specific thinking and performing (such as diagnostic reasoning) are shaped? The next chapter addresses these key questions, and more.

2 Metaphors, once down and out, make a comeback

Analogies, metaphors and similes/resemblances

An analogy is where one thing is compared to another for extra effect, explanation or clarification (such as: 'a fish out of water'), and is one of many linguistic tropes or 'figures of speech' (literary and rhetorical devices). Analogies include metaphors and similes or resemblances. A metaphor is a comparison of one thing to another whereby unlike things are shown to have something in common – such as 'a blanket of snow', 'a heart of gold' or 'drowning in money'. A simile or resemblance is where two unlike things are compared for effect (using 'as' or 'like') to make the sentence (and then the meaning) more vivid, such as 'timid as a mouse', 'bright as a berry' or 'a voice like thunder'.

> ('A voice like thunder' is famously employed in the first stanza of William Blake's poem 'Prologue to "King Edward the Fourth"':
> O for a voice like thunder, and a tongue
> To drown the throat of war! When the senses
> Are shaken, and the soul is driven to madness,
> Who can stand? When the souls of the oppressèd
> Fight in the troubled air that rages, who can stand?)

Similes or resemblances are self-explanatory ('the ball travelled like a rocket'), but metaphor requires more explanation. Metaphor (from the Greek *metapherein*) literally means 'to carry across' or 'transfer' – so, a term or phrase is applied to something to which it is not literally applicable in order to suggest a resemblance (such as 'time is money'). As Jeffery Donaldson (2015) suggests, A = B. Metaphor, then, has the important role in language of fuelling the imagination in its work against the mind (cognition or knowing) only taking things literally. A popular view is that the imagination distorts the senses, which otherwise receive the world in direct fashion. The French scientist and phenomenologist Gaston Bachelard (1977, 1988, 1989, 1992, 1994, 2002) wrote a series of books in which he challenged this view, illustrating how the imagination 'prepared' the senses so that the world is already 'seen' poetically (Stroud and Sardello 2015). Metaphors can bring colour and vibrancy to otherwise staid descriptions. Bachelard, moreover, argues that such imaginal perception is essential for scientific discovery, where the natural world is 'seen through' or seen afresh.

Metaphor potentially doubles conceptual capital through transfer from one conceptual platform to another: an economist describes a slight or weak economic upturn in medical terms, as 'an anaemic recovery' (www.bbc.co.uk/news/business-30208476). This is a compound irony – there are two subjects (the body and the health of the economy), and both are gently mocked. The metaphor simultaneously increases both our understanding or insight, and our appreciation.

However, metaphors do not always turn the ordinary into the extraordinary, or work to translate mundane things into something more imaginative. Metaphors can, as Shane Neilson (2015) suggests, 'close off thinking'. They can be negative, even destructive, in their effects. Neilson shows how medicine's use of both verbal and visual metaphors to describe and understand pain – such as neurology's use of 'wires', 'keys' and 'doors' – can restrict interpretations and opinions. On the other hand, literature offers a goldmine for metaphors of pain that open up thinking and imagination, such as the graphic torture scenes in Vincent Lam's (2012) *The Headmaster's Wager*, made all the more poignant as Lam is an emergency physician and must have witnessed pain on a daily basis.

In the following Chapter 3, I discuss the use of medical slang, which is highly insulting to the patients to which it refers; and, in Chapter 4, I discuss leading or didactic metaphors – 'big' metaphors that have historically shaped medical culture – as misleading or deleterious, closing down thinking. We have already seen from the previous chapter that Susan Sontag faced this dilemma head on by suggesting that we erase metaphors from talk of illness in case they turn nasty and stigmatize patients. Barbara Maier and Warren Shibles (2011), as we have also seen, start from a position in which metaphors could not possibly be erased from medicine, for they are an essential part of its fabric, both a permanent glow and a stain. Indeed, Shibles (1971) argues that to attempt to expunge metaphors from language is philosophically naïve and misguided.

'Big' metaphors include 'the body as machine' (mechanical metaphors) and 'medicine as war' (martial metaphors). Neilson's (2015) perceptive examples are from medicine's descriptions of pain as reductive of experience. 'Pain' is not just a neural pathway and cannot be encompassed by models of 'doors', 'keys' and 'wires' that can readily shut down thinking, rather than opening up possibilities. Rather, those who suffer from chronic pain in particular have a unique experience that cannot be reduced, as Elaine Scarry (1985) describes, to metaphors of weapons and damage (a subset of the 'medicine as war' didactic metaphor that is described by Elena Semino and colleagues (Semino *et al.* 2015) as a 'violence' metaphor).

Further, where tropes (such as metaphors) become overused, they may lose their impact. In Mark Antony's speech to the people after the assassination of Caesar in Shakespeare's (1599) *Julius Caesar*, the line 'Friends, Romans, countrymen, lend me your ears' (i.e. 'listen to me') has, arguably, become hackneyed through repeated use and no longer has the effect that it once had. (In a *Mad* magazine from the 1950s, the era of the Beat generation and 'hipster' vocabulary, Shakespeare is lampooned – Antony says: 'Friends, Romans, hipsters, let me clue you in'.) In contrast, where Antony in the same speech says 'I come not, friends, to steal away your hearts', the metaphor remains powerful, particularly because the heart is traditionally the locus of love, passion and courage. This could mean that Antony is persuading the crowd that he is not trying to agitate them, but rather, that he is encouraging each of them to follow their own passions and courage of conviction in the wake of the murder of Caesar.

The literary critic and rhetorician I.A. Richards (1965) described metaphor as 'a carrying over of a word from its normal use to a new use'. This plain definition underplays the impact of metaphor, where the shift in the 'carrying over' is often unexpected and, potentially, can turn the ordinary into the extraordinary. For example, in Homer's *Iliad* (lines 415–19, trans. Fagles 1998) the Greek fighters are compared to ravenous wolves: 'As ravenous wolves come swooping down on lambs or kids to snatch them away from right amidst their flocks/ ... / so the Achaeans mauled the Trojans.' The Greek soldier (the ordinary) becomes the swooping and mauling, ravenous wolf (the extraordinary). Potentially plain or bland description is turned into vivid and disturbing imagery through use of metaphor, so that the reader's emotions and imagination are engaged as well as the mind. Homer's description goes beyond inviting understanding to a full-bodied appreciation, engaging the reader's (visual) eye and (visceral) gut. Homer's poetry is the primary example of how metaphors are embodied and vivify.

Homer's language here – or this particular translation by Robert Fagles (1998, p. 424) – is even more complex, as one would not normally think of wolves as 'swooping'. This conjures up images, rather, of eagles or other birds of prey with their talons extended, adding to the power of the metaphor. Further, the use of 'wolves' in the plural conjures up a ravenous pack on the hunt, far more disturbing than the lone wolf (the latter a good metaphor for the *Iliad*'s Achilles).

In the first Western account of literary theory – *Poetics* – written in 335 BC, Aristotle argued that language gains 'distinction' by 'deviating' from 'the normal idiom'. He goes on to say that those who understand such exceptional use of language are themselves marked as exceptional – they are poets, for whom 'the greatest thing by far is to have a command of metaphor ... it is the mark of genius, for to make good metaphors implies an eye for resemblances'. Dennis Donoghue (2014, p. 62) suggests that Aristotle uses 'resemblances' here to mean going beyond comparing one thing with another. Rather, it is the ability to see 'likeness between relations involving them' – an underlying structural similarity that brings two things together unexpectedly, but forcibly, such that the imagination is fired and the world is seen anew. This is recognition of complex patterns below surface features, a 'seeing through'.

Aristotle noted that Homer could, as it were, bring the dead back to life through appropriate use of metaphor: 'making the lifeless live'. In other words, a metaphor animates. We are so used to analogies such as 'right as rain' (first recorded in 1894) that they now pall, but reflection on such analogies soon renews appreciation. The analogy works not just because of the alliteration but because rain falls straight, cleanses and makes things grow. What could be more 'right'? A further view is that, as the analogy first appeared in England, Britain is associated with rainy weather, or rain is the order of the day.

Metaphors release the mind and body from the prison of the literal. However, historically, under the hegemony of literalism, the Western mind has been imprisoned for some time, as it has refused the value of metaphor. Metaphor is seen as peripheral to everyday language and as ornament or embroidery – fine for poets, but not for everyday speech or for technical language, especially in the sciences. With the rediscovery of the Classical tradition during the Renaissance, studies of rhetoric flourished, with over 3,500 works published in over 15,000 editions between 1460 and 1700 (Mack 2011). This was a golden age of innovation and experiment in rhetorical theory and included many studies on metaphor. Indeed, personal identity and expression came to be seen as a metaphorical art of 'self-forming' (Greenblatt 1980), an early version of 'self-help' and 'identity construction'; for example, the cultivation of melancholy was seen as a sign of intellectual prowess and not a symptom of 'depression' – the latter a blanket term concealing as much as it reveals.

During the Enlightenment, however, metaphor was demonized as unnecessary clutter, serving the function of extending and prettifying language – as rhetoric or forms of persuasion, or as poetic devices. In the empiricist tradition, exemplified by the work of the seventeenth-century philosopher John Locke, rhetoric and figurative language such as metaphor should be avoided. Language should be logical, cleansed of any poetic leanings. Scientific language, above all, was valued for its supposed lack of rhetoric and metaphor. The value of metaphor was rediscovered during later interest in semantics or the meanings of language in context.

In *The Philosophy of Rhetoric*, I.A. Richards (1965) famously challenged the empiricist view of metaphor and suggested that metaphor's function goes well beyond its stylistic or rhetorical concerns to the heart of semantics and language's social uses. Where language fundamentally shapes thinking, metaphor infects that language. Indeed, cognition *is* metaphor. Thinking is the process of 'interaction between co-present thoughts' such that the analogy (metaphor or resemblance) moves thinking forward, generates insight and innovation, and provides adaptability. Without metaphor, thinking would remain static. Half a century after Richards, George Lakoff, a linguist, and Mark Johnson, a philosopher, both familiar with the contemporary landscape of cognitive science, wrote *Metaphors We Live By* (Lakoff and Johnson 1980), providing the evidence from cognitive science that was needed to justify Richards' claim. Lakoff and Johnson put metaphor at the centre of conceptual thinking and the understanding of cognitive conceptual systems.

For Lakoff and Johnson, the use of metaphors is not just a function of language and part of our cognitive process, but is the very essence of it – indeed, the architecture of conceptual thinking. We draw on a wide variety of metaphorical positions that have become second nature in speech acts – for example, metaphors of cutting: 'we need to slash the budget', 'she has a razor sharp wit', 'I can undercut his price', 'they cut my argument to ribbons'; or spatial metaphors: 'she fell in love', 'I shot him a sideways glance', 'it's downhill all the way', 'things are looking up', 'don't invade my personal space', 'there's room for manoeuvre'.

Metaphor, then, is where one conceptual domain is understood in terms of another – thus, 'time is money' involves Richards' 'interaction between co-present thoughts' to arrive at a new conceptual understanding or insight. This 'co-presence' of thinking can work at a larger level of conceptual complexity. For example, Bleakley (1992) shows how metaphors of human relationship, such as 'bond', 'security' and 'trust', familiar to proponents of John Bowlby's 'attachment theory' of mother–child early life interaction, are seamlessly transposed as metaphors to the world of economics and banking, where we buy 'bonds' and set up 'trust' funds in order to ensure financial 'security'. Heartless and cold economics is instantly transformed into fleshly warmth.

Richards describes this relationship between co-present thoughts as that of a 'tenor' and a 'vehicle'. The tenor is the original conception, which is given greater freedom and/or expression by the vehicle. For example, in 'life is an uphill struggle', 'life' is the tenor and 'uphill struggle' is the vehicle. Linguists interested in cognitive science have largely replaced these terms, so that 'tenor' is described as 'source' and 'vehicle' as 'target'. The source is often concrete and sense based, while the target is often conceptual ('love is blind'), although the target may be felt sensually, even more strongly than the source. The target 'blind' in 'Love is blind' hits you not between the eyes but right in the eyes. Most of us have keenly felt this blindness when the object of affection is idealized.

From isolated text to real world metaphors

In a shift away from cognitive science's recent dominance in metaphor studies, linguistics is once again staking a claim for a more nuanced study of metaphor emphasizing 'real world' metaphors (Cameron and Low 1999; Cameron 2003; Low *et al.* 2010). Here, abstractions in linguistics and studies of isolated texts are replaced by concrete social use of language extended to the non-verbal and performative realms. Such contextual use (for example, in everyday conversation, or in contexts such as school education) is subject to analysis at the macro level of discourse regulation and innovation, or at the micro level of the sentence or utterance. As noted, Richards' 'tenor' and 'vehicle' have been replaced by 'source' and 'target', but also by 'topic domain' and 'vehicle domain' when referring to conceptual or content domains, and 'topic' and 'vehicle' when referring to lexical items. (With singular exceptions – for example, Richard Gwyn (1999) – this literature does not touch the field of metaphors in medicine.)

Metaphors in real time and space lose their identity as objects or specimens for analysis when they acquire the status of 'process' as dynamic, complex, adaptive systems, whereby key metaphors act as more or less stable attractors to be potentially undone or replaced by other attractors in system adaptations.

This shift to historical, cultural and social contexts for metaphors – again, often referred to as 'real world' use (Low *et al.* 2010), taking them out of purely lexical and linguistic abstraction – has consequence for 'metaphor' itself. While a metaphor can be defined in the abstract, what counts as a metaphor in real world interaction is whether or not a communication – an utterance, a speech act, an exchange, a performative communication (or miscommunication), a virtual message or exchange such as in tweeting or sending an email or text message, an advert, and so forth – is either intended or received as metaphorical. (See Appendix 2 on how to decide whether or not a particular textual or spoken word or phrase, an image or an action can be counted as a 'metaphor' when researching the use of metaphors.)

What counts as metaphor, then, depends upon context and frame. Thus, common idiomatic usage such as 'you've really put the cat amongst the pigeons' is easy enough to pick out as metaphorical use of language. However, this may be taken literally by somebody who is autistic or schizophrenic. An ironic gesture, a sardonic smile, a subtle sleight of hand in language use may all be intended metaphorically but received literally where their potential impact is misjudged. A 'handoff' in an Emergency Department to a variety of in-patient services (Hilligoss 2014; Hilligoss *et al.* 2015) has the opposite meaning to a 'handoff' in rugby (where the opponent is pushed away – a 'stiff arm' in American football).

Cameron and Low (1999) discuss how metaphors may be identified and discussed by researchers in spoken discourse data as an issue of the validity of such data. It may seem obvious that spoken discourse can be validated, or not, for metaphorical usage by the speaker, but this proves to be difficult when speakers do not realize that they are using metaphor; the metaphorical use is 'dead' or habitual; metaphor is a flow of slang; or metaphors are artfully reinvented and deconstructed in spontaneous improvised art forms such as rap, hip-hop, poetry slams, action painting and modern jazz. Researchers tend to identify metaphor use intuitively from the overall flow of language.

If I say not that 'I opted out of the meeting today' (literal description), but 'I back-tracked from the meeting today', does this mean I am drifting into the realm of metaphor, however slightly? What if I say 'I avoided the meeting like the plague'? This is plainly a metaphor, but is it too tired to have impact or generate imaginative response? If a urologist says to a medical student at the bedside 'Benign prostatic hyperplasia is causing an obstruction of the urethra', how will Tom, the medically naïve patient, receive this as he overhears it? Will he hear only slightly meaningless or confusing metaphor? Will he be insulted if the urologist reverts to talk of 'there's something wrong with your waterworks'? How will the surgeon explain to Tom that he needs a trans-urethral resection of the prostate (TURP) without resorting to spoken and verbal metaphors? Will he explain that the first urination after the operation is commonly described as 'peeing through ground glass' or as 'peeing fire'?

As Cameron and Low (1999) note, what constitutes a metaphor may be an individual's response, but a discourse community shapes this. This may be a cross-cultural difference, or discourse within a specialist community such as medicine interacting with a general population. It may also be a generational issue – the elderly will not 'get' youth culture metaphors such as those derived from hip-hop or grime music; also, try talking to a child who is just acquiring language – despite his or her vivid imagination – about a 'traffic jam', or worse, 'kicking the bucket'!

Further, as Cameron (2003) notes – in an analysis of how children at school aged 10 and 11 discuss a child's science text describing the ozone layer and how the human heart works – the adult's and the child's uses of metaphors may differ to create misunderstandings. The biology text describes the heart as a pump, where the heart has 'walls' and is the centre of a 'transport system' for blood. The children, however, do not receive these metaphors in the way that the adults who devised the text intended them. The child's primary knowledge of a 'pump' is not based on a generalized abstraction of mechanics, but on specific objects – particularly the bicycle pump. As the heart drawn in the text does not correspond in any way with how a bicycle pump looks, it is difficult for the child to transpose the notion of pump (and pumped air) onto the imagined heart.

Finally, what constitutes a metaphor in living language and performed interactions – including a high level of the non-verbal – depends upon use, abuse and overuse of metaphors. Overused metaphors become 'dead metaphors' and have no 'meaning', or at least the meaning has been squeezed out of them through overuse and abuse, so that the tired and bruised metaphors are part of habitual language and offer no surprise or shift in cognition or imagination. Metaphors set up home in the unconscious or the tacit realm of knowing.

Blended and embodied metaphors: slow nightfall

Returning to the relationship between tenor and vehicle or source/topic and target, in the earlier Homeric example, the Achaeans (Greek soldiers) constitute the tenor/source/topic and the swooping and mauling, ravenous pack of wolves the vehicle/target through which the impact of the metaphor is achieved. Again, the metaphor 'works' because it suddenly undoes the conceptual nature of the vehicle or target by grounding it in the surprise or unimagined sensory and the active (or, the metaphor is 'embodied'). Thus, 'love is blind' again works because the concrete source (love) is dissolved in the abstract target (blind), whereby the target loses its abstraction in the pairing. You can once more 'feel' the blindness of love. The writer Jorge Luis Borges (undated www.brainyquote. com/quotes/quotes/j/jorgeluisb125297.html) described his progressive, hereditary deterioration of sight as 'slow nightfall', where 'Nothing is built on stone; all is built on sand, but we must build as if the sand were stone.' Here, the sighted can empathize with the blind thanks to metaphor.

Contemporary metaphor theory (Fludernik 2011) is suspicious of a sharp division between tenor/source/topic and vehicle/target, describing 'blended' metaphors in which there are emergent structures. This turns metaphors into active, fluid phenomena upsetting the supposed stability of the tenor as ground or source. Recall that Richards had already described the power of metaphor as 'co-present thoughts'. Returning to my example from Shakespeare's *Julius Caesar* above, 'lend me your ears' has neither tenor/source nor vehicle/target but is, rather, an interactive blend in which the hierarchy of source and target domains is dissolved or democratized. Brutus had, in fact, earlier used a formulaic oratory addressing the people: 'Romans, countrymen, and lovers, hear me for my cause, and be silent that you may hear' (lines 13–14). 'Be silent' is a plain, literal, cold command, where 'lend me your ears' is a warm metaphoric invitation, almost an embrace, in which tenor and vehicle dissolve into one. Mark Antony cleverly lampoons Brutus' earlier speech, and the use of metaphor gives the speech greater rhetorical or persuasive power.

Lakoff and Johnson (1999) insist that so-called 'conceptual' thinking is embodied. They completed their project of anatomizing metaphorical thought as an everyday cognitive strategy with *Philosophy in the Flesh: The Embodied Mind and Its Challenge to Western Thought.* This book challenges the Western Cartesian tradition of splitting body and mind and then disembodying reason and of assuming that most thinking, and scientific thinking in particular, is literal and logical. The authors reverse traditional thinking that metaphors are peripheral to conceptual thinking and metaphysics to suggest that metaphysics arises from a ground of cognition best appreciated metaphorically.

When the poet Wallace Stevens (1954) writes, in the poem 'St John and the Back-Ache', that 'the world is presence, not force', we sense precisely what this means. It is not just conceptual. It is as if 'the world' were sitting next to us, negotiating, rather than pressing on us or confronting us ('the weight of the world on his shoulders'). Where Burton describes the 'anatomy of melancholy', or better, Joseph Conrad confronts us with a 'heart of darkness', these metaphors slip straight into our limbic systems, creating tensions and emotional states. Conrad's metaphor enters us like a parasitic worm and burrows into our moral body – the novella begins at the mouth of the Thames, transports us to the Congo River, and takes us upstream to the source of darkness as the banks of the river begin to converge and oppress. Here, Kurtz, the ivory trader, has slipped into megalomania. High Belgian imperialism is embodied in these dark metaphors. Or perhaps these metaphors slip into the enteric nervous system that controls the intestines and digestion, so that a 'gut feeling' is really a knowing through metaphor; the enteric system has five times the level of neuronal complexity of the spinal cord, truly a 'sticky brain'.

While metaphors are embodied, metaphor making has a physical substrate in brain activity. Zohar Eviatar and Marcel Just (2006) used functional magnetic resonance imaging (fMRI) to scan the brain activation in 16 healthy participants when they were read stories of three lines that concluded with either a literal, an ironic or a metaphoric sentence. The brain responds selectively to non-literal language, with significantly higher levels of activation in the left inferior frontal gyrus (IFG) – an area that is important for language comprehension generally – and in the bilateral inferior temporal cortex for metaphoric utterances over ironic and literal utterances. There is, then, a differentiated functional cortical

architecture for the use of metaphor. Eviatar and Just suggest that dual processing occurs during metaphor comprehension, whereby the literal and the figurative are considered side-by-side and the literal comes to be abandoned for the
figurative as a resolution of Richards' 'co-present thoughts'. In other words, the
source is needed to grasp the more complex or imaginative target.

Douglas Hofstadter, a cognitive scientist and scholar in comparative literature, and Emmanuel Sander, a cognitive and experimental psychologist (Hofstadter and Sander 2013), have developed Lakoff and Johnson's work and
brought the field up to date. Importantly, they point out how metaphors are contextual and culture specific. They claim that conceptual thinking is not at all
abstract but grounded in the language of things, and best described as 'analogical thinking'. Indeed, analogy is 'the fuel and fire of thinking', as their book title
suggests: *Surfaces and Essences: Analogy as the Fuel and Fire of Thinking*.
Analogy includes both metaphor and resemblance. These are often collapsed.
When we say 'Richard Lionheart' (a metaphor), we mean that Richard is like a
lion (a resemblance). A metaphor such as 'it rained cats and dogs' is hard to
convert into a resemblance. A resemblance such as 'pug faced' is self-
explanatory – even descriptive. An analogy such as 'red mist descending' (a
sudden fit of anger) is literal enough for resemblance (the blood boils and then
goes off the boil, so it ascends and descends as a fine mist), but also complex
enough for metaphor, so that plain 'anger' is raised to another level of appreciation and complexity. Anger is poeticized. Achilles is invoked – not just 'lion-
hearted' but also 'breaker of men'.

What Hofstadter and Sander do is to keep us close to language itself and not
to activity (other than speaking or writing), to demonstrate that language does
work, creates feeling and sensations, fuels the imagination and makes creative
leaps. Language is not some abstract thing that is accessed to conceptualize our
embodied life, but rather, is a tangible medium through which we experience
and make sense of embodiment. Again, metaphors are tangibly felt, embodied
(such as 'we had the lion's share', 'it's water off a duck's back', 'her voice is as
smooth as silk') – you feel the metaphor's impact in your being as you say it or
read it. Metaphors are sensual or aesthetic.

Most importantly, Hofstadter and Sander move the philosophical basis of
understanding metaphor from a broadly structuralist to a poststructuralist basis.
Structuralists, such as the anthropologist Claude Lévi-Strauss, suggest that the
mind universally functions through the language of dualities such as the 'raw'
and the 'cooked', or 'nature' and 'culture' (others include male–female, adult–
child, human–animal). Poststructuralists suggest that such basic universal rules
(grand narratives) do not exist – rather, there are local rules and structures (small
narratives), so that thinking and behaving are social constructions contingent
upon historical context. There are no shared, basic frames, but a proliferation of
contextually defined habits as multiple voices.

Lakoff and Johnson veer towards structuralism, suggesting that the mind is
structured through three main metaphorical forms. These are 'metaphors we live
by' ('we' being all humanity): (i) structural metaphors such as 'time is money'

and 'argument is war', where one concept is metaphorically structured in terms of another; (ii) orientational metaphors, where thinking is structured spatially, such as 'happy is up' and 'sad is down', 'keeping our heads above water', 'we've got to get on top of this' and so forth (familiar from medicine, such as 'feeling on top of the world' or 'fell ill' and 'dropped dead'), or somebody is 'out there' or 'in control'; and (iii) ontological metaphors that shape experience in terms of forms such as containers ('she's in the clear', 'we are entering difficult territory', 'I feel hemmed in'). Lakoff and Johnson are not, however, fully committed structuralists – they note that some metaphors will be culture specific. However, they suggest that there are universal 'natural' metaphors, by which 'love', 'time' and 'argument' are expressed in terms of other domains of experience such as 'journey', 'money' and 'war'.

Following Richards' lead, these authors reject both subjectivist and objectivist interpretations of the world for an 'interactionist' view. Here, meaning is obtained through one perspective engaging with another, where the second usually raises the intensity of the first through conceptual transfer across domains. Meanings also change through time as new metaphors emerge. This is important for science and medicine, suggesting that:

1   Scientific 'truths' are culturally and historically defined meanings shaped metaphorically. This does not mean that 'facts' cannot be established, but 'truths' lead us into a different territory.
2   Medicine is essentially an interactionist practice, where the meanings brought by science meet the meanings brought by patients.

However, despite Lakoff and Johnson's interactionist view, they still hold that in the two terms of metaphor, the source and the target domains, there is a hierarchy. Target trumps source or replaces source as the thinking process is enhanced and transferred. You cannot play for two teams at once. For example, the superlatives 'over the moon' or 'it makes my blood boil' take us from the ordinary (source) to the extraordinary (target), where the source is now even omitted from the pairing.

In a new wave of thinking about metaphor, Fauconnier and Turner (2002) question the structure of the hierarchical interaction in a call for democratic pairings. This new turn in metaphor theory is away from cognitive metaphor theory towards a new kind of literary approach that rejects structures of hierarchy between target and source, or democratizes these terms to produce 'blended' metaphors. An example is 'this will put lead in his pencil' (restore virility). Source and target are meaningless terms here. Rather, there is a democratic conversation between 'lead' (suggesting gravity and weight, as well as inscription) and 'pencil' (suggesting penis, virility, stiff, erect).

Concepts are created by drawing on different domains of knowledge brought together as a collage. In the example 'life is an uphill struggle', framing 'life' as the source and 'uphill struggle' as the target does not really get us anywhere in terms of replacing a simpler concept with a more complex one. What could be more complex than 'life' itself or more simple, or explicit, than 'uphill' and 'struggle'? When they are conjoined, however, something magical happens in terms of a fresh meaning. Indeed, the jointed and 'blended' metaphor seems more powerful than the two, dis-jointed, component parts, and readily invites (often ironic) comparisons with other metaphors, such as 'it's downhill all the way'.

Four spaces are involved in any metaphor (Fludernik 2011). Take the simile 'bright as a button'. 'Source' and 'target' terms here are really meaningless, as both terms afford equal weight within the conceptual space. There are two input spaces: 'bright' (as both shining and intelligent) and 'button' (military buttons are shined). The third space is the generic space that links the two, and the fourth space is the blend. Meaning is created as these mental spaces come into democratic relationship with one another. The blended space is greater than the sum of its parts but is also a highly compressed version of the sum of the components.

An illustrative example from mental health is 'bipolar disorder', once known as 'manic depression'. Extreme cases show mood swings from depressive, suicidal 'downs' to manic, unrealistic 'highs' in which delusions can readily occur. Spatial metaphors in particular abound for these two states: 'down in the dumps', 'leaden', 'hitting rock bottom' for depression, and 'the sky's the limit', 'things are looking up', 'high as a kite' for mania. A generic third metaphorical space can link the two; let us imagine those preferred by psychiatry – 'mood stabilization' (drug therapies) – and psychotherapy – 'getting balance in your life' and 'talking it through' (talk therapies). A fourth, or blended, space might be the preferred metaphorical space of the person carrying the symptoms: 'I'm back on track.'

The new wave of interest in metaphor from linguistics working with cognitive psychology, then, dramatically challenges the popular misconception that analogies produce a kind of embroidered language or artistic conceit fit for poets and painters. Cognitive psychologists have reclaimed the ground of analogy as everyday. Hofstadter and Sander (2013) claim that everyday cognition is, in fact, analogical thinking. Analogy, again, is both 'the fuel and fire of thinking' (foundational to thinking), or the means by which everyday concepts are initiated, maintained and transformed: 'fuel' because metaphors are necessary for thinking, 'fire' because they animate thinking. To refuse the metaphorical is to go against the grain of everyday cognition and requires a good deal of unproductive burning of thinking 'fuel'. To resist or argue away the value of metaphorical life is like purposefully flattening affect – it is to squander a gift, that is, the texture afforded through human imagination (see Appendix 1 for a taxonomy of metaphors).

From everyday language to medical expression

The use of metaphor in medicine is not one of choice – metaphor is already embodied in medical language and practice. Indeed, to repeat the earlier metaphor, medicine is saturated in analogy (whether in language, use of artefacts or performance). The stethoscope and white coat 'stand for' the doctor (Mangione 2012). As with overused metaphors that lose their impact, so the white coat and stethoscope are both disappearing in medicine. The white coat is already a dead signifier (and metaphor) in the UK. It was phased out in 2007 because of infection issues where coats were not laundered properly. The stethoscope may lose traction for very practical reasons – doctors use stethoscopes less and less in bedside examinations because imaging techniques such as ultrasound are more reliable.

The use of metaphor may not always be 'positive' (used for good effect, such as meeting a very ill patient and commenting on how he or she is like a 'ray of sunshine today'). Metaphorical activity may be a way in which medicine – as physically and emotionally demanding, even draining – defends itself against potential attack, collapse, confusion, chaos or whiteout.

Hardy (2012) suggests that in medicine, 'metaphor may fill the space created by uncertainty'. Metaphors offer a way of embracing the value of uncertainty, dropping the façade of certainty about diagnosis and treatment (the scientific conceit) to embrace the reality of uncertainty and ambiguity as a resource. It is not that medicine needs more metaphors; it needs better metaphors, and a better ear for them from clinicians, especially in the metaphorical meshwork that constitutes productive patient–doctor communication. As Schwartz (2015, p. 734) suggests,

> Even in so-called hard science and medicine, metaphors are stuffed like old newspapers into the gaps of our understanding.... The task of the next generation is not to replace these metaphors with absolute truths, but to exchange them for more apt ones.

Some may argue that patients want to hear certainties, so medicine should constantly strive for certainty, and this is why the march of science informing medicine is important. However, research shows that patients do not necessarily want to hear certainties – rather, they want a good, trusting relationship with their doctor focusing on their 'chief concern' rather than just the doctor's version of the 'chief complaint' (Schleifer and Vannatta 2013). Further, despite the rise of evidence-based medicine, research shows that general practitioners do not resort to evidence bases in consultations but rely on what John Gabbay and Andrée Le May call 'clinical mindlines' – expertise-based, context-driven judgements (praxis) (Gabbay and Le May 2010).

Where medicine continues to refuse the value of metaphor, the surface of medicine may not be a great one upon which to gain traction for new metaphors. Take 'mindlines' above. Gabbay and Le May coined the term to describe 'internalised and collectively reinforced tacit guidelines' as opposed to 'written clinical guidelines' (Wieringa and Greenhalgh 2015). Mindlines are 'fluid, embodied and intersubjective' (ibid.) means of thinking medicine and diagnosing – in other words, they act just like metaphors, as connectors that raise deeper meanings.

Yet, in Wieringa and Greenhalgh's (2015) meta-narrative review of the literature on 10 years' reception of 'mindlines', they discovered widespread resistance to, and misunderstanding of, the term. The resistance may be grounded in discomfort with 'mindlines' as a term that reduces tacit knowledge to an overall category, rather than recognizing differences between forms of such knowledge. This may be likened to Lakoff and Johnson's (1980) popularization of the 'conduit' metaphor (things travelling from one place to another), which replaces a complex range of metaphors with a 'super metaphor' (Grady 1998).

Perhaps 'mindlines' does not resonate in the same way as 'songlines' (the Australian aboriginal term for sacred paths walked in the outback), or the now everyday 'online', or 'faultline'. It may not be a productive metaphor for what is a tacit web of knowledge, more a mycorrhizal structure than a linear track, which does not press for certainty but is able to soak up and tolerate ambiguity. The image that 'mindlines' conjures – in lines, on tracks – is not how the brain appears to operate tacitly, as webs of interrelated illness scripts. Do we need 'sticky' or 'fuzzy' mindlines?

Admittance of uncertainty makes medicine 'human', removes unnecessary 'heroic' status from doctors, invites collaboration to seek differing viewpoints, and engages the patient in realistic conversation. More, where intolerance of ambiguity is the central trait of the authoritarian personality (Bleakley 2014), as medicine reshapes its culture from an authoritarian and hierarchical historical form to a contemporary democracy inviting authentic patient-centredness and team collaboration, so tolerance of ambiguity will become the central value of medical practice (Bleakley 2014, 2015). Donald Schön (1983, 1990) describes how professional practitioners in a variety of fields, including medicine and healthcare, must negotiate between the messy realities of the practical 'lowly swampland' of the individual patient, which is full of uncertainty, and the rarefied, theoretical 'high ground' of evidence-based practice. Pedagogy, too, is enriched by such metaphors, and I have devoted Chapter 8 to this, focusing on medical education.

How does an evidence-based approach deal with the fact that in one study using a sample of 890 patients across two London hospitals in a cross-sectional survey (seven clinic specialties excluding psychiatry), around 50 per cent of patients presented with 'medically unexplained symptoms' – primarily in gynaecology (an alarming 66 per cent of the sample studied) (Nimnuan *et al.* 2001)? Eben Schwartz (2015) notes that

> Estimates of the prevalence of medically unexplained symptoms range from 5–65% in primary care to 37–66% in specialty clinics. It is difficult to pin down a solid approximation partly because it's hard to define what constitutes a medically unexplained symptom.

We need more than technical-rational thinking in medicine to deal with phenomena such as medically unexplained symptoms and complex and shifting symptoms such as those that occur in mental health contexts. The use of metaphor helps to better inhabit such landscapes. Indeed, as Neil Pickering (2006) argues, 'mental illness' itself can be read as a metaphor (see Chapter 7).

Just as doctors need to cultivate tolerance of ambiguity to better practice medicine, so we need tolerance of ambiguity to consciously and reflexively inhabit the world of metaphor. Within new 'blended' models of metaphor, the two parts – once distinguished as source and target as a way of resolving some uncertainty – must now be democratically held together and tolerated as a complex and unstable interactive unit. We also need high levels of tolerance of ambiguity to face the reality, mentioned earlier, that key, or didactic, metaphors that have historically shaped medical culture – such as 'the body as machine' and 'medicine as war' – are not productive, no longer turn the ordinary into the extraordinary, and will slowly be displaced. The historical context for the emergence of these metaphors is discussed below and in Chapter 4. They are, in fact, unhelpful to contemporary medicine, having shaped an heroic, masculine, hierarchical, 'dragonslaying' culture that runs against the grain of the contemporary desire for a democratic, feminine, patient-centred and team-based culture. Such negative and unproductive leading metaphors need to be actively transformed or ditched through attention to both the language we use in medicine and typical styles of performance. This is a challenging project for medical education.

Indeed, just how a metaphor changes, and what part human agency plays in this, is unclear. We attempt to grasp the evolution of metaphors through the metaphor of 'evolution' (natural selection, best fit, extinction), as Jeffery Donaldson (2015) explores. What part, then, does intervention play in shifting metaphors, such as policy decisions? Above, I talk about 'ditching' and 'transforming' metaphors, but are these appropriate metaphors in themselves? Greenhalgh and Wieringa (2011) ask if it is time to 'drop' the 'knowledge translation' metaphor from healthcare policy, where 'knowledge translation' is both a fuzzy and awkward notion; but is 'drop' the best metaphor to use? Can we really just 'drop' a metaphor at will, like dropping a player from a football team?

Dead metaphors exhumed

Ulrike Kistner (1998, p. 10) argues that metaphors in medicine are historically contingent and are continually being developed; 'different kinds of metaphoric constructions' have 'different kinds of assertive or explanatory power'. Kistner shows that metaphors operate at differing levels of rhetorical urgency (power to persuade) and sophistication in terms of explanatory power. The most sophisticated metaphors address issues of causality in diagnosis and treatment. The least sophisticated metaphors are descriptive. Kistner notes that Ernst Anton Nicolai, an eighteenth-century German philosopher, had, as early as 1756, written that medicine utilized language in ways that went beyond literal description (in the emerging scientific tradition) to include metaphor, but that such use had not been theorized or systematically explained. More, symptoms are read as signs where the meaning of the relationship between the sign and what it signifies is not explicated. In other words, the disease that the symptom points to remains hidden from the diagnostic process. Diagnosis is always dealing with the sign, rather than what the sign signifies, and so the meanings of diseases or illnesses actually remain a mystery to the doctor. Further, while every symptom is a sign, not every sign is a symptom.

Nicolai then argues that a semiotic medicine, where sign is equated with symptom, is uni-dimensional and does not represent the reality of illness. A truly diagnostic medicine does not work forward from sign as symptom to diagnosis, but rather, from the overall meaning of the illness (thus taking into account the context for illness, the individuality of the patient and the emergence of the illness temporally within that patient's lifeworld) back to the symptom(s). This is the mark of expertise in medicine (Schleiffer and Vannatta 2013).

Kistner notes that by the 1830s to 1840s, 'semiotic' medicine is eradicated from the textbooks, to be replaced by 'diagnostic' medicine. The doctor does not simply 'read' the patient according to a standard classification of frozen signs that fits all. Rather, the doctor 'reads into' every patient as an individual, 'seeing through' the surface semiotics to deeper meanings for disease and illness where symptom manifestation is appreciated temporally (what develops into what?). A metaphorical medicine is then born in the shift from signs to symbols as diagnostic indicators. Kistner (1998, p. 17) notes the 'semantic impertinence' (a term made popular by the philosopher Paul Ricoeur) of the metaphor in developing wider ranges of meaning in diagnostic work. Semantic impertinence describes words that could not, or would not, be used literally, but that have deeper and possibly disturbing figurative value.

Metaphors, however, can become 'dead' over time, whereby the target merely substitutes for the source and thus no new insight or meaning is generated. This reminds us that metaphors are historically sensitive. Didactic metaphors have tremendous staying power – they are 'big guns'. But these, too, must lose impact and may become dead over time. 'Paternalism' is one such metaphor, now dead on its feet in contemporary medical practice, where more feminine metaphors of collaboration ('patient-centredness', for example) are now established as showing 'semantic impertinence'. The level of impertinence can be road tested by tracking the level of resistance to such metaphors within traditional medical culture. For example, surgical culture in particular remains resistant to these more feminine metaphors (Bleakley 2014).

Another didactic metaphor that has surely lost any semantic impertinence is 'medicine is war'. When this metaphor emerged in the mid-seventeenth century with John Donne's and Thomas Sydenham's usage, it must have felt explosive and empowering – indeed, impertinent. However, now it feels tired, battle-weary, exhausted. Ludwick Fleck described the death of the military metaphor as early as 1935 in the context of bacteriology. Rather than infectious diseases being seen as the invasion by a microbial enemy, resulting in a war against that invading army (as a metaphor for treatment), Fleck suggests that infection and treatment must be seen, rather, as 'a complicated revolution within the complex life unit' (Fleck quoted in Kistner 1998, p. 26), where the 'invading' organism does not meet a foreign army of the body. Rather, the body already has immune system receptors able to meet the microbe. War metaphors are then replaced by negotiation and conciliation metaphors, where, in the latter, the conciliator is a morphological process.

Kistner's work reminds us that not all metaphors are equal – again, some are already 'dead' metaphors that do not provide rich conceptual ground in the target domain. Source and target remain largely interchangeable at a low level of stimulation. This is where metaphors are 'motherhood and apple pie', where everything about old times is good and should be retained. Paul Ricoeur's (2003) distinction between 'dead' and 'living' metaphors is that the latter produce higher levels of conceptualization than the former. Kistner distinguishes between base semiotic metaphors and higher-level semantic metaphors, the latter stacked with meaning, the former merely descriptive.

'Medicine as war', 'the body as machine' (the legacy primarily of Cartesian reductionism) and 'illness as a journey' may already be three didactic or master metaphors that are close to retirement, possibly dead on their feet. (Or, they may be ripe for exhumation and even revival in new forms – for example, combat metaphors applied to contemporary personalized medicine in which genomes are 'targeted'.) The first (medicine as war) has been replaced by patient-centred and team-based collaboration metaphors ('we're in this together'); the second (the body as machine) by a bio-psycho-immuno-socio-ecological model of medicine and healthcare (Pauli *et al.* 2000; Stineman and Streim 2010; Hatala 2012); while the third (illness as journey) has been trivialized by the New Age and self-help (pop psychology) cultures in the face of recent pleas by serious commentators such as Art Frank (2013) to treat such illness journeys as opportunities for 'reflexive monitoring', and not to be pulled into fads and fashions, such as 'doubling up' the metaphor (for example, 'journey' as 'growth').

'Medicine' as a master metaphor

The literature, then, suggests that metaphors in medicine help doctors to 'think medicine' better. Another historical body of literature suggests that 'medicine' itself – employed as a master metaphor, or one that is primary in shaping life – may help us to 'think life' better in terms of diagnosing and treating the health of a culture. This transposes 'medicine' from medical culture to everyday or lay culture as a metaphorical frame or a 'master metaphor' (Woods 2009). There is a tradition in modernism, from Samuel Johnson (Wiltshire 1991) and John Wesley (Ott 1995) in the eighteenth century, through Friedrich Nietzsche in the nineteenth century (Bleakley 2014), to Gilles Deleuze (1998) in the twentieth century, of writers and artists acting as 'physicians' of culture (Smith 2005) or 'symptomatologists' (Deleuze 1998). In other words, if culture is taken as a body or organism prone to symptoms, then one of the roles of artists and writers is to articulate such symptoms and suggest ways in which they may be addressed.

Kenneth Burke (1897–1993) – a literary theorist most famous for his studies of rhetoric – used 'medicine' itself as a 'master metaphor' or a 'reading strategy' in which culture is read medically (Burke 1959; Woods 2009). Burke was a close friend of the doctor and poet William Carlos Williams and developed his view of medicine as a master metaphor through correspondence with Williams. Carly Woods (2009) notes that Burke framed society in terms of health and disease, whereby most of us are 'anaesthetized', insensitive, for example, to the nuances of language use, such as how we are persuaded through rhetoric. Burke saw the study of language and literature as potentially curative of society's symptoms, as the desensitizing anaesthetic is lifted and a sensitizing occurs.

Burke, then, saw society as ill, and literature as able to offer a remedy. We can 'read' society medically, as a symptomatologist, and intervene. Burke offered three kinds of treatment for societal sickness: symbolic action, identification and rhetorical demystification (Woods 2009). In symbolic action, writers (or artists in general) generate metaphors that give succour to readers. Artists, drawing on their various rhetorical media, generate deep questioning and can offer radical provocations that appear to create further symptoms rather than cure. But the metaphor dose may be like immunization, creating illness in tolerable doses as it gives longer-term protection (against banality and anaesthetizing or dulling). This makes identification an important strategy to counter societal illness. One must know the disease one is fighting. Importantly, the arts and humanities prepare us to face the epic and tragic rather than the trivial. Rhetorical demystification refers to the conundrum that the artist, as effective rhetorician, may be a charlatan. How will we know? Well, literature itself provides the means for cultivating discrimination.

Models of the 'health' of culture – applying 'medicine' as a master metaphor – go back to antiquity, where, for example, the ancient Greek notion of catharsis involved audiences working through social issues, or assessing the relative health of a society, using the medium of theatre, where art offers a social medicine. Nietzsche again revived that tradition for modern Western audiences, emphasizing the value of the Dionysian (catharsis) rather than the Apollonic (reason) in writing, music and theatre. The revival of interest in antiquity during the Renaissance stressed Apollonic virtues and forms – the classical notion of fine lines in Greek statues and temples and rationality in thinking. However, the wilder, less tempered and emotionally tinged Dionysian was favoured by the Romantics in particular, recognizing the value of the passions. Greek statues and temples were painted in vivid colours – cold marble affords a false picture of antiquity's aesthetic, while theatre celebrated Dionysian fervour and Pan's natural impulses (Hillman and Roscher 2000). In this tradition, Nietzsche saw that the role of the artist is to question instrumental values of 'health'. What is regarded as healthy and ideal is reduction of life to a dogmatic monomyth of 'purity'. Rather, the cross-infections of pluralism and relativism are healthy.

Nietzsche (in Smith 2005, p. 152) described the 'great health' of a culture as the overall depth of sensibility in that culture. Individuals may themselves be medically ill, suffering from symptoms, as did Nietzsche himself, yet be acutely sensitive to broader cultural health, or to what extent the arts and humanities permeated, challenged and shaped the culture. For Nietzsche, the greatest diagnostic cultural capability was to track the historical conditions for the emergence of phenomena and to recognize that emergent values were historically contextual, transient and then relative. Following in the wake of Nietzsche, Gilles Deleuze (1998), in *Essays Critical and Clinical,* uses the metaphor of the clinic to re-vision cultural symptoms as in need of treatment through the 'critical' – pushing language to its limit so that it stands outside of itself and enters a state of delirium, a clinical condition. In this state, culture may be re-visioned.

Artists and writers are, of course, experts in metaphor. Just as the sensibility of a doctor is educated to diagnose symptoms and suggest cures, so the sensibility of an artist can be thought of as being educated to diagnose culture's ills and offer appropriate interventions. A common remedy for social ills is a dose of metaphor. Virginia Langum (2013, p. 7) suggests that 'metaphor *serves* medicine, even functioning *as* medicine', where metaphor is invigorating. Metaphor-infused medicine serves patients. Will metaphor-infused language and activity also serve life?

Philip Ott (1995, p. xx) describes the work of the eighteenth-century Methodist minister John Wesley (1703–1791) as based on the notion of medicine as a master metaphor, where 'Wesley moved through a sermon as if he were a diagnostician.' Wesley's sermons included 'the circumcision of the heart' and 'the cure of evil speaking'. Faith was equated with a 'recovery of primitive health'. Wesley had studied medicine at Oxford, where Thomas Sydenham was a formative influence. Again, it was Sydenham who first established the 'medicine is war' didactic metaphor, although the metaphor seems to have been first coined by the poet John Donne, who referred to disease as 'violent' (Alford 1739, p. 411). Wesley saw that illness was often psychosomatic or psychological in nature and that this was the soul calling to be tended. A salve to the soul is to regain wholeness or balance between the physical and the spiritual.

Wesley was influenced by the work of George Cheyne, who described the body as filled with a series of canals through which 'liquor of different nature' flowed. These canals could become blocked. Healing involved unblocking the waterways and allowing free flow for the various bodily fluids. Wesley described the body as having 'a thousand tubes and strainers', any one of which could get obstructed. Health entailed the free flow of air and fluid through these tubes under the impulse of 'fire' or spirit. Eating the biblical 'forbidden fruit' (a metaphor for sin) could clog up the vessels or 'adhere to the inner coats of the finer vessels', leading to symptoms. The fruit from the Tree of Life (a metaphor for Faith), on the other hand, was said to have an abrasive skin that could scour the vessels clean. Wesley's vision might be scoffed at technically, but in essence, the physical metaphors are still common in the talk of cardiologists who describe putting in a stent as a plumbing issue. For Wesley, gaining faith is equated with the discovery of Jesus as the great physician of the soul, who 'cuts away what is putrefied or unsound in order to preserve the sound part.'

Wesley did not formally systematize his worldview of medicine as a master metaphor or his role as a diagnostician of the human condition. The first to do this was Samuel Johnson (1709–1784), a contemporary of Wesley (Wiltshire 1991), in a series of essays – the *Rambler* – written between 1750 and 1752.

Known as 'Dr' Johnson, Samuel Johnson was not a physician. He did, however, surround himself with doctors as friends and collaborators, partly because he suffered from melancholy or depression, gout, alcohol dependency and tics, and cherished informed advice. Johnson, like Wesley, saw the body of culture as in need of care and transposed ideas and images from medicine onto society, using 'medicine as metaphor' (Wiltshire 1991, pp. 141–64).

Johnson mainly focused on shared emotional and psychological conditions that seemed to him to be an unwelcome yet persistent part of the human condition, such as 'sorrow', which he described in metaphorical terms as 'a kind of rust of the soul' and 'the putrefaction of stagnant life'. He focused on how terms such as a 'vice', 'corruption' and 'degeneration' can be used to describe the material world, but also human moral slippage. Just as a vice is used to grip and squeeze or hold, so a moral vice grips somebody. Johnson was loath to blame an individual, seeing us all as prone to being visited by these forces. Metaphors, then, served to transfer meanings across from the natural material world to the human moral world.

The duty of the moralist – the physician of culture who sets out to heal or address fault lines in social or individual character – is, for example, 'to set the heart free from the corrosion of envy, and exempt us from the vice which is, above most others, tormenting to ourselves, hateful to the world, and productive of mean artifices and sordid projects'. Johnson's symptomatologist (he is himself, as writer and commentator, a prime example) is, then, the forerunner of the psychologist, psychiatrist and social critic. Moral philosophy becomes medical counsel as the body of culture is addressed for its ills. Boswell, Johnson's biographer, writes of the collected editions of the *Rambler* moral essays that they offer 'steel for the mind' (Wiltshire 1991, p. 163), an interesting metaphor that may have taken on a rather different meaning in Johnson and Boswell's time. Boswell was living at the end of the great age of industrial iron production and just at the beginning of mass steel production, so 'steel' may have been used by Boswell to refer to refinement as much as strength.

Samuel Johnson may have been the first writer to formally set out that his moral duty was to address 'medicine' as a master metaphor for culture, treating the body of culture through diagnosis and intervention, but this has been a running theme in modern literature, summed up by the black writer Ralph Ellison's call, in an era of deep racism in the USA, for artists to adopt a 'sense of responsibility for the health of a society', even where 'You might not like society' (Callahan 2004, p. 330).

'Medicine' as a cultural master metaphor, in the sense described by Kenneth Burke, strays beyond the province of the arts and humanities to politics. A contemporary example is a study of the use of medical metaphors such as 'medicine is war' in Italian political language (De Leonardis 2008). Here, the politician-ruler is seen as a doctor endowed with the capacity to heal or cure society's ills. This technocratic concept has dominated recent Italian politics and shapes the spread of racism, when the 'other' is cast as an infection, destroying the purity of the national body.

In this and the previous chapter, I have discussed a number of approaches to defining a metaphor and rehearsed the argument that medicine is a flow of metaphors. In the following chapter, I suggest that there are serious negative consequences from not recognizing the importance of metaphor in medicine, and that it is the responsibility of medical education to pick up the baton of metaphor and run with it.

3 What do we know about metaphors in medicine and what are the consequences of resisting metaphor?

Medicine's metaphors: messages and menaces – Samuel Vaisrub

Soon before his death in 1980, Sam Vaisrub (1906–1980), a distinguished physician, wrote the first study of metaphors in medicine (Vaisrub 1977). Vaisrub was senior editor of the *Journal of the American Medical Association* (*JAMA*) and associate editor of the *Archives of Internal Medicine*. His interests and enthusiasms ranged beyond medicine to philosophy and the humanities. Since Vaisrub's pioneering work, the history of interest in metaphors in medicine can be summed up as a history of neglect. I will argue that such woeful neglect has had a knock-on effect for medical education. The repression of, or the refusal to acknowledge, metaphor in medicine has meant that metaphor has returned in a distorted form – misunderstood and capricious, even malicious.

Unfortunately, commentators on metaphor in medicine have often been their own worst enemies, writing partial and sometimes unconvincing accounts, or treating the field of resemblances in medicine (see Chapters 5 and 6), such as an 'apple core lesion' or a 'raspberry tongue', as mere curiosities or light relief. The rather forced alliterative title (*Medicine's Metaphors: Messages and Menaces*) echoes the mixed nature of Vaisrub's book – by turns light and descriptive and frustratingly shallow, listing medical metaphors rather than critically engaging with them; and then offering sections of serious study echoing a deep personal expertise with a vision of future medicine that is holistic and complex. We should remember that Vaisrub wrote this book at a time when academic study of metaphor was unfashionable; it was published by a small house (Medical Economics Company, New Jersey), must have had a small readership, quickly went out of print, and ran to only 124 pages. We can only guess at the extent of its impact and the nature of its reception.

The first chapter deals with the didactic metaphor of medicine as war in a little over four pages of descriptive rather than analytical text, but coming to the conclusion that metaphors of interdependence and coexistence, based on the symbiotic relationship between humans and bacteria, form an alternative to martial metaphors. This is an important and welcome insight. Chapter 2 notes an enrichment of medical metaphor through supplement from myth – but this again is treated uncritically and is more a catalogue of naming ('Adam's apple', 'Achilles heel') or invocation. Subsequent chapters link fiction with medicine – for example, the 'Pickwickian syndrome' describes the red-faced fat boy in Dickens' novel whose obesity signals potential early heart failure; the 'Lot syndrome' describes excess deposition of calcium in tissues of patients with hypercalcinosis, leading to literal petrification; while a 'Lazarus complex' describes resuscitated survivors of cardiac arrest – as if brought back from the dead.

Nearly 30 pages are devoted to three glossaries: (i) word origins for medically related terms from 'abdomen' to 'zygote' (hardly metaphors); (ii) 'commemoratives', from 'Achilles tendon' to 'Ulysses syndrome' (a trail of diagnoses of mental and physical disorders resulting from a trail of false positive laboratory tests, reflecting Odysseus' tortuous 10 years' long journey home after the Trojan War); and (iii) 'colloquials', from 'anatomic snuffbox' (describing the junction of the wrist with the first metacarpal where the thumb is extended) to 'thyroid storm' (describing the feverish, restless state of a person with acute thyrotoxicosis).

Vaisrub (1977, pp. 120–2) concludes that 'Disparagement of metaphor has become the dominant attitude of science-oriented physicians.' He notes, again importantly, that the leading and reductionist metaphors of medicine as war and conflict (martial metaphors), 'survival of the fittest' (biology is conflict) and 'the machine metaphor' are inappropriate and outdated (for example, 'the martial metaphor often results in simplistic approaches to the complexities of medical research'). Metaphors of complex 'holism' and interdependence are more appropriate to describe and shape modern medicine: 'Holistic medicine is based on the psychosomatic concept of the mind-body interaction, treating the whole man [*sic*]. It cannot be reconciled with the mechanical model.' Vaisrub further warns against the transfer of medical martial metaphors to the public sphere as 'a call to political violence', for example, where zealots call for 'cutting out cancers' in society. This may result in 'metaphor demonology', whereby 'cancer' is used negatively, echoing the well-known views of Susan Sontag on the misuse and abuse of cancer metaphors (later extended to AIDS metaphors) discussed earlier and throughout this book.

Vaisrub (1977, p. 124) argues that medicine has been stereotyped as cultivating negative metaphors 'of infirmity, dread, and despair' and wonders if these might be transformed through an emergent medicine of 'hope', in which 'triumph' and 'achievement' are prominent. 'Hope' is an important metaphor in medicine, provides a contrast to violence and conflict metaphors, and is particularly important in palliative care. Olsman and colleagues (Olsman *et al.* 2014) looked at the use of metaphors of hope by palliative care professionals (in Canada and the Netherlands) and describe four key metaphors: hope as 'grip', 'source', 'tune' and 'vision'. 'Grip' referred to 'safety', 'source' implied strength, 'tune' implied harmony, and 'vision' implied positivity. Doctors used 'grip' more than other healthcare professionals, whereas chaplains used 'tune'. Canadian participants put more emphasis upon spiritual metaphors than their Dutch colleagues.

Vaisrub (1977), reflecting on the metaphor of hope, suggests that 'Medicine itself may then become a metaphor of liberation from the bondage of determinism.' Vaisrub's book, the first on metaphors in medicine, thus becomes a manifesto for an optimistic, expansive and ultimately triumphant 'interactional' medicine. Vaisrub's optimism is admirable, if close to inflation. His condensed book does offer an argument: the landscape of medicine has been shaped by reductive metaphors of war, conflict and engineering, whereas emergent metaphors – such as complex holism and interactivity – can shape a new landscape of medicine. Forty years later, the tide has not turned in Vaisrub's favour, and here I consistently repeat his argument for a major metaphorical shift away from martial and engineering metaphors.

Metaphors in medical texts: Geraldine van Rijn-van Tongeren

Two decades after Sam Vaisrub's groundbreaking book, Geraldine van Rijn-van Tongeren (1997) published a systematic study of metaphors in medical texts, focusing upon three textbooks (in oncology, surgical oncology and vascular surgery), with a total of 33 chapters between them. While groundbreaking at the time, the text only analysed didactic (dominant or leading) metaphors mainly drawn from oncology, such as

1   Anthropomorphisms and personifications
    Diseases are talked about as human beings (for example, cells have a 'life history' and a 'lifespan'), sometimes with idiosyncrasies or personalities. The author does not note the irony that the disease may be personified while the person ('patient') is depersonalized. Diseases are often referred to as the Other person, the outsider and stranger ('foreign bodies' that are 'invasive'). Of course, the body is made of cells, but where diseased, these are described as if they had intentions ('malignant').
2   Society
    Cells are not only anthropomorphized, but also described as living in groups and communicating with one another.
3   Colonization and invasion
    Part of the wider 'medicine as war on disease' metaphor. Tumour cells in particular 'colonize' and 'invade' in an aggressive manner.
4   Defence and attack
    Completing the 'war' metaphor, tumour cells are enemies that attack or invade as 'killer' cells. Medicine seeks a 'magic bullet' for cancer to 'fight back' against the disease.
5   Machine and mechanism
    The body is (like) a machine with input and output of information. Machines can be fixed when they go wrong, or they may have irreversible damage.
6   Agents
    Causation is ascribed to infections, for example, and we look for re-agents to cure diseases.
7   Steps and stages
    Metastasis develops in stages.

8   Seeds
Metastases are sown from the primary tumour.
Metaphors 1–4 in particular group as a 'coherent network' (van Rijn-van
Tongeren 1997, p. 78): 'Human beings live in a society, where colonization
and war are typically human pursuits.' Van Rijn-van Tongeren notes also
that alternative labels could be applied to metaphor groups – 'communication' and 'text' labels could be used to describe the 'human' or 'personification' metaphors.

Van Rijn-van Tongeren argues that the metaphors she notes in medical texts
(which also appear in clinicians' talk) are not just descriptive, but also serve to
facilitate the forming of medical theories. While Van Rijn-van Tongeren does
not draw on examples from brain science, this field offers a good way in to
understanding how theory-making and metaphorical thinking link. For example,
while inborn capacity is described as 'hard wired', it is also 'plastic' or has great
adaptability. The 'plastic' metaphor serves to generate theories about adaptation
through learning. Plastic is not as malleable as, say, putty (then the brain could
readily turn to 'mush') but not as fixed as, say, metal (we talk about 'hard-
headedness' as fixity of ideas). Plastic also implies that the brain can receive
lasting 'impressions' (memory).
    That neurons 'fire' helps not only as a descriptive metaphor but also in
forming theory to understand tangible events. A synapse has 'potential' and this
builds up on one side of the synapse chemically until a threshold is reached, at
which point the 'firing' occurs and the synaptic gap is jumped or bridged. To
describe a set of cortical connections as a complex 'web' and 'network' helps to
model brain processes in a different way than thinking of linear, even if complicated rather than complex, connections.
    Metaphor generates theory – this is epistemological work. In parallel with
this, and fundamental to the appearance of metaphor in medicine, is ontological
work. Here, metaphors serve the purpose of medical students and doctors
making experiential sense of the world into which they are socialized and which
provides them with an identity.

Metaphors as defences against the pressures of work

Analogy (metaphor and resemblance) is fundamental to the landscape of medicine, or inescapable. Medicine, however, defends against the appearance of
analogy through tactics of literalizing and trivializing. The most obvious appearance of this in medical culture is the use of English for Medical Purposes (EMP),
or standardized medical-technical and medical-professional language, as reductive text and performance. Metaphor is seen as a symptom that must be
expunged, as it brings complications and moves medicine into the territory of
uncertainty or ambiguity.
    As noted earlier, Donald Schön (1990) describes this territory as the 'swampy
lowlands' of practice. Craving the 'high ground' of logic and certainty, doctors

often find themselves in practice in different territory, where metaphors abound and cannot be expunged. The poet, writer and doctor Iain Bamforth (2015, p. 147) sums this up in suggesting that medical students undergo 'a crammed, often dogmatic training ... which tends to hinder critical thinking', so that when they come to face real medical practice, they might panic in the face of deep uncertainty, afraid 'to lose face by admitting they don't know'.

Medicine's relationship with metaphor can be imagined metaphorically as driving a car with the brakes on (albeit another machine metaphor). The brakes equate to the refusal of metaphor and simile, or their reduction to trivia or pleasant distraction from the job at hand. The more one revs the engine with the brakes on, the greater the incidence of backfiring from the exhaust. The primary forms of refusal are intolerance of ambiguity and reduction of complex process to literal events (for example, the body is a machine and can be fixed). This is best exemplified by medicine's adoption of EMP, as discussed below.

Medicine resists metaphor: English for Medical Purposes (EMP)

Medicine is laced with metaphor, yet its public face refuses this, claiming plain language and concrete (non-metaphoric) thinking (rational, empirical, plain and scientific rather than poetic or embroidered). This suggests that medicine suffers from a split between its conscious public persona and its unconscious structure. This section explores this split, as symptom, through a discussion of medical language informing practice. While, for example, the public or 'frontstage' face of medicine is 'clean' and uses 'appropriate' language, as encouraged by recent intensive emphasis upon professionalism and integrity in medical education, there is a tradition of a 'backstage' of medical slang shared amongst doctors (Parsons *et al.* 2001; BBC News Channel 2003; Fox *et al.* 2003; Piemonte 2015).

Medicine prides itself in being a hands-on (or these days, 'machine-on'), interventional practice (surgery, drug therapies, physical examinations, taking blood, inserting a catheter or a central line, cleaning and dressing a wound, injections). However, much of what happens in a patient encounter – such as a consultation, or in team care such as ward work in a hospital – is talk and writing (including patients' notes and charts) with patients or between colleagues. This is particularly the case in general practice, mental health and paediatrics (involving parents as a go-between).

Language use in medicine is both descriptive and performative (Austin 1975). Austin described how words do things ('I feel for you') as well as describe things ('Mr P is a 67 year old man with stable angina'). Medical language in the English-speaking world is a well-developed, formal system of description and expression known as EMP (Allum undated; Maglie 2009; Skelton and Whetstone 2012). EMP is often thought of in a narrow way, as the medical language that is taught to medical students and doctors whose first language is not English, but the ramifications of EMP go far beyond this. EMP is a template for a global *practice* of medicine and not just a preparatory course for doctors who wish to work in English-speaking countries but who do not have English as a first language (see, for example, Allum undated).

EMP is, at face value, empirical, rational, technical, instrumental and economical or pithy. Such language is paralleled by its collection of speech acts – typical language usage, phrases or textual strategies to communicate knowledge and values. In consultations, doctors typically use prescriptive phrases, impersonal structures and the passive voice. Rosita Maglie (2009) points out that this is grounded historically in Latin scientific writing. Maglie sets out the landscape of 'frontstage' EMP vocabulary as:

1   Uses just one word for a particular concept and meaning (monoreferentiality and semantic univocity), avoiding periphrasis or convoluted language. EMP gets straight to the point but the descriptive word is technical, such as 'contusion'. Ironically, the patient may be just as blunt, thinking 'bruise' rather than the technical 'contusion' (readily distinguished from a haematoma where the latter is hard to the touch).
2   Is denotative rather than connotative. To denote is to give one precise, literal meaning. To connote means to imply several meanings.
3   Privileges certainty (the indicative) over uncertainty and ambiguity (the subjunctive mood).
4   Uses technical words that are precise and transparent to those who use them, usually derived from Greek or Latin roots.
5   Prefers shortness (to the point) to redundancy in the form of lexical and syntactic collapse (for example 'contraception' rather than 'contraconception'); acronyms (AIDS, HIV); abbreviations (fld for fluid, OT for operating theatre, BP for blood pressure); and stacked noun phrases (body mass index).
6   Uses truncated sentences and descriptions for precision. Medical students are taught to present 'cases' in a formulaic way.
7   Uses nominalization (processes and properties are described by nouns rather than verbs) to pack information into the smallest number of words and to provide objectification, or that something is taken for granted (language denoting certainty).
8   Employs 'necessity' modals ('must', 'should') in professional and academic communications, where 'possibility' modals ('can', 'could', 'may', 'might') are used in popular medical texts – again, indicative rather than subjunctive mood.
9   Employs the passive voice as a means of depersonalization – this places emphasis upon the effects or results of an action rather than upon the author of the action ('symptoms make Sue permanently tired', rather than 'Sue is permanently tired in the face of her symptoms').

Language use in medicine is, however, Janus-faced. Besides 'frontstage' use, there is a 'backstage' to performative language use in medicine. The above profile of projected certainty, authority and to-the-point brevity in EMP is the public face of medicine that greets patients in consultations. This prevailing modality is ideological: paternalistic, authoritative and specialist. Another face of medicine embraces uncertainty and ambiguity (the subjunctive mood of 'possibly' and 'maybe'), while its landscape is that of analogy (metaphor and simile or resemblance) and aphorism: tropes or figures of speech. A typical example cited by Maglie (2009) is the common usage of the term 'screening'. Borrowed from common English usage, 'screening' (to use a filter) takes on a particular usage in public health and medicine that has become naturalized. Yet, 'screening' is originally used as what Salager-Meyer (1990) calls a 'bold metaphor', one with – originally – strong stylistic flavour and colour that fade with use.

Ironically, EMP teaching may now be fused with teaching for 'communication' in medicine. Skelton and Whetstone (2012) describe this fusion with several examples of an opening to a consultation, including: 'Can I just have a little listen to your chest?' In the context of the sentence, 'little' acts metaphorically, standing for a brief or non-intrusive examination. The fusion of EMP with communication capability in this example then works against the general impulse to rid medical communication of its (stereotypically) ornamental tropes. Metaphor sticks its heels in and refuses to budge even in the bleaching-out process of EMP. The *British National Formulary* (BNF) best illustrates this bleaching out.

One of the main treatment aids used by doctors is a pharmaceutical handbook such as the BNF. A 'national formulary' is basically a list of drugs available in any one country, offering information and advice on prescribing, indications and contraindications, side effects, doses, legal classification, and names and prices of available proprietary and generic drug formulations. Such formularies make no attempt to be anything other than descriptive lists – they are purely informational. There could be no linguistic corpus more strongly diametrically opposed to creative literature than drug formularies. They represent medical culture's linguistic bottom line – the desire to be clear, succinct and informational, avoiding both embroidery and obfuscation. BNF Publications promise to offer: 'authoritative and practical information on the selection and clinical use of medicines in a clear, concise, and accessible manner' (www.bnf.org/about/). They follow the linguistic tradition of EMP described above, which encourages the use of specialist rather than lay terms but resists the use of tropes or figures of speech such as metaphor – preferring 'plain' speaking, but in technical language.

Medicine, then, refuses metaphor through its insistence on the importance of plain speaking (albeit using technical or medical language), flat affect, clarity, abbreviations and acronyms, information over debate, and certainty over ambiguity. This is the language of case presentation that senior doctors encourage medical students and juniors to adopt. In short, in terms of 'mood', again, indicative or imperative language is preferred to the subjunctive mode. Indicative language indicates what 'is' rather than what 'might be' (the subjunctive), and the imperative indicates that the speaker would like something to happen – an outcome.

Paradoxically, as already discussed, it was a writer and literary expert – the late Susan Sontag – who famously claimed that medicine should be cleansed of metaphor because it works against the dignity of the patient. Why, asks Sontag, should patients be seen as 'fighting' against an illness when their experience may be entirely different? They may not see themselves as combative and are then silenced, discouraged and shamed by the metaphorical wrap. Other comment-ators believe that Sontag is misguided in her critique where symbolic and meta-phorical language helps people to make meaning out of distressing experiences (Clow 2001), although the dominant metaphorical landscape (such as medicine as war) may not be appropriate.

There is extended discussion of the literature on the use of martial metaphors in the following Chapter 4. Here, my concern is to extend the debate about EMP. Is doctors' language really as bland and instrumental as drug formularies? While packed with acronyms and abbreviations, doctors' slang is far from bland; in fact, it is potentially insulting.

Medical slang: a consequence of the refusal of positive metaphor?

Guided by a moral rather than a technical code, medieval surgeons were urged to 'induce a light heart' in patients by joking with them and making them laugh. However, this must never become bawdy. Surgeons must avoid not only bawdi-ness, but also loquacity, scurrilous joking, boasting, backbiting, flattery, lying, insulting, sowing discord, grumbling, quarrelling, swearing and breaking confi-dences (Langum 2013).

The sociologist Erving Goffman (1959), in his 'dramaturgical' model of human relationships, in which we act roles shaped by scripts, described the 'frontstage' of a culture as the public and professional face. In medicine, frontstage language is that of the typical consultation with patients, and profes-sional and ethical teamwork with colleagues. Such language is stripped back, eschewing complex description and metaphor (and then colour and imagination). But there is also a 'backstage' to cultures such as medicine – what happens in the wings and behind the curtains. This includes offensive medical slang.

Coombs and colleagues (Coombs *et al.* 1993, p. 987) suggest that medical slang is typically first encountered by medical students in their third year and serves as a key socialization medium through clinical placements and into junior doctoring, where medical slang 'involved creating a sense of belonging; estab-lishing a unique identity; providing a private means of communication; exercis-ing creativity, humor, and wit; and softening tragedy and discharging strong emotions'. In an era of accountability, medical schools have introduced ethics and professionalism into the core curriculum, working against the tradition of pejorative medical slang encountered in the workplace.

Black humour, in general, especially in acute areas such as intensive care, is typically used as a method of catharsis and defence against the sometimes over-whelming intensities of the job, and can be seen as a necessary safety valve.

Black humour and medical slang, as 'dark metaphor', may, however, be a symptom of medicine not looking after itself more openly, and of the culture of medicine operating historically more like a secret society or a Masonic lodge than an accountable and transparent institution. Nicole Piemonte (2015) wonders whether gallows humour is the most appropriate way for medical students to learn how to distance themselves from the trauma they will inevitably face in their careers (see Chapter 10). Indeed, is such 'distancing' necessary? Can students not learn to live amid trauma in ways that neither objectify patients nor provide a supposedly protective distancing for themselves? Why should doctors not attend to the existential issues and suffering to which they are exposed both personally and politically?

Following Kathryn Montgomery's (2006) suggestion that medicine is misguided when it calls itself a 'science' (it is, rather, a 'science using' narrative activity), Piemonte suggests that medicine cannot profess authenticity when it lays claim to science's objectivity. Medicine has to include subjective accounting, even valuing the subjective as a measure of authentic feeling in the face of suffering. Perhaps the emergence of a culture of gallows humour and dark slang as a coping strategy – where malicious metaphor is purposefully manufactured – fills the vacuum created by an absence of adequate mentoring, support, counselling and psychotherapeutic services for medical students and doctors (Peterkin and Bleakley 2017).

Piemonte's plea is for medicine to drop the pretence that doctors should not be vulnerable (this includes the quasi-militaristic tactics of toughening them up) and to embrace the human condition, where vulnerability is an asset, as it breeds empathy for others who are suffering. Rather, we need to infuse the medicine curriculum with opportunities for learning reflection and unburdening. This has big implications for how we see the role of metaphors in medicine. Rather than sweeping metaphors into a dark corner where they go bad and stink – as slang and black humour – let us allow metaphors free play in the everyday life of doctors as vulnerable humans who are also imaginative amid such vulnerability; imaginative enough to invent authenticity, coping patterns and resilience.

'Doctors' slang' is referred to (perhaps tongue in cheek) as a 'dying art' in a 2003 feature from the BBC (BBC News Channel 2003). In an era of patient-centred care and greater chance of litigation, offensive medical slang is rapidly on the wane, although it is occasionally referred to in television medical soap opera scripts. Dr Adam Fox (Fox *et al.* 2003) of St Mary's Hospital London – who does not advocate the use of such slang, seeing this as unethical behaviour, but is fascinated by slang terms as historical curiosities – has collected over 200 examples of medical slang over five years, constituting a kind of underground or backstage culture of medical culture explicitly grounded in 'dark metaphor'. I approach this topic with caution, because it is unsavoury to repeat some of this slang, and I have chosen not to include the most offensive terms here. The http://messybeast.com/dragonqueen/medical-acronyms.htm website spills the beans for those who are interested, offering a comprehensive, international archive of medical slang.

Adam Fox and colleagues (Fox *et al.* 2003) list the top five most commonly used 'medical abbreviations' (slang) as: CTD (Circling the Drain – a patient expected to die soon); GLM (Good Looking Mum); GPO (Good for Parts Only); TEETH (Tried Everything Else, Try Homeopathy); and UBI (Unexplained Beer Injury). Others include NFN (Normal for Norfolk), FLK (Funny Looking Kid) and GROLIES (*Guardian* Reader of Low Intelligence in Ethnic Skirt). Fox tells a story of a doctor facing litigation on the basis of scribbling the expletive TTFO (Told to Fuck Off) on a patient's notes. Asked by a judge what 'TTFO' meant, the doctor said 'To take fluids orally'. Patients who are cognitively or intellectually challenged are the butt of a number of acronyms: LOBNH (Lights on But Nobody Home), CNS-QNS (Central Nervous System – Quantity Not Sufficient), and PP (Pumpkin Positive), implying that a penlight shone into the patient's mouth would light up the whole head because the brain is so small.

Other unsavoury terms include 'bagged and tagged' for the intake of a corpse at the mortuary. Elderly, confused ladies lying on a hospital bed clutching their handbags are referred to as Handbag Positive. The geriatric ward is termed the Departure Lounge. While in A&E, where regular visitors get to be known, a DBI (Dirt Bag Index) may apply: to estimate how many days since the patient last had a bath, the number of missing teeth is multiplied by the number of tattoos. But slang is not just used in this pejorative way to stereotype patients; it also serves as inter-specialty banter, where rheumatology and dermatology (often characterized as less busy specialties) are known to other specialties as 'rheuma-holiday' and 'dermaholiday'; anaesthetists are 'gassers', surgeons 'slashers' and psychiatrists the 'Freud Squad'. Further, there is celebratory slang such as 'champagne tap' for a perfect lumbar puncture.

Parsons and colleagues (Parsons *et al.* 2001) studied medical students' perceptions of dark humour and slang in hospital work-based settings. This is a world in which medical students can still experience what North American medical culture calls 'pimping': 'questioning with the intent to shame or humiliate the learner to maintain the power hierarchy in medical education'. Here, senior members of a medical team, usually on a ward round, ask purposefully difficult questions of students and junior members of the team in order to humiliate them as a kind of militaristic toughening-up socialization (Kost and Chen 2015). Within this now rapidly changing climate, Parsons and colleagues found that students could take on the perspective of both outsiders and insiders in the medical culture. They can identify with patients, who are the butt of the humour, but they can also see that the use of such humour provides a release for the tensions built into the job. Interestingly, given that the study is so recent, students find themselves participating in dark humour and slang, although often with reservations, as they seek to identify with their seniors.

Doctors' slang in a sense is diametrically opposed to EMP. Both serve a similar purpose of socialization into medicine and identity construction of the expert doctor, yet slang lives in the house of metaphor, whereas EMP inhabits the house of literal language. They are uneasy bedmates.

House, M.D.

Speaking of houses of metaphor, *House*, also known as *House, M.D.*, was an American television medical soap opera set in a teaching hospital in New Jersey, starring the British actor and comic Hugh Laurie. Dr Gregory House is portrayed as a psychologically unstable, irascible genius whose talent is brilliant diagnostic acumen. *House* frames medical diagnosis as a detective story. Kathryn Montgomery Hunter (1993) had previously used the same metaphorical frame, where the doctor is sleuth.

The series ran from 2004 to 2012. It was the most watched television show in the world in 2008. The scriptwriters are aware that diagnostic medicine, in particular, depends upon metaphors. Ironically, the face of medicine that the public ingests through the figure of Gregory House is the very stereotype that contemporary medical education wishes to erase – that of the male, rogue, aberrant genius (who is also a misanthrope, psychologically unstable and addicted to self-prescribed painkillers). Medical education now promotes common competence and collective responsibility.

House's original working title when it was pitched to Fox TV was *Chasing Zebras, Circling the Drain*, showing the scriptwriters' interests in metaphor and aphorism. 'Circling the Drain', as noted above, is medical slang for somebody approaching his or her death. 'Chasing Zebras' refers to a well-known aphorism: 'If you hear hoofbeats, don't think zebras' – in other words, go for the obvious diagnosis ('horses') and not for the unusual. *House* focused on the unusual.

Predictably, metaphors in *House* follow the contours of the dominant militaristic landscape of medicine, discussed at length in a later section:

> DR. HOUSE: The tumor … had already sent out a splinter cell … waiting to kill us all.
>
> DR. FOREMAN: Whoa, are you trying to say that the tumor threw a clot before we removed it?
>
> DR. HOUSE: … an excellent metaphor. Angio her brain, before this clot straps on an explosive vest.

Monika Cichminska and Marta Topolewska (2010) have analysed the use of conceptual metaphors in *House* and have come up with a predictable list:

1   The body is a machine ('the brain's like a big jumble of wires. MS (multiple sclerosis) strips them of their insulation').
2   The body is a factory ('lack of oxygen forces the body to overproduce red blood cells').
3   Medicine is war ('when the immune system attacks the infection').
4   Medicine is a detective story ('round up the usual suspects').
5   Disease is a puzzle to be solved ('what if there really are two puzzles?').
6   Illness is a journey/medicine is a voyage of discovery ('we wanted to explore all the possibilities').

7   Diseases are people/symptoms are personified ('little bugs that are now feasting on his brain move on to dessert').

Overworked, overtired and keeping metaphors over there

Is it any wonder that doctors suffer from stress and burnout in a culture that has been shaped around a pumped-up heroic value complex embedded in underresourced and dysfunctional organizational systems? Medicine carries an historical legacy of self-protective lack of transparency and denial under criticism. Where this is combined with paternalism, heroic machismo, literalism and intolerance of ambiguity, an authoritarian values complex continues to stubbornly hold at bay the more feminine values of authentic collaboration, patient-centredness and tolerance of ambiguity that must come to shape contemporary healthcare (Bleakley 2014). Medicine has been a culture that prides itself on pushing the Protestant work ethic to its limit, so much so that stress is a kind of badge of honour, yet self-care is poor and doctors are loath to admit to either physical or psychological incapacity, hiding symptoms and self-medicating (Peterkin and Bleakley 2017). This culture is changing under the influence of a shift in the metaphorical landscape from the 'steel' of competition, heroism and conflict to the 'softer' landscape of public, patient and colleague collaboration and positive self-disclosure.

In this chapter I have set out why I think that the repression, or refusal, of metaphor's presence in medical language and performance may lead to negative consequences – on the one hand, the entirely flat and humourless world of stripped-back medical language and case presentation, and on the other, the dark world of medical slang and humour that makes a mockery of the current focus upon 'professionalism' in medical education. Medicine's major blind spot concerning metaphor, however, is its continuing subscription to the historical legacy of meta-metaphors, or didactic metaphors, particularly medicine as war and the body as machine. I have already introduced these major shaping metaphors, and in the following chapter, I trace their history and trajectory from once powerful and useful 'guiding fictions' to potentially destructive metaphors that shut down thinking.

4 'Medicine as war' and other didactic metaphors

Parts of this chapter arose out of collaborative dialogue with Dr Robert Marshall. I am grateful for his insights and suggestions.

A sea change in medical culture

We have seen that metaphors are not just poetic devices restricted to literature, but part of the fabric of both everyday discourse and of specialist discourse such as medical practice (Wohlmann 2015). This is a result in particular of the groundbreaking work of Lakoff and Johnson (1980), who note that metaphors permeate both everyday and specialist languages, and are not reifications but embodied or *performed*, and Hofstadter and Sander (2013), who describe analogy as 'the fuel and fire of thinking' or the functioning of cognition to continually seek to break its own boundaries. Analogies (metaphors and resemblances) function to generate new ideas and transform practices. But we have also seen that metaphors can be unproductive. A metaphor may have a lifespan – from productive use, to overuse (as idiom), to a 'dead' metaphor. However, some metaphors start out as powerful gearshifts for appreciation, explanation and creative insight, but then the social context of their production, and productivity, changes. Yet they remain powerful, changing the forms of their impact to corruption, even malignancy. They also become stickier or more stubborn in the process, resisting change or banishment.

Metaphors are generally good to think with. Leading, or 'didactic', metaphors (van Rijn-van Tongeren 1997), also described as 'pervasive' (Hodgkin 1985), are so good to think with that they shape entire landscapes of cultures and practices, including the construction of identity. Lakoff and Johnson (1980) suggest that there are surprisingly few didactic, framing, or meta-metaphors, such as 'container' metaphors ('in trouble', 'out of reach', 'sandwiched', 'locked in syndrome', 'wrapped in cotton wool', 'banged up') and 'direction' metaphors ('under the weather', 'a rising star', 'left field', 'right wing', 'the height of arrogance', 'the depths of despair').

Discussion of didactic or leading metaphors in medicine dominates the literature, suggesting that such metaphors are active in shaping a landscape of practice and inculcating values, rather than being merely descriptive and passive.

This further suggests that the culture and associated practices of medicine may change as new didactic metaphors emerge. 'Emerge' is chosen carefully here, as the shifting of didactic metaphors can be modelled in terms of dynamic, complex, adaptive systems with emergent properties. Didactic metaphors can be thought of as attractors within state spaces. As the make-up of state spaces transforms (for example, the emergence of accountability and transparency in medicine, the establishment of authentic patient-centredness and interprofessional teamwork, and the introduction of more women doctors), so new attractors emerge. New attractors advertising feminine, holistic, collaborative and ecological values may eclipse the older attractors of 'medicine as war' and 'the body as machine' (Pauli *et al.*, 2000).

Indeed, I (Bleakley *et al.* 2011; Bleakley 2014, 2015) have argued previously that we are in the middle of such a sea change in medicine, where 'paternalism' – the doctor is a father figure, the patient a child – is a longstanding divisive metaphor disappearing from medicine, replaced by the more collaborative metaphor of 'patient-centredness'. I also recognize that big terms, or 'god terms' as the rhetorician Kenneth Burke calls them (equivalent to 'uncontested', 'charismatic' and 'rhetorical absolutes' – terms against which nothing can be said), conceal as much as they reveal. To address this, I have analysed 'patient-centredness' as a complex term with a variety of meanings (Bleakley 2014). It can be argued that along with this shift from paternalism to patient-centredness, a more negative complex of metaphors has arisen – that of patients as 'consumers' and 'customers' in a 'marketplace' (Beisecker and Beisecker 1993; Hudak *et al.* 2003). This offers a 'restaurant model' of medicine, where patients now order from Internet menus. This can be empowering for the lay public, but also frustrating for doctors, who may feel compelled to give patients what they want against their better judgement.

The two leading or didactic metaphors for Western medicine have been 'the body as machine' and 'medicine as war'. These are discussed in detail below.

The body as machine

Once the body is configured as a machine, suggests Cheryl Mattingly (2011), it becomes 'potentially fixable'. This is the primary mindset of doctors, especially surgeons. Bracketing out the difficult bits such as the mind and emotions – or leaving these to the oddballs, the psychiatrists – reduces the person to the body, the body to machine (albeit complicated), and the machine to related parts. Even the psychiatrists join in (see Chapter 7) as the mind is reduced to a physical brain, which in turn is metaphorized, first in terms of electrical engineering ('wiring'), and then in terms of the computer with its 'hardware' and 'software'. Sick bodies are a product of broken parts, often able to be mended; and sick minds a product of faulty wiring and then malfunctioning software. As more is known about the sympathetic and parasympathetic branches of the autonomic nervous system, and the enteric nervous system associated with the gut, so neural metaphors spread, whereby the body becomes an integrated network of circuits and signals, replacing metaphors of organ specificity (often culture specific) such as the liver as a 'chemical factory'. (Such organ metaphors linger – they are archived on the website metamia: analogy as a teaching tool (www. metamia.com)). But these modern metaphors of the body as machine have historical antecedents.

The ancient Egyptians viewed the body as a series of conduits for carrying blood and the 'humours' – the flooding and receding cycle of the Nile's movement was projected onto the human body, which similarly flooded or dried out to create symptoms (Osherson and AmaraSingham 1981). As noted previously, the 'conduit metaphor' (Grady 1998), according to Michael Reddy and reinforced by Lakoff and Johnson (1980), accounts for as many as 70 per cent of the expressions we use for talking about language. There are well over 100 such expressions in English, where:

• Ideas (or meanings) are objects.
• Linguistic expressions are containers.
• Communication is sending.

Examples of the conduit metaphor include: 'it's hard to get my ideas across', 'what she says seems hollow', 'his words do not carry any meaning'. The ancient Egyptians did not speak English. My point is that the conduit metaphor has a long history and is co-existent with the physical world. Just as the draining and flooding of the Nile suggests motion of fluids in the body, so other motions of fluids in the world will be mirrored in body mechanisms (such as Harvey's description of the circulation of the blood with the heart as a pump).

Marri Lynn (2012) traces 'the body as a machine' metaphor back to Vesalius' *Fabrica* (1543), probably the most influential Western anatomy text until *Gray's Anatomy*, first illustrated by Henry Gray in 1858. Lynn notes the dominance of mechanical and engineering metaphors in Vesalius' text, especially 'pipes'. Veins, arteries and nerves are described as hollow tubes 'like a pipe'. Lynn suggests that this was not merely descriptive use of metaphor but rather, a complex mnemonic, where arteries carried a 'vital spirit' and nerves an 'animal spirit'. These conduits supposedly worked through pneumatics, by which air gives motion to fluid. Vesalius wanted his readers to view his pictures and think of them in motion. Jacques Gleyse (2013) notes that the idea of conceiving the body as an energy-generating machine was common in Europe in descriptions of the value of physical exercise from the seventeenth to the nineteenth century. This metaphor remains powerful today, especially in areas such as sports medicine.

René Descartes (1596–1650) explicitly compared the arrangement of the organs in the body to that of an 'automata' or 'moving machine', declaring that 'the body is to be regarded as a machine' (quoted in Vaisrub 1977, p. 35). Georgio Baglivi (1668–1706), an Italian physician and scientist famous for distinguishing between smooth and striated muscle, deepened this metaphor. Baglivi, says Vaisrub (1977, p. 35), 'divided the human body into numerous smaller machines. He likened teeth to scissors; viscera and glands to sieves; heart and blood vessels to a waterwork; and the stomach to a flask.' Vaisrub reminds us that such metaphors still linger: the lungs are thought of as 'bellows', the urinary tract as 'plumbing', the liver as a 'factory', the heart as a 'pump' or a 'ticker', and various electrochemical mechanisms passing sodium or calcium ions across cell membranes, as 'pumps'. The rise of neurophysiology brought with it notions of 'circuits', 'switches' and 'transistors', and the brain is finally compared to a computer.

Personalized medicine, based on the genome, becomes a function of genetic 'engineering'. We have already seen that such medical engineering metaphors were in the public domain long ago, through, for example, the sermons of the eighteenth-century Methodist minister John Wesley (1703–1791), who had studied medicine at Oxford, where Thomas Sydenham was a formative influence (Ott 1995). Again, Wesley described the body as having 'a thousand tubes and strainers', any one of which could get obstructed.

Deleuze and Guattari: bodies as desiring machines and assemblages

It may be that I am stereotyping the 'machine' and 'engineering' as hard, cold and masculine. My point is that no patient wants to be objectified – reduced to a bare function or a set of mechanics. In *Anti-Oedipus: Capitalism and Schizophrenia*, Gilles Deleuze and Félix Guattari (1988a, pp. 1–2), in a typically counter-intuitive and purposefully challenging gesture, say 'Everything is a machine.' That, of course, is untrue, but Deleuze and Guattari are being rhetorical, opening debate, coining a kind of anti-metaphor by calling humans 'desiring machines'. They boldly and explicitly problematize literal and mechanical readings of the 'machine'. They extend machines to 'machinic assemblages' to show that bodies are not independent but interdependent: 'An organ machine is plugged into an energy-source-machine: the one produces a flow that the other interrupts. The breast is a machine that produces milk, and the mouth a machine coupled to it.' This seems both to be sexist and to objectify the body – but let us persist, because there is quality in the notion of machinic coupling and assemblage.

Medicine isolates the individual and treats his or her body as a machine, but the reality is that the 'machine' of the body is interdependent within a series of assemblages. Viruses and bacteria are transmitted; the major cause of illness is lifestyle, either chosen (overconsumption) or imposed (poverty); dislocations and broken bones occur because of falls or violence and abuse. These are not links in a chain, but rather, attractors within interacting dynamic, complex systems, where each system has multiple metaphoric expressions. Medicine has historically reduced the body to an isolated machine and often treated symptoms and not causes, because it has not embraced the more complex metaphor of machinic assemblages and couplings. Where the body is treated as a machine (a metaphor), reasoning about the body tends to be through metonymic links, like a chain, rather than metaphorically (potentially, transposition from the ordinary to the extraordinary).

Bodies as machines are also not closed, but open, systems, working by 'flows' and 'interruptions', and, again, are coupled. Above all, bodies are 'desiring machines' or, again, interdependent. The machine, in Deleuze and Guattari's own term, is taken out of 'striated' space (which reduces the machine to mechanics) and placed in 'smooth' space, where the 'machine' becomes organic and fluid, seeking connections often through eroticism and pleasure. Striated space is territorial and regulated. Smooth space is nomadic and deregulated. Deleuze and Guattari's 'machines' are anti-machinic.

In the sequel to *Anti-Oedipus*, *A Thousand Plateaus* (1988b, pp. 97–8), Deleuze and Guattari progress their model of the machine to 'machinic assemblages'. On the horizontal axis (the living world) is a machinic assemblage of 'bodies, of actions and passions' formed of 'content' and 'expression'. Content involves bodies responding to one another; expression involves 'acts and statements' or a 'collective assemblage of enunciation'. The first is corporeal, the second incorporeal and transformative. On the vertical axis (the world of ideas), the assemblage has two possibilities – territorializing or stabilizing tendencies, and deterritorializing or destabilizing and 'cutting edge' tendencies. Deleuze and Guattari again upset any literal reading of 'machine', as the machine metaphor 'assemblage' displaces the simple mechanistic reading of 'machine'. Their systematizing offers four metaphorical positions, which are summarized in Table 4.1.

To re-employ a machine metaphor used earlier, by sticking with machine and war metaphors, contemporary medicine operates as if driving a car with the brakes on. How will patients benefit from values, descriptions and practices that objectify and dehumanize them and place them in a war zone? Just as medical students learn 'communication skills' only to enter practice and interrupt patients on average within 20 seconds of the clinical encounter, so imagining the body as a machine needing an oil change or a tune up negates the body-mind reality of human experience. Further, how will a doctor tune the engine of somebody with a medically unexplained condition?

Table 4.1 Four metaphorical states of the body as 'machinic assemblage' described by Deleuze and Guattari

1 Territorialized body assemblages:	2 Territorialized enunciation:
A metaphor for socialized bodily health (e.g. using condoms; visiting the GP when ill; medicalization of symptoms)	A metaphor for socialized debate about health (taking notice of campaigns against excessive alcohol consumption)
3 De-territorialized body assemblages:	4 De-territorialized enunciation:
A metaphor for resisting socialized bodily health (not using condoms; sharing needles; recreational drug use; seeking alternative therapies)	A metaphor for resisting socialized debate about health (e.g. William Burroughs extolling the virtues of drug use; William T. Vollman extolling the virtues of visiting prostitutes and not using condoms)

Medicine as 'against' nature, or 'with' nature: Osler and Garrod

William Osler (1849–1919) is one of the most celebrated doctors in history. He was a brilliant teacher and famous for his aphorisms. However, Osler subscribed to an engineering model of medicine in which, if a person was ill, then the body should be fixed, 'against nature' as it were, where disease is a puzzle to be solved and not tolerated. A good illustrative example of this is the medicalization of childbirth and death, both of which became 'engineered' in the sense of greater use of technologies. This was within the frame of seeing the body as a reproductive machine, one that could potentially be fixed if malfunctioning, and one that would eventually run down (Osherson and AmaraSingham 1981). Osler was succeeded as Professor of Medicine at Oxford by Archibald Garrod, whose clinical practice was shaped by a different metaphor – that of environmental 'adaptation' or 'with nature' (www.med.uottawa.ca/sim/data/Models/Osler_Garrod.htm).

There is a big difference between the two guiding metaphors. The engineering model stresses normative 'typical' and 'best' examples of health, that health and illness can be clearly separated, and that the diseases causing illness should be conquered. Further, treatments are standard for all patients. The adaptation model looks at the individual person, why things occur, and sees 'health' and 'illness' as relative notions. Treatments here might differ between patients for the same illness.

While both the 'body as machine' and 'medicine as war' metaphors can be traced back to origins in the mid-seventeenth century, they were aligned and cemented in the era after the Second World War as part of a wider cultural 'military–industrial' complex. The body was 'attacked' by germs and 'defended' itself through the immune system. Emily Martin's (1994) history of immunity notes how the body in early twentieth-century medicine is configured as a fortress that must be protected from external penetration by germs, or defended from attack. Within the industrial–military complex, medicine is masculine and hierarchical (even militaristic and authoritarian) and paternalistic or doctor-centred; doctors are heroes and ambiguity is not tolerated – rather, there is a search for certainty and truth.

Medical education, too, has followed the 'body as machine' model. Osherson and AmaraSingham (1981) point out that Abraham Flexner's root and branch overhaul of the North American medical education system just over a century ago was based on an industrial model in which the engineer was adopted as the key model for professionalism. Flexner's model for medical education required a mechanical view of the body – which would be studied scientifically largely through dissection and reductive laboratory science in the first two years of medicine. The curriculum would be designed as if it were an engineering problem, to include efficiency and standardization as its key values.

Medicine as war and illness as a battle

Thomas (2003) describes the hospital as 'a particularly volatile environment' and 'a virtual war zone'. Abraham Fuks (2009) suggests that 'The war metaphor is so familiar and commonplace in our medical rhetoric that we easily lose sight of its militaristic origins and significance.' Virginia Langum (2013, p. 5) notes that 'war is considered to be the dominant rhetorical domain in medicine', and that such a view is commonly historicized, for example traced to the seventeenth century, the American Civil War or the advent of germ theory.

Why does it matter that 'medicine is war' is a leading, or perhaps *the* leading or didactic metaphor? We have seen that Susan Sontag stresses the outcome of stigmatizing the patient. Fuks (2009) notes that the individual patient is lost to the sight of the doctor when the overall field of conflict becomes the focus. The person is lost to the disease, and all the armaments available – drugs, imaging technologies, therapies – are mobilized despite side effects or individual intolerances. This leads, suggests Fuks (2009, p. 1), to 'the eradication of the patient's voice from the narrative of illness'; more, 'The military metaphors that pervade medicine undermine the ability of physicians and society to deal with the burgeoning burden of chronic illness.' This is a big claim.

A metaphor, again, works by transposition, whereby a particularly abstract or complex idea or object, such as the body, can be grasped in terms of a simpler or more familiar notion, such as 'plumbing', or a 'machine' – for example, the brain is a computer, or the heart is a pump. The metaphor mediates between what is unknown and what is known. Through metaphors of war, the complexities of medicine can be reduced for ease of comprehension. We can think of enemies (illnesses such as cancer, causes of illnesses such as viruses) on battlefields (the hospital, the operating theatre, the clinic) being attacked by commanders (doctors) of armies (clinical teams) with sophisticated weapons (drugs, surgery).

Medicine's latent 'hospitality' (sharing the same etymological root as 'hospital') has been forced to adapt to a tough-minded, masculine Procrustean bed. Arrigo (1999) describes medicine as 'anchored by martial images and saturated in war-making discourse'. In Greek myth, Procrustes was a blacksmith who made an iron bed to which he fitted people by stretching them or cutting off their limbs. Does the bed of martial metaphors force the practices of doctors, healthcare practitioners, and above all patients into fitting what can otherwise be seen as an arbitrary set of guiding metaphors? Phrases such as 'war on cancer' and talk of *combating* illness, where *invading* bugs are the *enemy* in the *battlefield* of the patient's body, which is under *siege* but might be treated with *magic bullets*, are taken for granted and then not actively changed in discourse, and discourse is the script shaping performance, or how medicine is practiced. Thomas (2003) describes how such metaphors extend to nursing culture, which is configured as adversarial; practitioners use phrases such as becoming 'fatigued by having to do all these battles', feeling 'sabotaged', 'getting flak', working 'in the trenches', while their supervisors had 'deserted the troops'.

It is not only the language and metaphors of the activities and sites of war that might shape medical practice, but also the language of emotions accompanying strife, such as 'exploding with rage'. Hodgkin (1985) notes that medical training includes a hidden curriculum of metaphors concerning the temperature control of emotions – when the patient is boiling, the doctor can reduce the emotional temperature through cold detachment.

That didactic metaphors change can be established from historical evidence. It was not always the case that medicine was described martially. For example, in early modern Europe, cancer was associated with impurity and rot, or with a corrosive acid (Stolberg 2014). The root meaning of cancer, as we have seen, is 'crab' or 'crayfish', and the disease was imagined as corrosively biting into surrounding flesh. In the late fifteenth and sixteenth centuries, military metaphors, by which cancer is configured as a hostile presence that has to be killed, were not common (Stolberg 2014). A more common metaphor was that of a rooting (and not a rotting) plant that was difficult to eradicate and produced seeds, referring to metastasis, from the Greek, meaning 'a change of position'. Virginia Langum (2013) notes that where medieval medical texts refer to 'fighting' metaphors, these are in the context of fighting sin, so that illness may be metaphorically contextualized as a moral problem – 'holy' and 'healing' stem from the same root, where a holy body is a whole body, balanced and well.

Notions of 'fighting' disease not as a moral struggle but as combat entered Western medicine through the works of Thomas Sydenham in England in the mid-seventeenth century. Sydenham described medical intervention as if he were vigorously using an assault weapon: 'I attack the enemy within', and 'A murderous array of disease has to be fought against, and the battle is not a battle for the sluggard.' Sydenham, the most famous physician of his day, summed up his approach as: 'I steadily investigate the disease, I comprehend its character, and I proceed straight ahead, and in full confidence, towards its annihilation.' Sydenham may have known the poet John Donne's reference in 'Devotions Upon Emergent Occasions' to his own illness in 1627 as a 'siege' and a 'cannon shot'. Donne thought he was dying from a fever 'that blows up the heart' (Penson *et al.* 2004). In *AIDS and Its Metaphors*, Susan Sontag (1989) reminds us that Donne describes an 'illness that invades'. I have already referred to Donne's use of 'violence' metaphors for illness in his sermons (Alford 1739).

Sydenham's metaphors, however, did not constitute a dominant discourse at the time. Such a discourse was established in modern medicine two centuries later through Louis Pasteur's 'biomilitarism'. Montgomery (1996) notes that while early nineteenth-century doctors often used passive language such as plagues 'lying' upon people, Pasteur mobilized an unashamedly active, militaristic language, in which diseases 'attacked' persons. Pasteur's description of germ theory displaced a previous language of bodily 'excess of vital forces' with a language of invading armies laying siege to the body, which becomes a battlefield. Over a century later, medicine as battle is now a naturalized notion, but it once had to be established with militaristic zeal. As Fuks (2009) further argues, the medical gaze can be equated with the martial gaze, as the battlefield changes through history from the sickroom of the eighteenth century, to the pathologist's bench of the nineteenth century, to the imaging room of the twentieth century, to the DNA sequencer's computer screen of today. This is compounded through the lens of gender; a male medicine may be treating a woman patient, for example, with breast (although males, too, can suffer from breast cancer) or ovarian cancer.

Sontag (1989) notes that the gross military metaphor gradually becomes more specific and refined through cellular pathology, as knowledge accumulates about the microorganisms that cause illness. Organisms then 'invade' the body, which produces its own 'defences', but sometimes these are not enough and must be supplemented or augmented. Medicine's supplement in some cases, specifically with cancers, becomes 'aggressive' treatment. In public health, diseases 'invade' societies, which must 'mobilize' health education and health practices to 'defeat the enemy', as alien other. Again, this whole process stigmatizes rather than cares. The patient, after all, is in the line of fire. Yet, suggests Sontag, it is the metaphors themselves that can kill.

A 'war against cancer' was first described in a lead article in the *British Medical Journal* in 1904 (Reisfield and Wilson 2004). This rhetoric was extended to identify the 'fight against cancer' as an issue of imperialist domination; the disease itself was described as 'darkest Africa' waiting to be discovered and conquered. Later, cancer cells were identified with Bolsheviks, as 'anarchic', threatening the stability of the body (ibid.). Cancer has continued to attract militaristic and imperialistic language. In 1971, Richard Nixon, then President of the United States, delivered a famous speech declaring a 'war' on cancer, by which science would 'conquer' the disease. At this time, bioscience was replete with martial terms such as 'killer' cells and 'invasive' species. However, to employ martial language against itself, there are casualties from this approach. Is illness to be eradicated before it is understood?

Martial metaphors have gained a purchase in medicine and surgery, and continue to be used by doctors and surgeons, possibly because they serve a purpose in maintaining the power of such doctors and surgeons at the apex of a militaristic hierarchy, where a meritocracy is misread as an autocracy. There is a long-standing argument in political theory that under a 'state of exception' or a 'state of emergency', such as a war, unusual steps may be taken to award absolute power to an individual or government (Agamben 1998). It is, then, a commonly used tactic by authoritarians to maintain a permanent state of emergency so that they can retain their powers.

When, for example, the surgeon wishes to maintain authority, surely a good tactic is to maintain a permanent state of emergency or unrest? This seems to be a tactic used by some surgeons, where the permanent 'enemy' in the war is not, however, disease or illness, but rather, 'management', 'bureaucracy' or 'protocols' (Bleakley 2014). The surgeon can then divert attention away from internal conflict by reminding his team that the real enemy, the interfering 'other', is 'management'. De Leonardis (2008) suggests that the widespread use of medical metaphors follows a similar logic of 'dehumanization' and 'reification of the enemy', whereby the 'governed must submit to the ruler with the same eagerness a patient entrusts his/her health to a physician'.

The language of war works within its own logic by eradicating its enemies, so that it is difficult to spot alternative metaphors. Reisfield and Wilson (2004) note that martial metaphors are inherently bullying – masculine, power based, paternalistic, and violent or violating. But patients may tire of this. Reisfield and Wilson quote a patient with colon cancer who said that seeing his relationship with cancer as a battle 'was less than palatable' because 'I had already experienced real war in Vietnam and was not anxious to repeat anything closely resembling that.' It may be exhausting for already exhausted patients to think that they have a battle on their hands, and the notion of victory may be far from the reality.

This again echoes Sontag's (1978, 1989) plea to abandon the language of war in medicine, by which patients are stigmatized: 'We are not being invaded. The body is not a battlefield. The ill are neither unavoidable casualties nor the enemy', and the martial metaphor should be given 'back to the war-makers'. Colleen Bell (2012) agrees with Susan Sontag, suggesting that drawing on metaphors of war for medicine is unethical, granting legitimacy to war itself and acts of war such as atrocities and rape. George (2010), meanwhile, brings us back to specific locations on the battlefield, noting that in care for dementia the common and unquestioned use of bellicose terms, such as 'fight' and 'arrest', is 'metaphorically rendering the brain a seat of violence', where the metaphor is unproductive.

Hodgkin (1985) points out that 'medicine as war' is readily twinned with 'the body as a machine' discussed earlier, further alienating patients through 'mechanistic hubris', rather than recognizing the organic individuality and humanity of each person. Hodgkin notes that fighting wars is primarily a masculine activity. Medicine as war may have been useful in reinforcing the demand for steel and stamina that doctors needed to work long hours within a militaristic hierarchy and code of honour, but such a culture – serving to work against the development of feeling tone and reflection in doctors' work – is outdated. Hodgkin (1985, p. 1821) suggests that medicine needs 'to incorporate new images' into its thinking, and 'Essential to this process would be new metaphors around which we can reconstrue both our present and our emerging knowledge.'

Alternative metaphors to medicine as war

In the previous chapter, I described Sam Vaisrub's view (now three decades old) that reductive and negative martial (conflict-based) and engineering metaphors were outdated and acted as a brake on an emergent positive medicine of complexity and interdependence. This recognizes an about-turn for didactic medical metaphors, a reversal of interests from pessimism to optimism, and a radical reshaping of the landscape of medicine.

From her own experience as somebody with cancer, Barbara Ehrenreich (2001) found it difficult to relate to the martial metaphor as the best description of the landscape of illness that she now inhabited. Imagining a war against cancer cast the illness as an evil predator that should be eradicated, rather than a part of her self that must be understood. Ehrenreich describes 'the fanatics of Barbaraness, the rebel cells that ... carry the genetic essence of me'. The proliferating cells are not her enemy but are certainly overzealous. She did not wish to see her body as a battlefield in which the army of medical intervention treatment invades the bad cells and beats up the disease. Rather, having the illness made her rethink her identity; the diagnosis signalled 'not the presence of cancer but the absence of me ... I have been replaced by it'.

Pranay Sinha (2015) suggests that metaphors can empower patients by making complex medical conditions more understandable and accessible. However, martial metaphors may work against this. Sinha points out that many of his patients are war veterans, for whom martial metaphors restimulate damaging memories. Yet, 'the metaphor endures'. Sinha notes that there seems to be 'no deliberate, large-scale effort to find alternatives', when even the 'microbiology textbook in medical school equated bugs and drugs with terrorists and missiles'. How can doctors exposed to this regime not 'reflexively resort to martial metaphors?'

Garth Nicholas (2013) ponders the possibility that if cancers are eradicated in the future by medical progress, then the 'war on cancer' metaphor will become obsolete and fade. But to buy in to this view is also to buy into the 'medicine as war' metaphor itself. The end point of eradication of the enemy remains. If military metaphors in medicine are historically transient, fraught with contradictions and conceptually weak, and fail to capture the patient's perspective, it is hard to understand why they have gained such a foothold and maintain traction. Again, it may be that they fit a broader cultural form of medicine as quasi-militaristic in its organization. Further, such metaphors dull the capacity for reflection where their rhetorical style is that of the insistent bully – yet medicine seems to like to take on the mantle of 'working against the odds' instead of doing something about the odds. Thus, anaesthetizing environments are tolerated rather than changed; typically, doctors do nothing about confronting chronic organizational paradoxes such as bad hospital food (never mind a stultifying management team, or brash and cynical colleagues).

Hodgkin (1985) recognizes the staying power of the militaristic-industrial complex of metaphors in medicine, suggesting that the introduction of new metaphors may seem 'precocious'. Helga Nowotny (2015, p. 98), discussing the current rise of personalized medicine, notes how genome sequencing in particular 'is used to launch "precision" attacks ... against different types of cancers'; 'the old military metaphors of combating disease are back' in a new guise.

Yet, medicine and illness can readily be imagined as collaboration rather than heroic struggle, or as exploration and a journey. Douglas Slobod and Abraham Fuks (2012) suggest four alternatives to 'medicine as war': (i) balance and imbalance (homeostasis and dystasis), (ii) flow and blockage, (iii) medicine as a journey, and (iv) medicine as a collaborative exploration. Living with cancer has been described as a chess match, a marathon, a drama and a dance (Skott 2002)

– four more alternative metaphors to the martial complex. While biomilitary metaphors are common for cancer, 'bioinformational' metaphors are common for neurology, where the brain and central nervous system are described as a communication device with 'receptors' and 'transmitters'.

Writing on pain, its treatment and its metaphors, Shane Neilson (2015) notes that metaphors used for pain are often negative, closing off thinking for patients. Typically, medical metaphors are of the instrumental bioinformational kind akin to the body as a machine, where 'locks', 'keys', 'wires', 'circuitry', and 'doors' or 'doorways' are commonly described. Elaine Scarry (1985) noted that pain is typically described in medicine through metaphors of weaponry and damage. Neilson suggests that use of schematic metaphors in neurology leads to the accumulation of large amounts of data masquerading as fact or certainty, hiding a good deal of use of metaphor admitting to high levels of ambiguity and uncertainty. Neilson (2015, p. 8) further argues 'that for pain outcomes to change, our metaphors must change first'. He concludes on a damning note that metaphors of pain as damage are themselves potentially damaging to those who suffer from pain, so that pain 'is more than neurological metaphor'; it 'is what we say it is over time'. Further, pain is 'the context in which we feel pain, and that context need not be a clinicoapocalyptical one of damage, weaponry or live wires'.

What, then, are the historical conditions of possibility for didactic metaphors to emerge? Again, as we move into an era of medicine when more doctors are women than men, collaborative or democratic interprofessional teamwork is the norm, and authentic patient-centredness is realized, will militaristic metaphors, such as the 'damage/weapon' metaphor for pain discussed by Neilson, fade?

Yet, such militaristic metaphors remain stubbornly in place, shaping thinking, recurring as 'precision attacks' of personalized medicine resulting from knowledge gained by genome sequencing, as noted earlier (Nowotny 2015, p. 98). Reporting verbatim a cancer care team meeting, Harden (2013) notes how the clinicians involved recognized that their language was shaped by martial metaphors, even when such metaphors did not resonate with the patients they were discussing:

C1: we use language … that is all about war …

C3: I had a patient say to me … 'I have heard about … this battle with cancer…. I am waiting for the battle.'

C1: they feel like they've been done short if … they've not been in their army gear.

Note how the C1 member of the team still attempts to position the patient within the militaristic metaphor complex in what appears to be either a misunderstanding or a misrepresentation of C3's comment.

As noted already, Susan Sontag argued that metaphors circumscribing illnesses – in particular cancer and AIDS – could stop patients from seeking appropriate treatments and may add to their suffering. She demanded that illnesses be stripped of their metaphorical clothing to reveal them simply as naked phenomena open to largely successful medical interventions. Using as a background an analysis of tuberculosis, an illness that did not carry the stigma of cancer but, indeed, was often cast in a positive light, Sontag argued that cancer is neither a stigma nor a curse that people bring on themselves; nor is it a punishment or an embarrassment. AIDS, in turn, carries stigma as a disease that punishes and plagues, offering retribution. Militaristic language frames cancer and its treatment as a combat zone, and prescriptive moral high ground language frames AIDS as divine retribution for unsavoury behaviour, a plague on the house of transgression. Of course, these are views that may not resonate with patients themselves, or that they may not feel up to engaging with. Uses of martial and punishment/retribution metaphors are then counterproductive. In summary, for Sontag, diseases should be thought of without recourse to metaphor, stripped particularly of militaristic associations.

But Sontag herself was a writer, and her absolute rejection of the relationship between metaphor and illness is surely too sweeping and in danger of throwing the baby out with the bathwater – a more productive argument may be to call for a shift in the focus of metaphors, away from martial images to other forms. Anatole Broyard (1990), dying of prostate cancer, also thinks that Sontag goes too far in rejecting metaphor, suggesting that 'Metaphors may be as necessary to illness as they are to literature, as comforting to the patient as his own bathrobe and slippers.' Metaphors are important in helping us to form meaning in, and for, illness. Switching from combative 'warfare' to collaborative 'welfare' metaphors may affect practices – for example, by turning attention away from a disembodied agent of illness that must be eradicated to an embodied person who needs care.

Unlike Sontag, Carola Skott (2002) sees value in illness metaphors where they create meanings and bind patients to supportive communities sharing the same metaphorical complexes. Skott, focusing on cancer narratives, does question the uncritical acceptance of martial metaphors; some patients see cancer as 'a thing in the air' rather than being 'invaded by a killer'. Our list of alternatives to medicine as war now grows: (i) Sontag's *via negativa* view that medical interventions should be stripped of metaphor altogether; (ii) illness as 'exploration' and 'journey'; and, as mentioned above, (iii) cancer as 'a thing in the air', (iv) a 'chess match', (v) a 'marathon', (vi) a 'drama' and (vii) a 'dance'. The relative weights of these metaphors differ. Sontag's scepticism towards simply trying to alleviate the burden of illness through 'lite' metaphors, as if calling cancer an 'exploration' would turn suffering into a virtue, is noted. A strong alternative to war metaphors is that of medicine as collaboration, where collaboration may even be framed as an art of war rather than a love of war – a matter of strategy rather than attack, of productive confrontation rather than head-on challenge.

From war and violence to journey, economic and ecological metaphors

While medicine has promoted the twin metaphors of 'war on disease' and 'the body as a (broken) machine (to be fixed)' (for example, by the mechanics of surgery or drug interventions), this has been doctor-centred. People who are ill (medicine's 'patients') – in particular those suffering from chronic illnesses – have characteristically had their identities shaped by the didactic metaphor of 'illness as a journey' (Lapsley and Groves 2004; Semino *et al.* 2015). This meta-phor offers rich cross-domain mapping (Reisfield and Wilson 2004), drawing on speed, progress, direction, goals and pursuit. It is not as aggressive as the martial metaphor, and for this reason it may be easier to accommodate for patients. Cer-tainly, it is the key didactic metaphor in self-help books about illness, now a major genre in literature. In researching end-of-life care, Elena Semino and col-leagues (Demmen *et al.* 2015; Semino *et al.* 2015) describe the 'illness as a journey' as the most used metaphor beyond 'violence' metaphors. This is dis-cussed in more detail later.

'Do didactic or leading medical metaphors shape the culture and landscape of medicine?' was a question asked by George Annas (1995) two decades ago in an article entitled 'Reframing the Debate on Health Care Reform by Reframing our Metaphors'. Annas argued that in health insurance financing, militaristic meta-phors had already been replaced by market metaphors, but both metaphors 'narrow our field of vision' and 'neither can take us where we need to go'. Annas suggested that militaristic metaphors dominated both the practice and the financ-ing of North American medicine in the post-Second World War era largely because many physicians had been in the military. However, militaristic meta-phors have a longer history than this, as already discussed.

Another danger of the dominant militaristic metaphor is that it engages medi-cine in a medical arms race, where the dominant fantasy is that all health prob-lems will ultimately be solved with sophisticated technologies. Further, this metaphor again encourages militaristic organizational structures such as hierar-chies with male dominance. Finally, the militaristic metaphor celebrates control and certainty, whereas much of medicine is, in fact, about tolerating ambiguity. These dangers have, suggests Annas, led to the demise of the militaristic meta-phor and the rise of the 'market' metaphor, where the focus has shifted from production of medicine (laboratory and clinical research, pharmaceutical research, medical schools as the force behind medical education) to consumption and the 'needs' of consumers or patients (patient-centred concerns and medical schools as shaped by clinical, work-based practices around patients' needs).

The 'bottom line' of the economic production-consumption model is a profit-able health economy rather than healthy patients cared for by vocationally ori-ented doctors and healthcare practitioners whatever the burden of cost (for example, the UK National Health Service constantly running at a widely toler-ated loss). Indeed, power now shifts to managers of hospitals and family prac-tices – which are run as businesses – who come to oversee even the most senior clinicians. Clinicians who want to 'succeed' have to become managers themselves. The market metaphor ultimately fails because the 'free' market is a myth. The customer in a healthcare market does not shape that market – rather, the major movers are pharmaceutical companies and health insurers seeking profit.

Annas (1995, p. 746) suggests that the militaristic and market metaphors have shaped dysfunctional healthcare systems. An alternative shaping metaphor is proposed – the 'ecologic'. We need, suggests Annas, 'a new metaphoric framework that permits us to re-envision and thus to reconstruct the American medical care system. I suggest that the leading candidate for a new metaphor is ecology.' Annas suggests that concepts from the ecology movement can readily be translated across to medicine, described by words such as 'integrity', 'balance', 'natural', 'limited (resources)', 'quality of life', 'diversity', 'renewable', 'sustainable', 'responsibility (for future generations)', 'community' and 'conservation': 'If applied to health care, the concepts embedded in these words and others common to the ecology movement could have a profound influence on the way the debate about reform is conducted.'

Importantly, the use of an ecological metaphor complex may shift medicine's primary concern from treatment to prevention, where population medicine becomes primary, while also shifting values away from waste to conservation, from maintaining life at all costs to facing death more realistically, abandoning false hope in technology as saviour, and replacing individualism with collaboration and shared vision. Further, the ethics of medicine might be shaped less by market concerns led by 'Big Pharma' and more by patients' concerns, with an emphasis on variety of individual needs.

Martial metaphors can be unproductive for patients

The overarching cultural and institutional shaping by dominant metaphors trickles down to finer-grain activity – in particular, doctor–patient clinical encounters. Elena Semino and colleagues at the University of Lancaster (Metaphor in End-of-Life Care Study: http://ucrel.lancs.ac.uk/melc/), working from empirical data, suggest that martial or 'violence' metaphors are unproductive for many cancer patients, who do not frame their cancer as a 'battle'. In fact, such war metaphors may make terminally ill patients feel worse, as they see themselves losing the battle, leading to feelings of guilt and failure. Many people also live 'well' with cancer diagnoses. However, metaphors of the 'fight' help other patients, so a blanket condemnation of the metaphor as negative should be resisted.

Semino first established, through computer-assisted corpus linguistic analysis, that violence and war metaphors are indeed common in cancer discourse (Demmen *et al.* 2015; Semino *et al.* 2015; Potts and Semino 2017). Data about individuals' relationships to such metaphors were gathered from patients, carers and health professionals through interviews and analysis of online blog posts. The 'journey' metaphor, characteristically associated with patients, was found to be less negative than war and conflict metaphors. In the context of palliative (end-of-life) care, battle or fight metaphors are inappropriate for some, who prefer, say, journey metaphors to describe approaching death. A 'good' death may be compromised if a person feels that they have to fight and struggle to the end.

The fine grain of Semino and colleagues' studies shows that a badge such as 'violence metaphor' – including martial metaphors such as 'battle' – must be used with an understanding of context: first, which discourse communities are utilizing a studied metaphor; and second, in what genres are the metaphors used? Their research studied the potential for miscommunication between discrete communities (patients, family carers, and healthcare practitioners) as a result of established metaphor usage within such communities, and within genres (such as interviews and online forums).

Further, 'violence' metaphor' is an umbrella term covering a range of meanings, such as:

- warfare (fight, battle)
- violent actions (blast, confront)
- damaging and destroying (destroy, shatter)
- violent/angry (hit, attack)
- helping (defend, protect) or hindering (fight as a noun)
- trying hard, engaging (struggle).

These nuances are important, as they shade meanings in language. For example, a term such as 'hard as nails' implies a much tougher 'violence' than 'she put up a struggle'. 'I want to crack this' has a problem-solving feel, where 'I'll crack its head open' is a confrontational violence. What Semino and colleagues' nuanced work shows is that violence and journey metaphors are complex aggregates, that they are contextually sensitive, and that they are 'productive' or 'unproductive' in use dependent upon whether they empower patients or not. We cannot simply dismiss the use of violence metaphors when there is evidence that for some patients it appears to offer an appropriate frame for understanding and for resistance or recovery.

There are, then, potentially didactic alternative metaphors to 'medicine as war'. Only time will reveal whether one or more of these, such as a 'collaboration' or an 'ecology' metaphor, gains a foothold. Certainly, there is no lack of voices in the literature claiming that the 'war is over' as far as violence or martial metaphors are concerned. Vogt and Mach (2015) ask medicine to abandon competitive, martial metaphors and work collaboratively. Miller (2014) sees the doctor as transforming from the martial doctor 'at war' to the pacific doctor 'washing feet' or committed to patient service. Lane *et al.* (2013) ask whether we are 'battle weary yet' in the 'war against dementia'.

As noted earlier, we might ourselves be getting weary of the failure of such critiques to have an impact on the peddling of violence and war metaphors, especially for cancer, since Sontag, Penson and colleagues (Penson *et al.* 2004) called for an end to war metaphors in cancer care well over a decade ago.

Wiggins (2012) repeated this call in the *British Medical Journal* (*BMJ*), and McCartney (2014) reinforced this in the same journal. As already noted, Hardy (2012) had suggested, again in the *BMJ*, that 'metaphor may fill the space created by uncertainty' – a slightly tangled idea, which misses the point that metaphor in fact purposefully creates uncertainty, with an emphasis on 'creates'. Metaphoric uncertainty is an imaginative construction aiming to open up inquiry rather than offer closed outcomes. Medicine resists uncertainty while dealing with it at every turn. Metaphor is a key tactic in managing this dilemma.

We are still a long way from understanding how didactic metaphors that shape discrete discourse communities such as medicine come to be displaced by other metaphors or metaphor clusters. Given that metaphor use is contextually sensitive and occurs in differing genres (such as medical talk rather than medical texts), it is too simplistic to imagine that an historical process will unfold in which the two dominant metaphors of 'the body as machine' and 'medicine as war' will be replaced or erased. It is clear from personalized medicine, as discussed earlier, that 'target' metaphors will stick around for some time as the 'battle' metaphor is refined.

Metaphors seem to mutate like genes or adapt like aggressive pathogens – thus, the 'war on dementia', for example, mutates to a contemporary 'war on terror' (George and Whitehouse 2014). 'Shock' metaphors adapt historically, creating new epistemic objects through time – from Victorian psychopathological 'nervous shock' to current 'post-traumatic stress disorders'. The same concerns apply to the patient-oriented 'illness as journey', reinforced by the dominant healthcare discourse around patient 'pathways'. Further, the notion of 'dead' metaphors must be made more complex. Indeed, commonly used metaphors become a tacit part of everyday discourse rather than a skin that is shed; and we may be surprised by the rebirth of what we thought of as dead metaphors, returning to haunt us or stalk the streets as 'zombie metaphors'. Everyday slang from the hipster or Beat generation of the 1950s ('hip') morphed into hippie talk in the 1960s ('cool', 'far out') and returns today as zombie metaphors ('awesome', 'totally unreal') – see Chapter 11 for more on zombie metaphors.

In this chapter, I have critically discussed the current standing of overarching or framing metaphors that have historically shaped medical culture, particularly the body as machine and medicine as war on sickness or disease. A number of alternative leading metaphors have been scanned. It may be that the days of a grand narrative metaphor are gone and that what will emerge is a range of differing small narratives. In the following chapter, I move away from classic metaphor to look at the functions and meanings of resemblances in medicine – often treated flippantly, or as 'light entertainment', or as the lyrical element in medicine's normally epic and tragic world.

5 Medical metaphors as resemblances
Putting aesthetics to work

A feast of resemblances

Some years ago, my prostate enlarged so that it was difficult to urinate. The diagnosis was benign prostatic hyperplasia (BPH). A biopsy later shifted the diagnosis away from the 'benign' end of the spectrum to what the urologist referred to as some 'displacement' of cells suggesting 'low-grade' prostate cancer, echoed by a low Gleason score. At the time of writing, I inhabit a world familiar to many older men, that of 'watchful waiting' through regular prostate-specific antigen (PSA) blood testing, which my urologist admits is a 'bit hit and miss'. Another 'non-invasive' biopsy may be on the horizon, but at the moment I am 'relaxed' about it. What a sackful of metaphors we 'patients' must carry! We must be patient. We must learn to live with tepid uncertainty, in a fog of non-specific language – 'benign', 'low-grade', 'watchful waiting', 'hit and miss', 'non-invasive' – where the metaphors have ditched their roles as transformers of the mundane into the imaginative and have, rather, come to haunt or shadow us as mildly venomous.

'Patient' entered the English language in the fourteenth century. It is akin to the Greek *pema* (suffering) and derived from the Latin *pati* – 'to suffer'. The Middle English *pacient* gives us the noun that describes the one who is suffering – the patient. 'Patience' is derived, then, from putting up with suffering: either carrying a personal burden (my PSA results come around every three months) or world-weariness (the community of those who engage in 'watchful waiting' to see if symptoms develop). Metastatic activity of prostate cancer cells is often referred to as a 'migration'. Both 'displacement' and 'migration' for me immediately bring to mind movement of people around the globe, driven out of their native countries by war or strife, and so produce an uncomfortable reaction. Probably, there was more 'displacement' on my part, emotionally, than on the part of my irritable, potentially migrating cells. But birds migrate, too, to find warmer climates; and I am familiar with another common metaphorical use of 'displacement' from psychoanalysis, in which uncomfortable feelings or thoughts are substituted by acceptable ones as an unconscious defence mechanism. Commonly, we call this 'changing the subject' when the topic becomes too hot to handle.

My prostate, or what's left of it, has been expertly insulted. I underwent a surgical procedure – a trans-urethral resection of the prostate (TURP), in which (turn away now if you are squeamish), entering through the urethra, the surgeon pares away a section of the prostate to relieve pressure on the urethra. I was, of course, under a general anaesthetic. A pathologist friend and colleague told me that, although he had no first-hand experience of the procedure, a couple of friends of his had undergone the operation with great success. The drawback, he noted, was that straight after the operation, before the lining of the irritated urethra had healed, the first few urinations felt like 'peeing through ground glass'. Oddly enough, this analogy fitted the experience like a glove. I say 'oddly' because the resemblance is hardly exact. Yet it fits. And, believe me, it was the opposite to the sensation of slipping on a glove; more like being sandpapered from the inside.

The resemblance, too, is rather confused – a closer description might be 'peeing fire' rather than 'peeing through ground glass'. There is an established 'ground glass' metaphor in radiology. 'Ground-glass opacification/opacity' (GGO) refers to a hazy area of increased attenuation in the lung with preserved bronchial and vascular markings. The metaphor is non-specific with a possible range of causation: infection, chronic interstitial disease and acute alveolar disease. The two aligned metaphors of ground glass illustrate how a common image can work across differing senses – in this case, haptic (urine flowing through the urethra) and visual (the radiology image shows an area that looks like ground glass).

Some time later, I had an episode in which a gallstone strayed from my gallbladder into a bile duct, temporarily blocking the duct. The pain I encountered was like nothing I had experienced before. The young and extremely attentive doctor who treated me in the emergency unit said that the closest comparison on the pain scale would be childbirth. I was unsure how he – as a male doctor – could be so confident of the comparison, and certainly, as a male patient, I could not make the comparison myself.

By coincidence, I knew the young doctor – he was a graduate of the medical school from which I had recently retired as a full-time professor of medical education and medical humanities. I asked him how he could be so confident about the relative level of pain of childbirth, and he said he had never really thought about it; he was just applying a rough and ready scale that he had learned at medical school. This was a language of metaphorical comparisons acquired through rote learning – rote, because there was no reflective awareness of the use of metaphor in making comparisons of pain levels. I felt both aggrieved and embarrassed about this: aggrieved, because this kind of reflective learning of language used in consultations – such as a pain scale and its comparative components – is vital in medical education; embarrassed, because I was instrumental, along with Dr Robert Marshall, in introducing the medical humanities into the core medicine undergraduate curriculum at this medical school, and it is in this stream of the curriculum in particular that medical students should learn about the place of metaphor in medical language and practice, particularly consultations and diagnoses.

Both analogical resemblances – 'peeing through ground glass' and 'just like childbirth' – are actually in the imagination, and both are completely unnatural – the first because it is such a bizarre notion, and the second because I am a man. Yet, the first resemblance hit home (I could feel the analogy even before I had the operation), whereas the second remained abstract; 'peeing through ground glass' – for me – was what is described as an 'embodied' metaphor. Meanwhile, the second resemblance just did not make an impact emotionally or physically – it remained a cold and distant idea. Metaphors that hit the mark are at once both powerful and mysterious.

But metaphors can also miss the mark. When the same young, male doctor asked me to rate my gallstone pain on a scale of 1 to 10, I told him about the work of the artist Deborah Padfield (Padfield 2011; Padfield *et al.* 2003, 2010). I know about Deborah's work particularly because I examined her doctoral thesis. Frustrated by miscommunications between doctors and patients in explaining pain, Deborah set out to produce a series of visual images representing pain, like a deck of cards. These image metaphors can be used to illustrate and discuss the kind of pain the patient is experiencing, moving well beyond the limitations of a 1–10 scale. Deborah developed this work with a facial pain specialist doctor, Professor Joanna Zakrzewska.

Dedre Gentner and Arthur Markman (1997), writing about the psychological processes involved in the use of analogy and similarity, suggest that the long-standing view that these are differing cognitive processes should be challenged. Analogy has been viewed as a far more sophisticated process than mere similarity. A person is caught by a breaking wave in the shorebreak of a beach and is tumbled over – 'it's just like being in a washing machine!' she says. This is a fairly sophisticated analogy requiring an imaginative leap from observing the clothes going around in a washing machine to the current beach scenario. Actually, the analogy rests purely on the perceived motion of the clothes tumbling – and perhaps the white foam. The important thing is that this match is not simply coincidental. It is structural. Waves will always tumble you, and washing machines will always tumble their contents. However, the solid metal structure of the washing machine is nothing like the open seashore. The analogy has limits.

In supposed contrast, a jellyfish beached on the shoreline looks and feels just like an edible jelly, although consciously we know we should not try to eat it. Both have similar features, especially texture. The difference between this example of similarity and the example of analogy above is that while analogy is more sophisticated cognitively, similarity is less complex and has a greater number of shared attributes (Gentner and Markman 1997). Resemblances (X is like Y) are usually taken to be the same as similarities and are kinds of analogies.

There is a known brain region that deals with analogical reasoning. Damage to the left rostrolateral prefrontal cortex of the brain impairs the ability to reason by analogy (Urbanski *et al.* 2016). Further, analogical reasoning is not conceptual but embodied (Schaefer *et al.* 2015). Conceptual representations are, in fact, grounded in sensorimotor experiences and coded as such in relevant parts of the brain. In an experimental context, participants experienced rough or smooth touch and were then asked to judge the quality of an ambiguous social inter-action. Those who had experienced rough touch gauged the social interaction to be unsettling and adversarial, while those primed by smooth touch judged the social situation to be productive. Neural correlates to this embodied metaphor performance included primary and secondary somatosensory cortices, amygdala, hippocampus and inferior prefrontal cortex. Sensorimotor grounding seems to be intrinsic to metaphor-enhanced cognition.

The resemblances discussed in the section below (mainly food resemblances) move the sophisticated and conceptually rich 'peeing through ground glass' to more mundane connections. A radiological image 'looks like' an apple core (Figure 5.1). A bright red tongue 'looks like' a strawberry, while the next day the resemblance is more like a raspberry. But more is going on here than meets the eye as these mappings occur. The radiological image is of a cancerous colon, which is, in a sense, in a state of decay, like the apple. It is 'bitten into' or con-stricted as if the disease has a grip. The strawberry and then raspberry tongue – both 'hot'-looking fruits – afford a sign of scarlet fever. The bacterial infection causes a scarlet rash and the onset of fever – the hot colours of the fruits are part of the cognitive mapping across from the disease category's symptoms (source

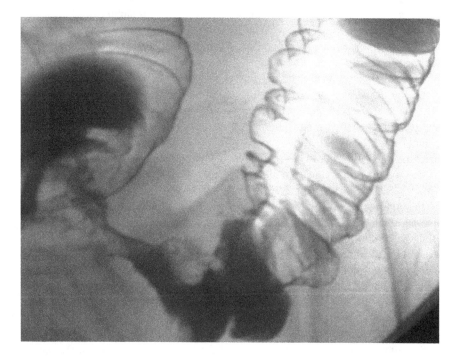

Figure 5.1 Apple core lesion.

Source: with permission: Dr Richard Farrow, Royal Cornwall Hospital, Truro, UK.

domain) to the fruit resemblance (target domain). The swollen tongue is fleshy like the fruit. There are, then, multiple dimensions to the similarities that turn them into analogies.

Analogy and similarity both foster insight, but with differing emphases – analogy requiring greater cognitive leaps for more sophisticated insight, similarity or resemblance relying on a mapping across of shared attributes that offers a sensory and emotional experience beyond a mere mnemonic. Medicine should be seen, touched, tasted, heard and smelt, not just on the ward but from the textbook and the teacher's mouth also. Working imaginatively with metaphors is central to an embodied medical pedagogy, discussed in full in Chapter 8.

Here is a composite teaching story that could be included in all undergraduate medical curricula. There is a remarkable set of passages in *Leviticus* 13 in the Old Testament – written around 400 BC – on 'how leprosy is to be recognised':

> If the priest, looking at the place on the skin, finds that the hairs have turned white and the skin of the part affected seems shrunken compared with the rest of the skin around it, this is the scourge of leprosy....

> If the skin is marked by a shiny white patch, but is not shrunken, and the hairs have kept their colour, the priest will shut him away for a week, and on the 7th day examine him....

> [If the priest] finds a white swelling that has turned the hair white, and shows the raw, live flesh, then it must be pronounced leprosy inveterate, deeply rooted in the skin.

Rabbis were taught to compare symptoms against a range of natural referents of over 30 shades of white, including 'wool', 'quicklime' and 'the skin of an egg' – a remarkably detailed monochromatic colour chart (Bleakley *et al.* 2003a, 2003b). Around the same period that these passages from *Leviticus* were written, the so-called 'father' of medicine, Hippocrates, noted symptomatic chest noises 'bubbling like boiling vinegar', and that a person with acute jaundice had skin 'the colour of pomegranate peel' (Volk 1990). So, medical analogies (metaphors and resemblances) have a long history. With the seed sown by Hippocrates, food resemblances in particular have a special place in medical lore.

Culinary concepts, or eating the menu

Almost forty years ago in the *BMJ*, S.I. Terry (a gastroenterologist) and Barrie Hanchard (a pathologist), from the University of the West Indies in Kingston, Jamaica, coined the tongue-in-cheek term 'gastrology' to describe the use of culinary metaphors in medicine, referring particularly to their use in gastroenterology (Terry and Hanchard 1979). Drawing on food metaphors themselves as a rhetorical style, the authors describe how they have 'culled 99 items of food and distilled 22 beverage-related items from various publications, and present an analysis of this harvest'. Unfortunately, no references are given, so we do not know the sources for the authors' catalogue – and their article is nothing more than a bare list, with no attempt to explain the purposes of these metaphors. The only critical engagement is a conclusion warning that metaphors are both time and culture based, so that the coining of new metaphors should bear in mind universality, accessibility and (my metaphor) perishability. (One of my favourite metaphors is 'long life' milk.)

Terry and Hanchard list fruit- and vegetable-based resemblances such as blackcurrant rash (xeroderma pigmentosum, a hypersensitivity of the skin to sunlight); mulberry molars (abnormal teeth caused by congenital syphilis); and spinach stools (caused by, well, eating too much spinach, so no cause for concern!). Not all are visual resemblances – percussion of the skull of a person with Paget's disease sounds like pinging a coconut. Not all are food metaphors either; alongside a sago spleen, nutmeg liver, strawberry gallbladder, apple core lesion and chocolate cyst (amongst many other food metaphors) are spoke wheel carcinoid (tumour of the small bowel as it appears on an X-ray); cobblestone mucosa (a characteristic radiologic and gross appearance of the intestinal mucosa in Crohn's disease, due to submucosal involvement); lichen planus (disease of the skin resembling lichen); treebark aorta (in syphilis, a diffuse thickening of the wall of the ascending aorta, where creases and radiating scars give a tree bark appearance); sabre tibia/sabre shin (malformation of the tibia presenting as a sharp anterior bowing or sabre shape, for example from Paget's disease of bone and from syphilis); rat's tail oesophagus (on a radiological image, the tapering of the inferior oesophagus in achalasia, where the muscles of the lower oesophagus fail to relax, not allowing food into the stomach); and rose thorn ulcers (radiological image showing extensive and deep mucosal ulceration in the small bowel). The resemblances are carried by the nouns, or by 'things' – cobblestone, lichen, treebark, rat's tail, and so forth – increasing the sensible power of the analogy or offering embodiment. (See https://radiopaedia.org for an archive of images.)

To return to the historical development of culinary metaphors in medicine, Volk (1990) notes that the Romans named the biconvex lens of the eye after the similarly shaped seed of the lentil plant. Fruit metaphors were particularly popular – cheekbones, bulging like apples, are *poma facies* ('face fruit'). In the seventeenth century, the anatomist Marcello Malpighi likened glands to bunches of grapes on a stalk. The uvula hanging at the back of the throat and the opening to the bladder comes from the Latin for grape, *uva*. Volk notes that Queen Victoria's surgeon, Sir Benjamin Collins Brodie, collected food analogies in the 1800s, offering these through a series of lectures at the Royal College of Surgeons in London. His anatomical observations referenced a range of foods: peas, chestnuts, walnuts, horsebeans, oranges, egg whites and pigeon eggs. For example, small fibrous masses lying loose in joint cavities or tendon sheaths were described as 'melon seed' bodies.

A few years after these lectures, the German biologist Dr Ernst Haeckel described a stage of cell division in a fertilized egg as 'mulberry-like'. I distinctly remember embryology lecturers using the same mulberry fruit analogy when I studied Zoology at university in the mid-1960s, and 'morula' – the Latin name for mulberry – is still used to describe the three-day-old fertilized ovum made up of 16 cells, and on to 64 cells after five days. Maintaining the analogy, embryology texts often show the morula in a bright, mulberry colour, somewhere between purple and red, although in the wild it is the shape of the developing embryo, rather than the colour, that is the distinguishing feature.

Prior to the development of the sophisticated imaging and testing devices available to doctors today, the human sensorium of the doctor was the instrument for physical examination, had to be well developed, and also had to flex to accommodate less savoury testing. The British surgeon and physiologist Herbert Mayo (1796–1852) wrote from experience that 'diabetic urine is almost always of a pale straw or greenish colour. Its smell is commonly faint and peculiar, sometimes resembling sweet whey or milk', while its taste is 'always decidedly saccharine'. The celebrated British surgeon John Hunter (1726–1793) wrote of semen that it 'would appear from the smell and the taste, to be a mawkish kind of substance; but when held some time in the mouth, it produces a warmth similar to spices, which lasts some time'. We assume that he was also the donor of the specimen. 'Mawkish' in Hunter's time meant having a faint sickly flavour (like warm beer), but now means cloying, saccharine, sickly, syrupy and even nauseating.

Hunter worked at the height of the European Enlightenment, a period characterized by an obsession with classifications – as if naming in its own right guaranteed knowledge. Classification demanded analogical reasoning, whereby resemblances between things (family resemblances), rather than things in themselves, provided the logic of knowledge. Analogical reasoning has driven science, and this has bled into medicine. Paul Thagard (1997) wrote the first systematic account of analogical reasoning in medicine, distinguishing between six types:

1   Theoretical: Pasteur's theoretical basis to the germ theory of infection was based on analogical thinking about the fermentation of milk, beer and wine. Pasteur wondered whether or not human wounds 'ferment' in the same way.
2   Experimental: just as fermentation of milk, beer and wine can be observed and controlled, so, by analogy, the theoretical notion of wound infection might be empirically tested.
3   Diagnostic: a patient has a disease with a configuration of three major symptoms. A second patient presents with these three major symptoms. By analogy, the second patient probably has the same disease as the first patient.
4   Therapeutic: the first patient above was treated successfully with drug A. By analogy, the second patient should also benefit from treatment with drug A.
5   Technological: Laennac describes the invention of the stethoscope through analogical thinking. When he wished to listen to the possibly diseased heart of a young woman, decorum stopped him from placing his ear against her

chest, while palpating with his hands led to little reward because of her obesity. The thought came to Laennac of how the sound of a pin scratching one end of a piece of wood could be heard, amplified, at the other end. By analogy, he made a cylinder from a quire of paper as the prototype stethoscope.

6 Educational: analogies are commonly used in medical education. For example, Donald Schön (1983, 1990) describes the 'swampy lowlands' of practice infected by uncertainty as opposed to the 'high ground' of practice shaped by certainty. Much clinical judgement occurs in the 'swampy low-lands' – a landscape of ambiguity (see Chapter 8).

Second helpings

Masukume and Zumla (2012, p. 55) note that 'Over the past century, over 450 metaphors have accumulated in the medical literature related to fruit, vegetable, cereals, seafood, dairy products, fauna, astronomical bodies, weapons, dining table utensils, laboratory equipment, drinks and colours' (see www.improbable. com/about/people/GwinyaiMasukume.html). The authors claim that 'These continue in use today', although many perhaps as archived historical curiosities. For example, it is hard to think that today's medical students would readily relate to a 'sago spleen' or 'hobnail cells'. Importantly, new metaphors (such as 'coca cola coloured urine' – a sign of acute glomerulonephritis or renal dysfunction due to inflammation, or sometimes after the consumption of diclofenac) – are relatively rare, suggesting either saturation of the field or loss of appetite for this way of thinking and recognizing.

Persistent culinary resemblances include a 'strawberry tongue', indicating an early stage of scarlet fever, whereas a 'raspberry tongue' is a late stage. A 'strawberry cervix' (Gholipour 2014) is a result of inflammation with a tri-chomonas infection, while a 'hot-potato voice' comes with inflammation of the epiglottis. There is 'red currant jelly' sputum as a result of pneumonia, 'pea soup' stools in typhoid and 'peach fuzz' skin in anorexia. An 'apple core lesion' or 'napkin ring sign' seen by a radiologist on an X-ray can indicate cancer of the colon, as previously noted. Tumours with large holes are 'Swiss cheese', vitamin B deficiency leads to 'goose skin', and swelling skin stretched to show the pores is like the skin of an orange (*peau d'orange*). 'Chocolate cysts' are endometrio-mas within the ovaries – although benign, they can cause infertility. A polycystic ovary has cysts covered with a pearly white capsule, hence the 'oyster ovary'. Amongst skin conditions are 'caviar spots' (small black lumps from vessel dila-tions), 'apple jelly nodules' and 'salmon-patch' benign skin lesions. There are 'chicken-liver' blood clots, for example in menstrual blood.

Again, these are examples drawn from a large and well-documented larder of food metaphors, many of which are already historical curiosities (Terry and Hanchard 1979; Volk 1990; Battistatou *et al.* 2000; Masukume and Zumla 2012; Cheng 2014; Lakhtakia 2014; MacGill 2014; Milam *et al.* 2015). Archiving such resemblances across cultures is vital as older generations of doctors, who had first-hand knowledge of their uses in diagnoses or at post-mortem, give way to new generations of doctors who may have little interest in what they may see as an historical footnote in medicine.

Amongst many food metaphors listed by pathologist Ritu Lakhtakia (2014) in an article in *Medical Humanities* are 'lardaceous spleens'. Enlarged spleens – caused by amyloidosis, an accumulation of misfolded proteins – have a wax-like discolouration resembling pork fat. Where pericarditis (an inflamed heart) leads to a whitish plaque forming on the outer membranes of the heart, this looks like 'milk patches'. A 'nutmeg liver' resembles the colour configuration of a cut nutmeg as a result of right-sided heart failure. Vaginal yeast infections result in a discharge resembling 'cottage cheese'. After bleeding, the stomach lining can resemble the striped rind of a watermelon (a 'watermelon stomach') as a result of gastric antral vascular ectasis (GAVE). Under the microscope, the nucleus of a spindle-cell schwannoma, a non-cancerous tumour that develops on the peripheral nerves, looks like a croissant.

As Lakhtakia notes, while such resemblances are striking and fire the imagination, they are, of course, indicators of pathology. Twinning often disgusting bodily suffering, such as exuded infections and bleeding stomachs, with gustatory treats, such as strawberries and cottage cheese, creates a living paradox – particularly for medical students, who are not yet professionally anaesthetized to the intimate bodily functions of perfect strangers. It is, perhaps, the juxtaposition of suffering with, for example, healthy, swelling fruits that makes these resemblances so striking and memorable or 'good to think with'. This juxtaposition of juicy metaphor with disease also creates an ethical conundrum ('uncomfortable to think with').

Food metaphors operate in sense modalities other than the visual, such as the fruity-smelling breath (to double the metaphor: like nail polish remover) that is the result of the production of the ketone acetone, warning of the onset of a diabetic coma. The type of tissue removal known as curettage is described as feeling and sounding like scraping a raw pear. Fibrinous pericarditis (inflammation of the two layers of membrane around the heart) is called 'bread-and-butter' pericarditis, as the two layers resemble buttered bread when separated during surgery.

In auscultation, listening to crackling lung sounds (rales) indicating various pulmonary disorders, the particular condition may be diagnosed through discriminating a range of sounds, from coarse to medium to fine, where the pitch becomes higher. These sounds – archived by René Laennec (1781–1826) as he developed and became more adept at using the stethoscope – were first mapped against naturally occurring sounds such as the cooing of the woodpigeon and crackling of salt in a heated pan (at the low end), and the sound of wood burning in a fireplace (at the high end). To illustrate the continued, if limited, production of new resemblances, contemporary auscultation metaphors include comparing chest sounds to those made by opening a Velcro strap, and to that of crumpling cellophane.

A group of Brazilian doctors, including José de Souza Andrade-Filho, a pathologist from Belo Horizonte, have catalogued a number of medical analogies within the specialty of tropical diseases. These appear in an ongoing series of letters to the editor of the journal *Revista do Instituto de Medicina Tropical de São Paulo* (Andrade-Filho 2011a, 2011b, 2012a, 2012b, 2012c, 2012d, 2013a, 2013b, 2013c, 2014a, 2014b, 2014c; Andrade-Filho and Pena 2001, 2010). These are not all food based – for example, 'violin string adhesions' describes a configuration of adhesions between the liver capsule and the parietal peritoneum caused by gonorrhoeal infections in women, first spreading from the fallopian tubes to the peritoneum, then healing as fine ('violin string') adhesions. This is known as Stajano–Fitz-Hugh–Curtis syndrome.

Food-based analogies include a 'spaghetti and meatballs' pattern on a skin biopsy diagnosing pityriasis versicolor, a common skin condition caused by a yeast infection. Tapeworms are described as 'intruder noodles'. Common in the tropics and subtropics, an infection of the liver by parasites carried there by the portal vein results in what is often termed a 'liver abscess' but properly is an amoebic liver necrosis that looks like anchovy paste. (I am not sure that medical students today will be familiar with anchovy paste such as 'Gentleman's Relish', a Victorian speciality.)

Such resemblances are widely described. For example, in the field of cytopathology, Rana and Syed Hoda (2004) describe a number of similes: 'chewing gum', 'cornflakes', 'Orphan Annie nucleus', 'strawberry gallbladder', 'mercury drops' and 'spider legs'. The Hodas' textbook *Fundamentals of Pap Test Cytology* (Hoda and Hoda 2004) contains a large number of specialty-based metaphors: bird tail, feathering, flat sheet and strip adenocarcinomas; ball-like, bamboo-like, and bean-shaped cells; blue balls; blue blobs; brown and brush artefacts; cannibalism; cannonball; cheesy; cigar-shape; clinging; clock-face; clue cells; cobblestone; collagen balls; comet-like; corkscrew; corn flakes; crowded cell; daisy-like; dark cell clusters; dirty; disordered honeycomb; dust ball; ferning; fishy smell; flailing; folded cell; giant cell; ground-glass (mentioned earlier); hair-like; halo; hand-mirror; histiocytes shower; hobnail cell; pap smear; pear; pearl; peg cell; pencil cell; perinuclear halo; picket-fence; polka dot; pomegranate; raisin-like; ratty; rosette; salt and pepper; scavenger; school of fish; sheets; signet ring; smudge cells; snake-like; snowshoe; soap bubble; spaghetti and meatballs; spider-like; spindle cells; and spindly cells. Of these, we might question why 'pap smear' is seen as a resemblance when it is literally a smear on a microscope slide. (Also, note how easy it is to resort to lists, without critical commentary.)

Such resemblances populate the three primarily visual specialties in medicine: histopathology (Lakhtakia 2014), dermatology (Milam *et al.* 2015) and radiology (Baker and Partyka 2012; Baker *et al.* 2013). Baker and colleagues (Baker *et al.* 2013) have written up a history of metaphoric signs in radiology over the last century. The first sign was published in 1918, and such resemblances increased in number up to the 1980s, when a monograph was published in 1984 listing such signs. Since the 1980s, there has been a rapid decline in naming radiological signs, as the specialty has evolved from one of descriptive naming to an analytical medicine. Baker and Partyka (2012, p. 235) describe reasoning through resemblance recognition as a use of metaphor central to gaining radio-logical expertise (and then identity as a radiologist). The authors describe how thinking with resemblances is central to radiological discourse and pedagogy: 'The inherent nature of radiologic images as simulacra of both normal anatomy and disease entities makes imaging findings well suited to explanation by means of named patterns borrowed from other realms of knowledge.'

The resemblances discussed above are often listed or archived (see, for example, a regularly updated archive of radiology signs on the website 'Radio-paedia', developed by Frank Gaillard, a neuroradiologist: https://en.wikipedia. org/wiki/Radiopaedia). They are, however, rarely critically investigated or theor-etically modelled – with the exception of Andrade-Filho and Pena (2001), Frieden and Dolev (2005) and Pena and Andrade-Filho (2010). These authors go beyond cataloguing and describing such resemblances merely as mnemonic devices stimulating recognition. Also, Masukume and Zumla (2012, p. 55) point out the historical imperialism of medical resemblances developed by Western medicine and transported to, for example, Africa – where metaphors may be employed that are not 'locally or culturally relevant'.

Analogies, even at the 'lighter' end of resemblances or similarities, have deeper cognitive and cultural and identity construction work to do, as already noted. I suggest below several reasons for the value of 'thinking with resem-blances' in medicine that progress this theoretical work. Such medico-cultural imperialism had been noted a decade earlier by Ahmed *et al.* (1992, p. 423) in a study of medical students in Africa grappling with Western 'culinary meta-phors', where 'the vast majority of medical students and young resident doctors are not familiar with many of the European foods, fruits and beverages that are commonly used in medical textbooks to describe disease conditions'.

In this chapter, I have introduced how resemblances appear in medical dis-course, as aesthetic objects for appreciation or as 'minimal cognition' diagnostic pattern recognition. I have noted the tendency for such resemblances to be treated as 'medicine lite' – either putting some fun into learning, or archiving historical curiosities. Already, the aesthetic framing discussed in this chapter raises an ethical conundrum, as we have seen: images of suffering can be beauti-ful, sublime and of great interest to medical students, especially if they are rare, but behind such images are suffering persons. In the following chapter, I chal-lenge the view that resemblances afford a 'medicine lite', setting out functions of resemblances in medicine.

6   Functions of resemblances in medicine

'Food for thought'

Good to think with or 'food for thought'

Why are medical metaphors, such as food analogies, 'good to think medicine with', or rather, 'good to sense with', moving beyond whimsical entertainment to serve serious and necessary functions? As we have seen, Douglas Hofstadter and Emmanuel Sander (2013), drawing on the latest research in cognitive science, suggest that analogy is 'the fuel and fire of thinking'. Analogy is not just good to think with, but necessary to think with, and this has been documented in medicine (Altoona Family Physicians Residency undated; Kanthan and Mills 2006; Ginn 2011; Shenoi 2011). Analogical reasoning keeps the process of thinking from bogging down; new associations afford innovation, so that thinking constantly outgrows its boundaries.

I.A. Richards (2001), in *The Philosophy of Rhetoric*, described the mind as 'a connecting organ' that prefers to connect 'two things belonging to very different orders of experience'. Resemblances or likenesses have often been considered the weak end of the analogy spectrum in relationship to metaphor, but resemblances are the workhorses of cognition, and both resemblance and metaphor work on Richards' principle of connecting differing orders of experience. With resemblance, the denominator is common (the strawberry tongue looks like a strawberry); with metaphor, the denominator is displaced (a blanket of indifference).

Rather than worrying about classification of kinds of analogies, we should be more concerned, first, about configurations – how metaphors appear and the aesthetics of such appearances (metaphors as startling, beautiful, challenging, ugly, sublime); and second, about explanations – what functions do metaphors serve (such as heuristic or pedagogical)? Where metaphor is a form of knowledge representation (Way 1994), in what sense might metaphor transform the ways of thinking and performing across an entire culture such as medicine, in principle transforming the landscape of that culture?

Gil Pena and José de Souza Andrade-Filho (2010) suggest that analogies or resemblances in medicine serve four functions: (1) naming, (2) remembering, (3) analogical reasoning and (4) learning. As already outlined, an analogy describes a structural relationship between two or more things so that sensory and conceptual knowing may be passed from one to the other as a form of enhancement, vivification or deepening of understanding ($A = B$, where $B = A+$, or $>A$). Again, where analogies are very close in form, they are described as 'resemblances'. For example, in the early stages of scarlet fever, a white coating appears on the tongue, only to peel back to reveal a red and swollen tongue resembling a strawberry in its colour and surface form. In the late stages, the tongue resembles a raspberry. This, in Pena and Andrade-Filho's model, is the basic function of resemblances as 'naming'. But, of course, the tongue in both cases is not a fruit. Again, the fruit (real or mirrored) is the common denominator.

We have seen that cognitive psychologists would refer to the original illness symptom (red and swollen tongue in scarlet fever) as the 'source', while the referent (the strawberry or raspberry) is the 'target'. The source is *in vivo* or a living thing, while the target is *in vitro* as mirror symbol or concept (Dunbar and Blanchette 2001). To progress the explanation already given, while resemblances and metaphors are both kinds of analogies, resemblances differ from metaphors in that they are based on object similarities rather than relational structures. The tongue in the early stages of scarlet fever 'looks like' a strawberry. It is not a strawberry, of course (literal identification), but uncannily resembles one. A far closer resemblance is the 'strawberry gallbladder' – a benign, diffuse cholesterolosis (fatty deposits) (Figure 6.1).

A metaphor works through relational structures ('she has the patience of a saint' or 'as right as rain'), offering conceptual links rather than object similarities. Pena and Andrade-Filho (2010, p. 611) suggest that while 'Mere appearance matches are limited in their predictive or explanatory utility', nonetheless,

> Similarity and mere appearance matches are extensively used in medicine, particularly in specialties dealing with high amounts of image information, in which they have an important role, not only in learning, but also describing, naming and retrieving pieces of information.

The authors' apparent lack of faith in the power of similarity matches is then swiftly contradicted. Such matches are already useful in condensing information into a shorthand sign not only for purposes of describing and naming, but also for purposes of retrieval or remembering. Further, as the authors note, such remembering is not necessarily rote but active and transformative, where resemblances act as 'advance organizers' – cognitive strategies that prepare the learner to move from what is known to what is unknown through 'scaffolding'. Here, the learner is still grounded in what is known, and what is unknown is not so distant as to be incomprehensible, but is readily related back to the known (see Chapter 8 for more on 'scaffolding'). Stepwise 'scaffolding' (itself a useful analogy) is typical of structured learning in a spiral curriculum. A spiral curriculum (another useful analogy) describes a process in which learning spirals around core topics that are repeatedly visited as knowledge and skills are accrued, as a deepening to those key topics.

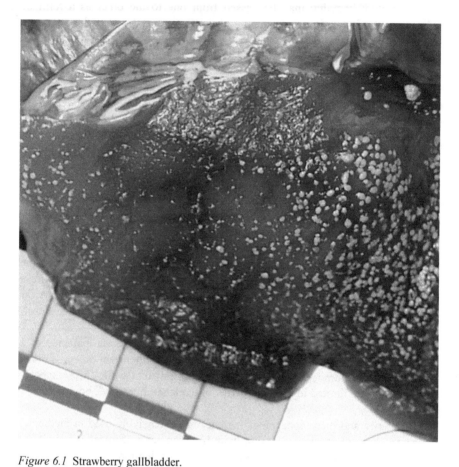

Figure 6.1 Strawberry gallbladder.

Source: with permission: Dr Joe Mathew and Dr Robert Marshall, Royal Cornwall Hospital, Truro, UK.

'Scaffolding' learning suggests that analogies must be within the learner's experience to be at all useful. Thus, a 'sago spleen' (amyloid degeneration of the organ, in which a cross section shows scattered grey translucent bodies resembling sago) or a 'nutmeg liver' (a perfusion abnormality of the liver, usually as result of hepatic venous congestion, causing dark red congested areas resembling a cut nutmeg) mean nothing if the targets (sago, nutmeg) are not in the learner's experience. Learning then becomes rote, or hollow ('rote' is an adequate yet mechanical descriptor, where 'hollow' is a metaphor). The same danger of rote learning may occur if the learner makes the connection from an *in vitro* source example (a photograph in a textbook) to an *in vitro* reference example (at worst, an unknown quantity, such as sago to a person who has never seen sago). These are issues of learning primarily for novices, such as medical students. However, as I related at the beginning of the previous Chapter 5, rote learning of pain metaphors ('childbirth', 'passing a stone', 'intercostal muscle strain/tear', 'gall-stone in bile duct'), paradoxically expressed on a numerical 1–10 scale, can be carried through from medical school to early clinical practice.

Analogical reasoning through resemblances

How does analogical reasoning through resemblances or surface similarity across source and target work for experts? Here is a verbatim diagnosis by a radiologist looking at an X-ray image where he sees a readily recognizable fruit resemblance – an apple core lesion, described in the previous Chapter 5 (Figure 5.1): 'There is an area of narrowing in the sigmoid. The undercut edges give an apple core appearance. This is colonic carcinoma.' (The sigmoid is the last part of the colon, which, in turn, is the main part of the large intestine.) Computerized tomography (CT) scanning is rapidly replacing such imaging, following the metaphor of polyphony or the capturing of many voices. CT scanning combines many X-ray images taken from different angles to produce virtual 'slices' of a body part.

The radiologist's judgement above is made without doubt creeping in: no 'maybe' or 'possibly', but 'certainly'. This is an example of Type 1 reasoning or pattern recognition. It appears to occur intuitively and rapidly but requires complex cognition at an unconscious level. A specific feature (source) is highlighted and matched unconsciously and rapidly against a referent that is actually a whole series of similar cases as exemplars of a diagnostic category seen before and stored in long-term memory. Remembering requires recognition of key features. At the same time, scanning quickly checks that there are no competing features that would call for a differential diagnosis.

The alignment between the pattern on the X-ray image and an apple core is not coincidental. Again, analogies have the characteristics of similarity, structure and purpose (Genter and Markman 1997). The similarity between a source and a target must be striking for the resemblance to have impact. However, there should also be structural and processual (purpose) resonances. The apple core is the residue of a healthy apple, while the apple core lesion is a stricture in the colon that is residual of cancer; the swollen tongue resembling a strawberry looks ripe and juicy; a 'bamboo spine' seen on an X-ray indicating ankylosing spondylitis – a form of spinal arthritis – signifies rigidity (Figure 6.2).

Resemblances work best when they are not only striking but also precise. Metaphors for cancer are rife, most commonly based around martial images such as cancers 'invading' and the 'war on cancer', as discussed in Chapter 4. These 'landscape', didactic or encompassing metaphors are perhaps both too broad and too vague to be helpful for anything other than rhetorical purposes. In terms of a metaphor that may help in diagnostic work, Guiot and colleagues (Guiot *et al.* 2007, p. 613) point to the 'splashing water drop' image that models tumour 'invasion' (another martial metaphor – 'invade' has its roots in late Middle English describing an 'assault' or an 'attack'). This metaphor of a splashing water drop does not stigmatize, but appears neutral. The splashing water drop

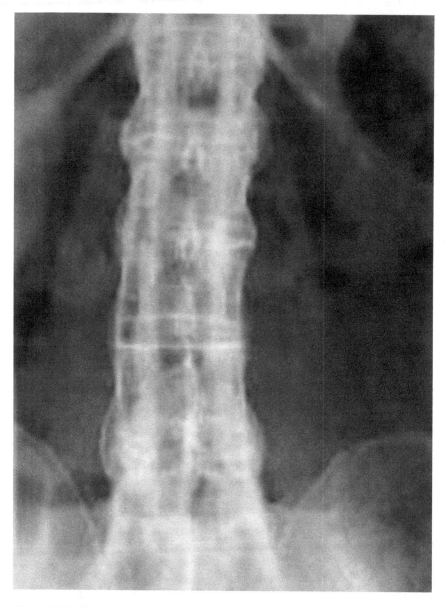

Figure 6.2 Bamboo spine (ankylosing spondilitis).

Source: with permission: Dr Richard Farrow, Royal Cornwall Hospital, Truro, UK.

produces a 'crown' that resembles the extensive branching systems of cancer cells, where droplets are dispersed in an unstable environment and take hold through surface tension above a critical level.

Through a martial mindset, we cannot help but see this cellular level process as 'invasive', but of course, the tumour cells have no such anthropomorphic designs. Shifting the metaphor through using the analogy of the splashing water drop can suspend the martial metaphor's grip to allow other ways of describing tumour 'invasion', for example through metaphors of 'surface tension'. Patients with cancer diagnoses or proto-diagnoses may feel that living with 'surface tension' in the broadest sense better captures their permeating psychological state than 'going to war' or 'preparing for combat'.

Analogies serve anticipatory functions in learning, preparing students for situations that are not readily experienced but may be simulated. For example, in the tactile senses, palpating the intestines in Crohn's disease is described as like palpating eels in rigor mortis (Rosai 2004, p. 721) – but it is highly unlikely that medical students, doctors or surgeons have had this first-hand experience with dead eels!

In summary, Pena (2007) argues that in order to make inferences, one has to map relational similarities and not mere similarity attributes. Thus, a similarity attribute (apple core shape) is sufficient for naming (the first function of resemblances), but not for remembering, analogical reasoning and learning. The latter three require mapping of relational similarities or disjunctions (apple core as perishing apple; luscious, juicy strawberry in contrast with fatty gallbladder). Below, I expand the four functions of resemblances described by Pena and Andrade-Filho (2010) to nine possible functions, with a strong degree of overlap between them.

Nine functions for resemblances in medicine

1 As emblematic of medical culture

Analogies in medicine are paradoxical in that they celebrate aesthetically uplifting images that refer to suffering and death. While medicine does not fetishize illness, its litany of metaphors and resemblances serve as objects of fascination. Further, such metaphors are central to medicine's history and advertise its cultural biases (Ahmed *et al.* 1992) (see point 7 below).

The literature on medical metaphors itself is biased towards historical archiving, where, for example, food metaphors may be treated as little more than historical curiosities to be catalogued. Little reference is made to critical issues of archiving, such as bias in selection as a result of a prevailing ideology. For example, as noted already, metaphors may be culture specific and then exclusive.

Gwinyai Masukume (Zimbabwe) and Alimuddin Zumla (London) (Masukume and Zumla 2012) and Ritu Lakhtakia (Oman) (Lakhtakia 2014) have recently revived interest in the use of food metaphors in medicine. However, this work tends to see the value of such metaphors as light relief from medicine's heavy load. Gwinyai Masukume in particular continues to do a remarkable job of archiving 'food related medical terms' through an extensive and beautifully illustrated blog (http://foodmedicaleponyms.blogspot.co.uk), but parallels this with tongue-in-cheek descriptions. Masukume and Zumla (2012, p. 55) talk about how food metaphors 'bring light humour' to medical education and are interesting as 'aide memoirs'. A commentary on Lakhtakia's article by Anna Almendraia (2014) in the *Huffington Post* is entitled 'The Whimsical Way Medical Students Learn about the Body'. Hoda and Hoda (2004) describe how resemblances 'serve to translate microscopic images into memorable catch-phrases, enhancing the learning experience and alleviating its tedium'.

Perhaps the tedium of learning in medical education is the fault of teachers within the field who prefer old-style instructional methods such as mass lectures to a more enlightened facilitative and small group inquiry method. In eating terms, the former is cramming (with its bulimic symptoms) and the latter is grazing. Kathryn Montgomery Hunter (1997, p. 167) coins the term 'the alimentary metaphor' for learning as ingestion in medical education, where 'students are spoonfed, forcefed; they cram, digest, and metabolize information; and they regurgitate it on tests', but, paradoxically, this leaves them 'metaphorically starving'. Hunter suggests, as any good educationalist would, that medical education should be a student-centred experience, where learners plan meals collaboratively with teachers 'and periodically check that information for freshness'.

As noted earlier, Frank Gaillard, a neuroradiologist, has developed 'Radiopaedia', an online radiology resource (https://en.wikipedia.org/wiki/Radiopaedia). A host of resemblances are posted here, showing how these bloom particularly in the visual specialties according to culture and historical period. Thus, food-inspired resemblances include a 'cervical hamburger sign', a 'mesenteric hamburger sign' and an 'oreo cookie sign', showing that resemblances continue to be generated. This also continues the tradition that such resemblances are fascinating, and then ethically troubling, as symptoms are turned into menus. On a medical student's blog from 2015 (http://medicowesome.blogspot.co.uk/2015/02/study-group-discussion-food-analogies.html) is a 'study group discussion' on 'food analogies in medicine', where symptom is curiously turned into desire for the edible:

> I came to know about the Oreo Cookie sign today! It's seen on a chest x ray (lateral view) when there is a pericardial effusion! The anterior most layer (the chocolate part!) is the epicardial fat. The mid layer (the cream part … yumm!) Is the fluid. And the posterior layer (again, the chocolate part) is the pericardial fat!

Established analogies in radiology include celery stalk anterior cruciate ligament (a mucoid degeneration of the ACL leads to an appearance of a celery stalk), a banana fracture (due to softening of bone in Paget disease) and a honeycomb lung (the lung develops air spaces patterned like a honeycomb as a symptom of diffuse pulmonary fibrosis). The Radiopaedia site, where possible, traces the historical origins of resemblances. For example, the honeycomb lung is thought to have originated in the nineteenth century in Germany and to have first appeared in a 1949 study (http://radiopaedia.org/articles/honeycombing).

As part of a project studying a century of metaphoric sign naming in radiology (Baker *et al.* 2013), Stephen Baker and Luke Partyka (2012) studied references to metaphors in general medical dictionaries and texts from the following specialties: radiology, dermatology, pathology, internal medicine, orthopaedics, paediatrics and general surgery. Of the 375 metaphoric signs, 66 per cent (249) were culled from radiology. Radiology has more metaphoric signs than eponymous signs (named after persons), while other specialties have a predominance of eponymous signs. Pathology (42) and dermatology (38), the other two 'visual' specialties, were second and third, respectively, in raw numbers of references to metaphors – as might be expected. The authors suggest that radiology is unusual in dealing with simulacra (images) of symptoms rather than physical symptoms themselves, and this has bred a culture used to transferring between knowledge domains.

Baker and Partyka (2012, pp. 237–8) suggest that as anatomical detail is necessarily sometimes obscured or accented by radiological media, this has led to the need for a metaphoric language for what is seen. They remind the readers of the tradition of naming bodily parts in terms of resemblances – for example, the thyroid is from the Greek meaning 'to resemble a shield'. This frequent use of metaphors in radiology 'makes their value for discourse and instruction readily apparent'. Metaphors then extend beyond diagnostic categories – where '[v]isual metaphors enhance perception by increasing a person's sensitivity to important features that may otherwise get overlooked' – to offer pedagogical possibilities. Baker and Partyka (2012) archive 37 metaphoric signs in radiology.

As noted above, José de Souza Andrade-Filho and colleagues in Brazil are cataloguing pathology resemblances through an ongoing series of letters (currently 14) to the editor of the journal *Revista do Instituto de Medicina Tropical de São Paulo*. Meanwhile, a medical student-led study group referred to above – inspired by a metaphor-loving pathologist – has archived one of its 2015 sessions on 'food analogies in medicine' (http://medicowesome.blogspot.co.uk/2015/02/study-group-discussion-food-analogies.html). The pathology department has a chart saying 'Pathology restaurant'. The discussion included 'apple peel sign' – intestinal atresia, 'bread crumbs' appearance in complicated cataract, and 'onion skin' appearance – Ewing's sarcoma.

Emily Milam and colleagues (Milam *et al.* 2015) have recently collected culinary metaphors in dermatology (http://archderm.jamanetwork.com/article.aspx?articleid=2168932). They, too, cannot help but engage with food language, boasting 'a descriptive buffet of visual signs' and drawing from 'over 450 analogies documented in the medical literature', of which 'those pertaining to food are the most plentiful'. They note that 'Dermatologists especially relish culinary analogies.' Port-wine stains, *café au lait* macules and honey-coloured crusts of impetigo remind us of the importance of colour in symptom presentation, while signs of texture include cauliflower ears, *peau d'orange* skin and the cheesy secretions of thrush. Aromas include the smell of stale beer in scrofula, and the sweet, grape-like scent of pseudomonal infections. Patient education, too, relies on the use of food analogies, such as applying a 'pea-sized' amount of dermatological cream.

Masukume (2012) lists nearly 30 analogies in obstetrics and gynaecology, while Kipersztok and Masukume (2014) list nearly 40 analogies in paediatrics. Such archiving of food metaphors, however, cannot be read at face value. First, we are hardly ever (apart from the Radiopaedia site) given historical or contextual information about a resemblance, such as its origins and possible date of origin. Eponyms related to their founders are common across medicine and then easily historically contextualized, but this is not the case with resemblances. Rather, the metaphor remains historically free floating. Second, the archive is presented as an authority, but many resemblances are fuzzy, ambiguous or even forced. Third, the archive material is often learned virtually – from textbooks – and not seen in the flesh. This makes sense for many pathology resemblances, for example, that are revealed only through microscopy or at autopsy, and for rare examples.

Fourth, Jacques Derrida (1998), in *Archive Fever*, argues that the process of archiving (such as electronic inscribing) determines the structure of the archived material. With the exception of Radiopaedia and Masukume's blog, medical metaphors are archived loosely, mainly orally. The limited number of peer-reviewed articles and the grey literature of websites discussing those articles surely provide a flimsy archive for the use of resemblances in medical work, and cannot match the oral archive that should be collected as a matter of urgency, as a key element in the history and anthropology of medicine. Practitioners interested in teaching – particularly dermatologists, radiologists and pathologists – are keeping an oral archive alive, but not formally archiving. Online inscriptions tend to archive according to blog and electronic rules concerning brevity and potential entertainment rather than serious scholarship.

Fifth, archive 'fever' itself, as Derrida (1998) suggests, is a compulsion not only to complete an archive (an impossibility) but also to get at some kind of 'truth' that emerges from the archive. Actually, the archive speaks in its own, necessarily contradictory, voice. There is no ultimate 'truth' to be gleaned from archiving medical metaphors, and there is no discovery of an 'original' voice (much as my Levitican 'Ur' examples in the previous chapter seem to demand such status). Rather, the archive must remain incomplete and must offer contradictions and paradoxes. There is no one use for food resemblances in medicine, and they do not reveal a secret code. As Abraham Verghese (2009), discussed below, shows, food metaphors can be used just as well as literary devices for the wider reader as for medical diagnostic aids within the closed circle of medicine.

Medical metaphors as resemblances, then, characterize medicine as an apprenticeship, largely an oral one. They advertise a face of medicine that readily captures the interest of medical students and is central to medical education: how experts (their seniors) make clinical judgements through pattern recognition. Further, resemblances are emblematic of medicine in direct proportion to their rarity – most medical students want to hear of the odd, idiosyncratic and rarely seen species of symptom, as an expression of their natural history bent or learning clinical knowledge in the wild. Under the wing of the best teachers, medical students come to resemble those teachers; the analogy is one of unripe to ripe fruit. The medical student wants to know how to ripen quickly, or to be 'hothoused' into expertise, and then into the identity of 'trainee doctor' rather than 'student'.

2 Ritual and identity: further emblematic purposes

'Thinking with metaphors', then, situates students in an historical stream as a primary element in ritual identification with medicine (see point 1 above) and in the forming of identity within a specialty. As point 1 argues, analogies (metaphors and resemblances) act as emblems for medical culture, so that learning the codes of resemblances is also to partially learn the code of medical culture. Metaphors are part of the historical fabric of medical culture into which students are integrated (inclusion), while interested non-medics – such as non-medical academics who are medical educators – are refused or vetted (exclusion) as 'medicine watchers'. This is a process of socialization leading to an identity construction, associated particularly with gaining legitimate entry into a community of practice as expertise develops.

A 1992 edition of the literary magazine *Granta* (on 'The Body') introduced a physician writer – Abraham Verghese (http://abrahamverghese.com/home/faq/) – to a wider international literary audience. Verghese's essay 'Soundings' made a passionate plea for the value of hands-on bedside physical examination skills (auscultation, percussion and palpation) for doctors. Such skills were, and still are, being eroded in medical education as they are replaced by reliance on diagnostic imaging techniques. Verghese is Professor for the Theory and Practice of Medicine at Stanford University Medical School and Senior Associate Chair of the Department of Internal Medicine, medical educator, and established fiction and non-fiction writer working at Stanford University, California. He argues that learning and executing such hands-on clinical capabilities with patients and teachers goes beyond their immediate diagnostic value. They are part of the ritual of building trust in a doctor–patient relationship and of gaining an identity in entering the culture of medicine (both an educational and an experiential rite of passage that is performative). They serve, then, both to improve patient care and to socialize doctors. Besides, they are, says Verghese, 'low hanging fruit' in the skill set of doctors – so why not pick them? (See Verghese 2011, 2014a; Brockway 2015.)

One of Verghese's earliest published stories, 'Lilacs', appeared in the *New Yorker* in 1991 and was, in his own words, 'a very dark AIDS story'. Working as an infectious disease doctor in Johnson City, Tennessee, in the mid-1980s, Verghese treated people for AIDS in a period of ignorance about the illness. This is recounted in *My Own Country: A Doctor's Story of a Town and Its People in the Age of AIDS* (1994). This period plunged Verghese into unusually intense relationships with his patients and their families in an atmosphere of denial and repression, coping with a disease with no cure as an unfurling stigma. Passionate about literature himself as both reader and writer, Verghese was developing a medicine informed by a literary sensibility. Storytelling (and listening) paralleled the findings of the laboratory, and metaphor was seen as central to a medical imagination.

In *Soundings*, Verghese (1992, p. 89) notes that diagnoses can draw on analogies working across the senses, continuing the Hippocratic tradition of 'gastrology' but extending beyond foods:

> There are many distinct smells in medicine: the mousy, ammoniacal odour of liver failure – an odour always linked to yellow eyes and a swollen belly; the faecal odour of a lung abscess; the fruity odour of a diabetic coma.

In his best-selling novel *Cutting for Stone* (Verghese 2009, p. 223), one of Verghese's characters says:

> Take the food metaphors we use to describe disease: the nutmeg liver, the sago spleen, the anchovy sauce sputum, or currant jelly stools. Why, if you consider just *fruits* alone you have the strawberry tongue of scarlet fever, which the next day becomes the raspberry tongue. Or how about the strawberry angioma, the watermelon stomach, the apple core lesion of cancer, the *peau d'orange* appearance of breast cancer ... and that's just the fruits.

In recent TED (Verghese 2011) and TEDMED (Verghese 2014b) lectures and journalistic writing in particular, aiming for public involvement in medicine, Verghese (2015) has again argued for diagnostic resemblances as 'good to think with', as part of the ritual performative element of medical practice.

As doctors gain expertise in the transition from medical student to junior doctor, and then entry into a specialty, their clinical reasoning process shifts from Type II (logical and analytical) to Type I (pattern recognition), where repeated exposure to symptom cases leads to easier pattern recognition. As educators, experts find it difficult to teach novices what such pattern recognition is like, because by definition it is tacit and not explicit knowledge. Verghese (1999, p. 299) says: 'I taught students to avoid the "blink of an eye" diagnosis ... the snap judgement. But secretly, I trusted my primitive brain, trusted the animal snout.' For Verghese, then, pattern recognition is what the philosopher George Santayana called 'animal faith'.

In a series of articles, my colleagues and I (Bleakley *et al.* 2003a, 2003b; Bleakley 2004, 2006) have articulated the dynamics of such pattern recognition diagnostic reasoning in both medicine and nursing, placing emphasis upon its aesthetic rather than its technical or instrumental aspects, such as appreciation and connoisseurship, discussed below as point 6. In this research, I paired an experienced consultant pathologist, radiologist and dermatologist (the visual specialties) with three experienced visual artists. The pairs visited each other's practices and exchanged ideas about how they 'looked' and what they 'saw'. This collaboration was then extended to a public presentation and debate. What emerged from this study were new ways of thinking about the use of resemblances in medical judgement and reasoning:

- Doctors tend to reduce visual configurations such as pathology slides, radiological images and *in vivo* skin conditions to technical information rather than aesthetic images through an objectifying, trained clinical gaze. Artists tend to see even (and sometimes especially) informational images as having aesthetic worth.
- Doctors attempt to reduce uncertainty through diagnostic work, where artists tend to generate uncertainty and ambiguity. Doctors do not tolerate ambiguity that well, whereas artists are tolerant of ambiguity.
- Education of the senses for connoisseurship must be a part of medical education. In wine tasting, 'advance organizers' enhance appreciation. The teacher asks the student to distinguish 'dry peach with smoky pear and lemon' tastes and smells in a Californian Viognier, a particularly aromatic white wine. Not only can students quickly learn to enhance their senses in this way, but also this para-connoisseurship is transferable. It is an education of the senses through resemblances. Elliott Eisner (1998, p. 6) sees the educator's task as 'to function as a midwife to perception', where students learn 'to see, not just to look'. If this sounds a little left field for medical education, at Peninsula Medical School, where I was instrumental in developing a radical medical humanities programme with Dr Robert Marshall, a consultant pathologist, the latter ran a Special Studies unit with an oenophile and perfumer to teach medical students how to develop their senses of taste and smell.
- There are various kinds of expert practice: (i) habitual practice is where the expert sees what she expects to see and not what is there; (ii) saturated practice is where the expert eye becomes tired through exposure to everyday material and needs to be refreshed; (iii) restricted practice is where the expert eye is inflexible under conditions of ambiguity – collaboration with other experts is required to form a judgement; (iv) aesthetic practice is where the instrumental eye is extended to include appreciation and development of connoisseurship; and (v) ethical practice is where doctors always appreciate that while they are looking at 'images', they are actually looking at persons.

Stephen Greenblatt (1980) suggests that aesthetic structures govern the formation of identity. In other words, identities are shaped or sculpted. Such shaping implies a cultural hands-on art and connoisseurship. A doctor's identity is shaped through socialization into a specialty as particular ways of 'looking' and 'seeing' come to be developed. Thinking with resemblances and metaphors is a key part of this process. Michel Foucault (1988) suggested that forming an identity in the modern era is not accepting what is given but resisting convention to shape a new sense of self as both an aesthetic and ethical 'self-forming'. There are various ways in which identity may be formed through thinking with resemblances in medicine, as forms of resistance to habitual practices.

First, informational images can be viewed as having aesthetic or poetic worth and then appreciated as well as used functionally. Such images might educate the imagination, and doctors might become connoisseurs of informational images. This sounds rather depersonalizing, as such 'images' are, in fact, persons who present as patients. Connoisseurship must carry a deep humanity. This is an ethical practice. Second, while pattern recognition seems on face value to be an act of certainty in judgement, the whole business of plunging oneself into the world of metaphor educates for tolerance of uncertainty and ambiguity. This challenges habitual practices.

3 Making medicine more imaginative: continuous transformation of activity or changing a cultural landscape

Again, food metaphors such as 'red currant jelly' sputum in pneumonia, 'pea soup' stools in typhoid and 'peach fuzz' skin in anorexia are widely described (Lakhtakia 2014; Masukume and Zumla 2012), but rarely critically investigated or theoretically modelled (Bleakley *et al.* 2003a, 2003b; Bleakley 2004, 2006). This fails to connect the longstanding and continuing use of medical metaphors in both clinical practice and medical education with wider debates about the values and purposes of linguistic tropes.

Bleakley and colleagues (Bleakley *et al.* 2003a, 2003b) draw on the work of the scientist and phenomenologist Gaston Bachelard, who suggests that the imagination precedes and prepares perception, turning ordinary 'looking' into extraordinary 'seeing' (Stroud and Sardello 2015). Specialty experts, particularly as diagnosticians, are connoisseurs, and live through a medical imagination attuned to their specialist field. Just as William Osler lived and breathed the medical aphorism or maxim (Levine and Bleakley 2012), so one can see the same enthusiasm and depth of imagination in some doctors' engagement with metaphor – in this section I cite in particular Abraham Verghese, Ritu Lakhtakia, Gwinyai Masukume, Frank Gaillard and José de Souza Andrade-Filho. Where the imagination prepares perception, not only does 'looking' deepen 'to 'seeing' (these words are used as a metaphor to refer across the senses), but also memory is improved. In a classical education, memory was considered to be a virtue, not a skill, and was rigorously educated through mnemonic devices discussed in point 4 below (Yates 1966).

Medicine would become sterile and crystallize if it were not for continuous, imaginative or innovative transformation of the culture. The shifting landscape of medical metaphors is central to such transformation. The permeating use of metaphor is the primary means by which medicine as hard biomedical science is transformed into medicine as art and the practice of artistry. The continuing historical presence of catalysts, such as metaphors, that turn literal medicine into something more imaginative encourages innovation and educates for tolerance of ambiguity, which is central to good clinical practice (Bleakley *et al.* 2011; Bleakley 2014, 2015).

What, then, is the everyday practice as a mutative force within medicine that can transform it from science reasoning into a poetics of appreciation? Again, medicine is a metaphorizing activity, including widespread use of analogy, resemblance and maxims (pithy sayings), affording an internal mechanism of the transformation of a culture from active science to reflective poetics. Importantly, this implies an identity and identification shift for the doctor – from scientist to poet (see Chapter 9), identifying with the cultures of both biomedical science and the arts and humanities. But the use of food metaphors has, historically, been less grounded in poetics and more in mundane, concrete opportunity for diagnosis. As Masukume and Zumla (2012) note, prior to the development of microscopy and microbiology, a major part of diagnosis would have been the investigation of human stools. This would automatically be linked to digestion and food. The authors note 'rice water' stools of cholera, 'pea soup' stools of typhoid, 'red currant jelly stools' of intussusception (where part of the intestine has folded into another part) and 'anchovy sauce' stools of amoebic dysentery.

Salvatore Mangione (2012) suggests that the use of metaphors in clinical practice and medical education is part of an historical legacy of the 'humanist' doctor that should be maintained and cherished in the face of a dehumanizing medicine increasingly reliant on technologies and at-a-distance testing, rather than bedside expertise and hands-on physical examination capabilities. This has been a stance long espoused by Abraham Verghese, as discussed above. Mangione (2012) sees the stethoscope as a metaphor for the humanist doctor (and its disappearance from common usage as a metaphor for the dehumanizing of patients). He notes that brilliant diagnosticians such as Charcot, Laënnec, Bell and Osler were also artists and humanities scholars and would not separate the science of medicine from its art.

Mangione (2012, p. 546) describes the rise of scientific medicine and its divorce from the arts and humanities as a product of the shift in influence from French medicine to German medicine in the 1870s, when the outcome of the Franco-Prussian War 'shifted the axis from Paris to Berlin, and medicine went the German way'. Where the French way privileged the bedside, the German way privileged the laboratory. Medical education was stripped of its interest in a liberal education, so that the early socialization (and consequent identity construction) of doctors was shaped as anatomists and bench scientists. This was largely due to the influence of Abraham Flexner, the son of German immigrants to the USA, whose 1910 report on medical education shaped the next century of medical practice (Flexner 1910). Mangione (ibid.) further notes, following William Osler, that the arts and humanities in medical education (including the education of sensory or perceptual acumen) 'may increase our tolerance of ambiguity, a trait sorely lacking in modern medicine'.

4 Diagnostic purpose: heuristics and beyond

Metaphors are used as heuristic devices in clinical reasoning and diagnostic acumen through pattern recognition (Type 1 reasoning) – useful for experts (resemblances are 'good to think with').

Again, as expertise develops within a specialty in medicine, so diagnostic acumen becomes more acute, as the ground for clinical reasoning shifts from 'Type II' reasoning to 'Type I' reasoning (the two types constitute 'dual process' or 'dual systems' reasoning). Type II reasoning is the logical process of working out a differential diagnosis through systematic exclusion of possibilities from the presenting symptoms augmented by physical examination and/or tests. Certain presenting symptoms are seen so often that they become familiar to the doctor, and a logical cognitive process of selection is replaced by instant pattern recognition (Type I reasoning), which appears to be intuitive. It is based on how tacit or stored knowledge is organized cognitively and how it can be accessed.

Experienced doctors learn to use their senses in highly defined ways. This is particularly true for the visual specialties – radiology, dermatology and histopathology. Type 1 reasoning can be subdivided into (i) heuristic reasoning (using rules of thumb such as aphorisms, or clear resemblances such as an 'apple core lesion' or a 'strawberry gallbladder') and (ii) intuitive reasoning or 'hunches', the latter a kind of educated guesswork.

General analogies give us *general principles* about diagnosis. For example, apple and pear shapes are resemblances commonly used for predominant fat distribution in the body. Smaller tumours can be sized according to their resemblance to peanuts or walnuts; larger tumours resemble oranges and lemons in size. The kidney is bean shaped, while the biconcavity of the red blood cell brings to mind a doughnut shape (Lakhtakia 2014).

Type I reasoning always involves a shift from observation to reasoning. The historian of medicine James Bradley (2014) notes that 'the senses remain vitally important to the practice of medicine and medical education. ... For like all sciences, medicine must not only observe but describe, and in shifting from observation to description, metaphor becomes crucial', adding that 'metaphor will only get you so far'; doctors are 'unlikely to sip the urine (of a diabetic) for a sugar-like taste; much easier – and safer – to test for glucose levels in the blood. And more reliable, too.' Embodied metaphors are historically contingent.

Resemblances, then – often striking or memorable – are not just 'good to remember with' for novices, but generally 'good to think with' and 'good to sense with' for experts and in developing phases of expertise. Resemblances do operate across the senses, although there is a large bias towards visual resemblances, and many of the resemblances that are and have been used in medicine are again food-based (hence the pun 'food for thought'). This is not so surprising; 'thinking with food' is fundamental to human existence. The anthropologist Claude Lévi-Strauss (1969) suggests that the transition from nature to culture can be summarized in the metaphors of the 'raw' and the 'cooked'. A raw observation is cooked as it is turned into a diagnosis.

Such resemblances, again, are, of course, historically contingent, and many that are catalogued would have no currency with contemporary medical students – while contemporary students might not readily relate to 'oat cell carcinoma' (a particularly aggressive form of lung cancer named for its appearance under the microscope), they would surely resonate with *café au lait* brownish splotches on the skin – where seven or more *café au lait* spots at birth suggest von Reckling-hausen's disease (neurofibromatosis, or Elephant Man's disease). I doubt that many, if any, of today's medical students are port drinkers, yet port drinking is such an historically and culturally stable phenomenon that they will relate to the port-wine stain birthmark, which is a vascular anomaly; and seeing *port-wine coloured amniotic fluid* could clinch the diagnosis of placental abruption – a life-threatening condition in which a normally sited placenta (which means a 'flat cake') separates prematurely from the womb (which is inversely pear-shaped). But are these signs, again, a lingering part of the matrix of Western imperialism, and exclusive?

Diagnostic purposes are closely linked to pedagogic purposes (see below), which, in turn, are linked to identity constructions of doctors. A clinical teacher may use a memorable resemblance but is insistent that medical students gain expert clinical descriptive language. As Lakhtakia says, what is described informally as 'creamy pus' – a wholesome metaphor – is formally 'the unwhole-some attribute of an inflammatory exudate composed of necrotic tissues, white blood cells and bacteria'. This again raises the ethical conundrum that presenting symptoms affording fascination for medical students are markers of suffering for patients.

5 Pedagogical purposes: mnemonic triggers and beyond

Patricia Volk (1990) argues that resemblances in medicine were developed as mnemonics – easy ways to remember facts. Over two decades later, a patholo-gist, Ritu Lakhtakia (2014), suggests that food analogies in medicine 'make memorization of difficult facts child's play'. Lakhtakia notes that '[f]ood imageries that have inspired and embellished medical learning are, distressingly, vanishing from medical writings.... It is time to revisit this powerful tool and secure its place in medical teaching and records.' Resemblances such as foods work, suggests Lakhtakia, as mnemonics, when the symptom is twinned with a memorable image such as 'spaghetti and meatballs'.

For something to be memorized, however, learning has to be meaningful. The principle of pairing something to be learned with a co-stimulus that is easily remembered, because it is unusual, bizarre or imaginative, and thus makes an impression, is a Classical rhetorical device. It was reanimated through the Ren-aissance technique of the 'Art of Memory' (Yates 1966), developing memory, like muscle, through exercise. The exercises consisted of twinning everyday objects or ordinary facts with extraordinary, bizarre or even revolting images, so that the memory is jolted. In medicine, what could be more memorable than twinning an outwardly disgusting symptom with a delicious fruit in order to turn suffering into potential healing, inverting the traditional Art of Memory method? The Art of Memory, then, situates itself right at the heart of the ethical conundrum that twins medical fascination with distressing and often painful symptoms with patients' suffering.

I mentioned earlier that some commentators see medical resemblances in particular as affording a learning 'lite'. Anna Almendraia describes cataloguing resemblances as 'The whimsical way medical students learn about the body' (Almendraia 2014). Kipersztok and Masukume (2014, p. 51) review food-related medical terms in paediatrics, but cannot stop themselves making light of a serious study through food-related puns. Thus, food metaphors are clinically useful, as they 'allow for rapid diagnosis of classic presentations'; but examples are 'cherry picked', provide 'a better taste for interpreting pathology', make medical education 'more appetizing' and provide 'a menu of possible medical maladies'.

Again, resemblances do more involved and interesting cognitive work than such views suggest. For example, the fact that foods rot serves as an important analogical principle, as mentioned earlier with the apple core lesion radiological resemblance. A symptom (tenor, source) is compared to a healthy fruit (vehicle, target), but that food is already rotting over time and then itself becoming diseased as the diagnosis is made that may heal the symptom. Thus, a transformative transfer occurs not only between the source and the target, but also backwards from the target to the source. Further, the resemblance works as an advance organizer in learning – preparing the student for the value of further resemblances. Once one is in the habit of utilizing resemblances, they become a familiar and helpful method for learning.

6 Medical-cultural and medical-historical markers

The development of food metaphors in particular signals the danger that the use of such metaphors in medical education can be both a form of cultural imperialism (Ahmed *et al.* 1992; Masukume and Zumla 2012), and historically situated. The former is a hangover from Western dominance of medicine. The latter refers to historically important but no longer current forms, which have been called 'consecrated' terms – still reproduced in textbooks, but no longer resonating with contemporary culture. For example, schistosomiasis is a liver infection – a fibrosis of the liver caused by the eggs of the schistosoma. In 1904, William Symmers, an English pathologist working at a hospital in Cairo, first described the appearance of a liver at post-mortem as 'white clay-pipe stem cirrhosis' (Andrade-Filho 2014c). It is not, in fact, cirrhosis but fibrosis. Symmers saw a configuration that looked like a number of clay pipe stems that had been cut through. The terminology has stuck, although nobody smokes a clay pipe any longer – again, a consecrated term.

As for remnants of cultural imperialism, the key voices in the renewal of interest in resemblances in medicine and medical education now form an international group. Abraham Verghese was brought up in Ethiopia by Indian parents.

His novel *Cutting for Stone*, from which I quoted earlier, illustrates the interplay between differing cultural readings of medicine from his own life experiences. Gwinyai Masukume is an epidemiologist and biomedical researcher from Zimbabwe, who has also trained in obstetrics (www.improbable.com/about/people/ GwinyaiMasukume.html).

As noted above, Masukume has developed an extensive and beautifully illustrated blog 'Food related medical terms', preferring the term 'eponym' to 'resemblance': http://foodmedicaleponyms.blogspot.co.uk. He has, with tongue firmly planted in cheek, developed the Group for Research and Advancement of Palatable Eponyms (GRAPE) at the Cuisine Research Institute (CRI) to archive medical food metaphors, and is seeking international collaboration (personal correspondence). (Eponyms are usually thought of as being named after a person, but they can also be named after a thing, such as a fruit.) Ritu Lakhtakia (2014) is the head of the Department of Pathology at the College of Medicine at Sultan Qaboos University, Oman. José de Souza Andrade-Filho is a consultant pathologist and co-ordinator of the pathology laboratory (surgical pathology) and cytopathology of the Felicio Rocho Hospital, Belo Horizonte, Brazil. This international picture bodes well for challenging historical cultural imperialism in medical education.

7 Analogical thinking in medicine encourages a Romantic biology

Analogical thinking offers a different way of approaching medicine than logical thinking; it is holistic and integrative rather than linear and fragmented. There is a tradition extending from the Renaissance to the eighteenth-century Romantics in which natural life is seen in terms of interconnections and resonances and is not atomized to specific phenomena. In this worldview, analogies are 'good to think with' as they uncover structural relations between human illness and natural forms. Pena and Andrade-Filho (2010, p. 609) suggest that analogies 'involve structural alignment or mapping between domains' where 'inferences' and 'new abstractions' may be learned.

Analogies serve first as a tool for classification, but their use goes beyond this, as already noted. Analogies uncover structural relations common to the target (tenor) and the source (vehicle). Again, an example is the life cycle of the fruit or vegetable analogy and the disease to which it refers. The healthy fruit or vegetable refers back to the disease from which the individual suffers. It may be that this disease can be treated or cured (made healthy) as the fruit or vegetable 'decays' (its use as a diagnostic form complete) in memory or imagination. At the same time, the image of the referent food remains stored as an unconscious trigger for future reference. The use of analogies, then, runs against the grain of reductive scientific medicine, in which patients are reduced to diseases, and diseases to informational images, test results, and genetic or biochemical markers. Such atomizing tears through the metonymic connective tissue of resemblances that places the patient within a web of diagnostic associations.

8 To stimulate an ethical dilemma

A primary purpose of analogies is surely to saturate clinical thinking in ethical dilemmas, keeping doctors on their toes ethically. I have already rehearsed this scenario – 'healthy' fruit and vegetable images, for example, are applied to persons suffering from symptoms. These resemblances may help with diagnosis and treatment and then 'decay' as the patient, in turn, may receive treatment and proceed to possible recovery or respite. This cycle is ultimately positive for the patient, but it does present an initial dilemma – that of medicine's fascination with disease in its own right preceding the desire to cure. One would hope that the ethical imperative is for the desire to cure to precede the fascination, although this fascination in its own right is a stimulus for interest in the place of metaphors in medicine.

Three major ethical dilemmas remain: (i) the postimperialistic legacy of using culturally specific metaphors that may alienate medical students; (ii) the continued use of heroic, masculine dominant metaphors that have shaped the medical landscape, such as martial analogies, at the expense of more feminine or collaborative metaphors; and (iii) the use of abusive medical slang. These issues have already been discussed in earlier chapters.

9 Analogies may be used to explain things to patients

As Ilona Frieden (a dermatologist) and Jacqueline Dolev (a paediatrician) (Frieden and Dolev 2005, p. 863) suggest,

> Dermatologists practice medicine at a fast pace. Patient visits may last only a few minutes, and physicians must find techniques to optimize doctor-patient communication. Many dermatologists use analogies, whether deliberately or intuitively, as a technique for communicating medical concepts to patients.

Analogies are helpful in (i) doctors explaining things to patients – particularly in translating technical medical into lay understanding (Frieden and Dolev 2005) – and (ii) patients helping each other, for example in online support communities. Hoybye and colleagues (Hoybye *et al.* 2005) identified different ways in which women in online support communities talk about breast cancer. Besides writing about experiences and sharing ways of educating about issues such as lifestyle, women shared imaginative acts in which embodied metaphors frame new ways of dealing with symptoms and what the future may hold.

Jaideep Shenoi (2011) describes the 'art of analogies in the clinic', where metaphors are used to connect with patients. This is framed largely as the translation of medical terminology into lay terms. Shenoi, as 'a busy hematology/oncology consult fellow', is consulting with an elderly Vietnamese male patient 'grimacing in pain' in a frenetic emergency medicine environment. Shenoi had to tell the patient the diagnosis of metastatic pancreatic cancer. He suggests that translating clinical information into human terms benefits from 'the effective use of analogies'. However, Shenoi's choice of analogies goes against the grain of the argument I have been making in this book for a shift away from blanket reliance on dominant martial and violence metaphors to a more tailored and discriminating consultation. Thus, continues Shenoi, 'white blood cells, red blood cells, and platelets represent the armed forces, the Navy, and the Air Force. All three are needed to fight disease', and 'Lymph nodes are like security guards at multiple checkpoints or roadblocks in the body', normally recruiting 'backup to swell their numbers', but 'If they are overwhelmed, metastasis occurs'.

Shenoi also mobilizes tired 'body as machine' analogies. Getting regular check-ups for non-malignant haematology patients is likened to an oil change. Paradoxically, Shenoi warns against overuse of metaphors and resemblances using an overused analogy: 'analogies are like cars – if driven too far, they will inevitably break down!' Again, it is vitally important that doctors use appropriate analogies to help patients to better understand their illnesses, and do not resort to blanket metaphors, or metaphors that may stigmatize.

In this chapter, I have been concerned with physical disease and often with diagnostic or post-mortem markers at the microscopic level. Let us now take a major turn – into medicine and the mind, exploring the use of metaphors in psychiatry.

7 Metaphors in psychiatry

The embodied mind at its limits

Laced with metaphor?

In a previous discussion of Mara Buchbinder's (2012, 2015) seminal ethnographic study of the interactions in a paediatric pain clinic between multidisciplinary clinical team members, adolescents with symptoms of chronic pain, and their parents, we saw how metaphors are key to framing interactions and hypostatizing otherwise rudderless concepts. Metaphors such as 'smart neurons' provide a positive twist to a symptom expression. 'Sticky neurons' and 'sticky brains' describe more difficult or negative symptoms of perseverative language and behaviour – unusual attention to detail – also implying that some chronic pain symptoms may be 'all in the mind'. 'Stickiness', says Buchbinder, is an 'idiom of distress' that can be applied not only to children and adolescents labelled as displaying pervasive developmental disorder (PDD), but also to their parents, and sometimes to their doctors.

Buchbinder notes, however, that in the current edition of the *Diagnostic and Statistical Manual of Mental Disorders* (DSM-5 2013), the diagnostic category of PDD has been dropped. 'Stickiness' as a neurological metaphor will now lose its traction, modelling the fate of many metaphors in having a life cycle – birth, development to a high point, neutrality and then disappearance. Metaphors flourish and then expire, sticky or not. In Buchbinder's account, she asks whether the metaphor of 'stickiness' is 'in' the brain (reductive explanation of symptoms) or 'in' the social situations in which children and adolescents with symptoms of abnormally perseverative behaviour find themselves – for example, where one or more parents display similar symptoms (expansive explanation of symptoms). The notion that these symptoms are 'all in the mind' takes on a different complexion according to whether you plump for a neurological or a social explanation. In the latter case of the social explanation, 'it's all in the mind' is a negative judgement; in the former case of the neurological explanation, 'it's all in the mind' becomes an apt descriptor. Actually, it is neither in the social context nor in the brain – it is 'in' the metaphor. What, then, happens to these symptom profiles when the metaphor explodes and expires?

The most fervent critics of modern psychiatry as an institution have suggested that 'mental illness' is all in the mind of the psychiatric community (Szasz 1974), or is an historical accident based on a 'civilizing' impulse that excluded those on the fringes of society (Foucault 1964). This would make 'psychiatry' a metaphor. Certainly, perhaps more than any other medical specialty, psychiatry might be thought of as laced with metaphor. (As I wrote this, three options went through my mind: 'soaked in', 'shot through' and 'laced with' metaphor. I chose 'laced with' as this implies a fragility not captured by the other two options. 'Shot through' refers us back to tired martial metaphors, while 'soaked in' implies, on the one hand, a solution – and there may be no 'solution' or 'resolution' to mental illness – and, on the other hand, a kind of limpness. Lace is fragile without being limp, and this is central to its exquisite beauty.) For example, at the level of treatment, Lorna Rhodes (1984, p. 49) notes that the use of medications in psychiatry constitutes a discourse whose motions are oiled with metaphor, such as a spectrum relating to 'clarity' and 'opacity'. Thus, a patient refers to a medication that 'fogs my mind', and a psychiatrist suggests a change in medication that 'will clear it up'.

Writers have possibly described mental illness better than the psychiatrists and psychologists who constitute the therapeutic community, with certain exceptions such as Sigmund Freud, who won the Goethe Prize for Literature rather than the Nobel Prize for Science, and Adam Phillips (for example, 1994), who today continues the tradition of fine literary representations of psychoanalysis. A favourite topic with novelists has been depression – 'my head is in a vice' – perhaps best described metaphorically in the title of William Styron's (1992) autobiographical *Darkness Visible*, where we also find clinical depression described as 'a bed of nails' and 'a storm of murk'; the sufferer is 'like a walking casualty of war', with 'anguish devouring his brain', where 'psychic energy throttled back close to zero' resembles 'the diabolical discomfort of being imprisoned in a fiercely overheated room' – and here, 'the weather of depression is unmodulated, its light a brownout'. The word 'depression' itself is a depressing washout for Styron as the weakest of descriptions and metaphors, where ' "Melancholia" would still appear to be a far more apt and evocative word for the blacker forms of the disorder.' Styron argues that melancholia – 'black bile' – 'was usurped by a noun with a blank tonality and lacking any magisterial presence, used indifferently to describe an economic decline or a rut in the ground, a true wimp of a word for such a major illness'.

Space metaphors ('up in arms'; 'your ideas are out there') are amongst the most commonly used embodied metaphors in everyday speech, according to Lakoff and Johnson (1980). Here, commonly, time is referred to in spatial terms ('out of time'; 'let's see where we stand in a month or so'). In psychiatry, space and place metaphors are commonplace: 'displacement' or 'out of place', 'spaced out', 'down in the dumps', 'feeling low', 'just keeping my head above water'; and similar metaphors also infect the medicines that deal with these spatial symptoms – such as 'uppers' (amphetamines or stimulants) and 'downers' (antidepressants or mood stabilizers).

Certainly, a hard-nosed orthopaedic surgeon would claim the fuzzy logic of many of psychiatry's diagnostic categories listed in the DSM – now in its fifth edition (2013) – as evidence of the ubiquity of the metaphorical in the specialty.

That surgeon might also recognize that he (only a very small percentage of orthopaedic surgeons are female) fits some of the criteria for a profile of attention deficit hyperactivity disorder (ADHD), such as 'often does not seem to listen when spoken to directly'; 'is often "on the go" acting as if "driven by a motor"'; 'often has trouble waiting his/her turn'; and 'often interrupts or intrudes on others (e.g. butts in to conversation or games)'. Wen Shen (2014), a surgeon, notes that the culture of surgery is changing rapidly, so that where many surgeons would once have been thought to exhibit traits of sociopaths (Dutton 2012), they now are better described as 'action-oriented perfectionists with little tolerance for ambiguity'.

Psychological studies tend to focus on the personality profiles of individuals as they move into medical specialties, but other disciplines, such as performance studies, focus on how the historically established performative elements of a discipline ('scripts') shape identities. These are best captured through metaphors. Stereotypically cast as the polar opposite to psychiatry in medical circles, orthopaedic surgery best advertises the playing out of masculinized spatial metaphors through strict spatial hierarchies that Karen Davies (2003, p. 732) describes in performative terms as 'doing dominance' and 'doing deference'. A woman orthopaedic surgeon suggests: 'We have to adapt to their [male surgeons'] rules. We're only allowed in as guests.' So, through hierarchy, orthopaedic surgery is shaped by spatial embodied metaphors, as is psychiatry.

An encounter with Pan

Some metaphors in psychiatry have long histories – mythological rather than historical. For example, 'panic' ('panic disorder' or 'panic attack' in DSM-V) derives from the Greek goat god Pan. Pan's German 'biographer', Wilhelm Heinrich Roscher (1845–1923), was a Classics scholar of the highest reputation. Roscher (in Hillman and Roscher 2000) describes how Pan, the smelly, hairy goat god, sneaks up on you at midday, when the sun is highest, everything is illuminated, and you are feeling sprightly and well. Just as your shadow disappears as the sun is directly overhead, so Pan jumps on your back and you experience a pan-ic attack. In other words, panic attacks come out of nowhere when you least expect them. They ride in on the back of a metaphor embodied as a beastly, pungent nature god.

It has been known for some time that classic 'Type A' personalities, such as ambitious and controlling orthopaedic surgeons – and heart surgeons also – are prone to suffer from anxiety and panic attacks. The surgeon Wen Shen (2014), introduced above, notes: 'Many surgeons are abrasive, abusive, and wildly self-centered – so much so that observers have speculated that they suffer from psychiatric disorders.' Shen cites psychologist Kevin Dutton's (2012) *The Wisdom of Psychopaths: What Saints, Spies, and Serial Killers Can Teach Us about Success* as 'a controversial book arguing there are certain benefits to being ruthless, cunning, and indifferent to the feelings of others'. Dutton's list (based on an Internet survey) of professions with the highest proportion of psychopaths includes surgeons at number five. This suggests that controlling personalities may be putting the lid on anxiety and panic that would show them as weak. This repression either sneaks out sideways as passive aggressive behaviour, or builds up and explodes within as panic attacks and cardiac failure.

Is the Pan story above not richer and more apt than the DSM-V version below? Here is that version for 'panic disorder':

A Recurrent unexpected panic attacks
B At least one of the attacks has been followed by 1 month (or more) of one or both of the following:

  1 Persistent concern or worry about additional panic attacks or their consequences (e.g., losing control, having a heart attack, going crazy).
  2 Significant maladaptive change in behaviour related to the attacks (e.g., behaviours designed to avoid having panic attacks, such as avoidance of exercise or unfamiliar situations).

C The Panic Attacks are not restricted to the direct physiological effects of a substance (e.g., a drug of abuse, a medication) or a general medical condition (e.g., hyperthyroidism, cardiopulmonary disorders).
D The Panic Attacks are not restricted to the symptoms of another mental disorder, such as Social Phobia (e.g., in response to feared social situations), Specific Phobia (e.g., in response to a circumscribed phobic object or situation), Obsessive-Compulsive Disorder (e.g., in response to dirt in someone with an obsession about contamination), Post-traumatic Stress Disorder (e.g., in response to stimuli associated with a traumatic event), or Separation Anxiety Disorder (e.g., in response to being away from home or close relatives).

This is to be distinguished from a specific 'panic attack':

An abrupt surge of intense fear or intense discomfort that reaches a peak within minutes, and during which time four or more of the following symptoms occur. The abrupt surge can occur from a calm state or an anxious state:

 1 *Palpitations, pounding heart, or accelerated heart rate*
 2 *Sweating*
 3 *Trembling or shaking*
 4 *Sensations of shortness of breath or smothering*
 5 *Feeling of choking*
 6 *Chest pain or discomfort*
 7 *Nausea or abdominal distress*
 8 *Feeling dizzy, unsteady, lightheaded, or faint*
 9 *Chills or heat sensations*
 10 *Paresthesias (numbness or tingling sensations)*

11 *Derealization (feelings of unreality) or depersonalization (being detached from oneself)*
12 *Fear of losing control or going crazy*
13 *Fear of dying*

NOTE: Culture-specific symptoms (e.g., tinnitus, neck soreness, headache, and uncontrollable screaming or crying) may be seen. Such symptoms should not count as one of the four required symptoms.

What is not a concern here is whether or not the person experiences these symptoms – panic attacks are 'real', but they are also metaphorical, as the ancient Greeks understood, and the medicalization of the story of Pan's antics somehow denatures and depersonalizes the condition. When I say that the panic attack is metaphorical, I mean this in terms of how meaning is made of the experience. The 'attack' (there is another metaphor, a martial one again, doubling up the metaphors as it rides in on the back of Pan, who, in turn, is metaphorically jumping on the back of the person experiencing the 'attack') must be thought about and talked about retrospectively. But such talk is also prospective, shaping one's 'defences' (another militaristic metaphor) against future attacks.

Certainly, for the purposes of contemporary diagnosis, DSM-V does something that would be considered rather strange to the collective Greek mind. As Ruth Padel (1992) shows, in the ancient Greek account, sensations and feelings, especially something unexpected like a panic attack, were accounted for as a visitation from the outside by a god or a natural force – hence pan-ic as the hairy goat god jumping on your back (and this is progressed into the metaphors of 'a monkey on my back' and 'get off my back'). Now, 'panic' is focused inward as a physiological response, a condition of psyche expressing to the world, and not, as the Greek mind would have it, the world impressing on psyche. While separating phobias from panic attacks does recognize the external stimulus, something like a 'free-floating anxiety' – a familiar modern condition – cannot be thought of as having a mental or physiological origin. It is a response to a cultural and environmental condition. The cure, then, is not to fix the person's mental state or physiology, but to 'attend to' the environmental and cultural problem ('therapy' has its roots in the Greek *therapon*, 'attendant'). People must once more recognize the presence of Pan in nature. But, just a minute, isn't that a sign of a delusional disorder, seeing gods in nature? In DSM terms, yes, but what I am arguing for here is to think not literally, but metaphorically, about the appearance and dis-appearance of 'Pan'. Surely panic is inevitable amongst us all as we inhabit a world that is so full of surprise and shock, or natural and cultural disasters – an expressive world that we can no longer 'contain'? One of our commonest metaphors is 'to hit the panic button', meaning to overreact.

'Pan' is derived from the Greek for 'all' or 'everything'. To 'pan' with a camera is to get the bigger, or panoramic, view. Again, is a cultural repression of this holistic view, this grasp of the gestalt or complete picture, this glimpse of a complex system, creating a free-floating anxiety as we are bogged down all day in details, planning rather than panning? We are afraid of the pan spilling over and of being panned. And this demand in contemporary life is, for many, overwhelming, leading to the return of the repressed Pan as symptoms of free-floating anxiety and panic attack, located somewhere 'out there'. Psychiatry, already panned by other medical and surgical specialties, seeks legitimacy in scientific grounding for its speculations and increasingly turns away from fuzzy psychoanalytic speculations to underlying neural mechanisms as explanations for symptoms of mental illness.

Indeed, some of this work has been on metaphor comprehension itself. Persons diagnosed with schizophrenia-spectrum disorders are known to display an inability to process (recognize, paraphrase and generate) metaphors (Mossaheb *et al.* 2014). Zeev-Wolf and colleagues (Zeev-Wolf *et al.* 2015) used neuroimaging (magne-toencephalography) data to show that people who had been diagnosed as schizo-phrenic showed atypical early right cerebral hemisphere overactivation during tests of metaphor comprehension in comparison with a control group. Those diagnosed as schizophrenic jumped quickly to 'remote' conclusions about the meaning of novel metaphors, leading to bizarre meanings or 'disorder-loose' associations. The control group showed ability for fine semantic processing of metaphors – giving them cognitive meaning – through left hemisphere processing involving delibera-tion and resistance to wilder associations.

Pies (2015) notes that as 'neuropathology' replaces 'psychopathology' in mapping mental illness, some claim that the term 'mental illness' itself will become redundant, although Pies argues that neuropathology and psychopathol-ogy will remain as interpenetrating domains.

Returning to DSM-V, such as the lists cited above for panic disorder and panic attack, these are versions of what I previously discussed in Chapter 3 as English for Medical Purposes (EMP), explicitly anti-metaphorical and reductive. But, of course, these descriptors paradoxically fail the EMP test: 'being detached from oneself', colloquially described as 'free-floating anxiety', and 'fear of … going crazy', colloquially described as 'cuckoo', are indeed metaphors and not stripped-down literalisms.

An encounter with wolves

In her autobiographical account *A Road back from Schizophrenia: A Memoir*, Arnhild Lauveng (2012, p. 21) describes her vivid encounters with imaginary wolves. She refuses to call them 'hallucinations' because they were so press-ingly real. She also refuses to consider their origins in terms of a faulty brain mechanism or repressed childhood memories or trauma: rather, 'I knew that the wolves were not a mistake.' They had a peculiar logic – that of metaphor:

> just like dreams, they also needed to be interpreted in order to give meaning. But in order to interpret them, I first needed to be clear that they were true and real, even though it was a metaphoric truth and not a literal one.

Yet the danger remains that the metaphor was indeed literalized.

Does 'mental illness' work as a metaphor?

When Neil Pickering (2006) says that mental illness is a metaphor, he is not disparaging psychiatry. Rather, he is trying to honestly answer Thomas Szasz's (1974) infamous critique that psychiatry has no medical or scientific basis, but is purely descriptive, grounded, rather, in legal, ethical and philosophical issues. Pickering disagrees with Szasz's view that a diagnosis such as 'schizophrenia' is a medical fiction and is, rather, a label for a set of behaviours and experiences that are not widely tolerated. Pickering says that, of course, something important is going on with, for example, schizophrenia or ADHD, which is very real for those who suffer from the symptoms. Further, the incidence of such symptoms is striking: one in four people in the UK suffer from a mental health episode each year, and this attracts poor resourcing for intervention in comparison with high-profile physical illnesses such as heart disease and cancers. Mental illness still attracts stigma and is hidden in the fabric of culture.

For Pickering, this reality, however, is not best appreciated or understood through a positivist scientific lens. A metaphor is a more imaginative way of grasping mental illness, where a metaphor itself – in a sense – is a mental illness, or at least an irrationality, as the ordinary world is shifted to another level of meaning such as 'his goose was cooked'. The paradox is that those with the most severe mental illnesses, for example living in the delusional world of a schizophrenic, fail to distinguish the metaphorical from the literal world. Lauveng's wolves are embodied metaphors experienced in a disembodied state. For this reason, they are hyper-real, pressing. The schizophrenias may be collectively defined as taking metaphor literally, or embodying metaphor while in a disembodied state. Psychiatrists, in turn, must enter the world of metaphor to empathize with the psychoses.

For Pickering (2006), psychiatry's troubles with metaphor are grounded in its historical origins, when psychiatric language borrowed from the established language of organic pathology to describe mental experiences. In the current trend to reduce psychological phenomena to neural substrates, Pickering wonders whether the transposition is possible. Established terms from organic pathology, grounded in didactic metaphors such as 'the body as machine', become the metaphors by which many psychiatrists now make sense of their patients' experiences. Ironically, a symptom reported by patients suffering from schizophrenia is that machines place thoughts into their heads by 'thought insertion' (Mullins and Spence 2003).

In the evolution of psychiatry as a medical specialty, complex nosologies promised understanding but merely hid ignorance. The very imaginative qualities we associate with literary use of metaphor, transferred across to rational human behaviour, were seen as abnormal. Freudian psychoanalysis added another twist through mapping mental territory as if it were a literal rather than a metaphorical landscape, reinforced by Freud's imaginative topographical maps (id, ego, superego; consciousness and the unconscious). With the arrival of the DSM, now in its fifth edition, conditions became hypostatized. Metaphoric adaptations of disease imagery were no longer provisional, but were set in stone, and these stones were flaked like flints to produce ever more baroque classifications.

Critics of this approach suggest that a kind of fantasism had overcome psychiatry. More, as psychiatry's interest in locating mental illness in the brain became more pressing, a contradiction appeared. Neuro-psychiatry displayed the very symptoms it noted in schizoid personality disorder – a retreat from the social into the cocoon of the inner world. In danger of getting sucked into the black hole of solipsism, we had to invent the notion of the 'extended mind' (Clark and Chalmers 1998) to link self-serving cognition back to the social world in which language and metaphor are exercised. Meanwhile, the DSM became more florid as it attempted to classify a messy social world of complex and context-dependent psychological behaviours, while the same behaviours were systematically reduced to commonly shared brain mechanisms that collapse the historical, cultural, social, and local or idiosyncratic. This is not to say that neuroscience has simplified brain mechanisms. Rather, the simplification comes with the reduction of difference in the social world to selfsame in the brain's anatomy and functioning.

Psychiatry has been described as using a system of knowledge 'that is not a copy of facts but a representation of them' (Martinez-Hernaez 2013, p. 1019) – a culturally specific 'folk knowledge' disguised as objective science. In the process, actual folk inflections of patients – which may seem bizarre but are rich in metaphor that can aid understanding of the patient's perspective – may be lost to both a diagnostic formula and a brain location. Martinez-Hernaez (2013, p. 1021) describes an example of such a folk knowledge and cultural metaphor – an Igbo (Nigerian African) 'idiom of distress for the somatic manifestations of a mental disorder': 'Things like ants keep on creeping in various parts of my brain.'

How are we to receive such a remark without intimate knowledge of its cultural context? And, in light of what I have just argued above, is it not strange that the idiom also reduces symptoms to an itch in the brain? What the psychiatric establishment presents as concrete, non-ideological, and truth spoken without power is actually abstract, ideological and saturated in sovereign power. The language of DSM makes claims for an asocial and universal character of mental illness categories (at the same time as it multiplies up those categories, or fine-tunes them), and for clinical practice and judgement as neutral and non-moral. Categorization of mental illness then proceeds, paradoxically, as 'the concealment of metaphor' (Martinez-Hernaez 2013).

Metaphors shape psychiatry (as with other medical specialties) at various levels. At the cultural level, psychiatry has bought in to the general metaphors of the body as machine and medicine as aggressive and competitive ('let's beat mental illness'). Rosenman (2008a, p. 391) suggests that a category such as 'depression' cannot be properly conceptualized without metaphor, which 'dictates not only the description of the condition but also its treatment and research'. Bjørkløf and colleagues (Bjørkløf *et al.* 2015) researched older persons' experiences of coping with severe depression and summarized their accounts through the commonly used metaphor of 'being stuck in a vice'. Patten (2015) suggests that several competing metaphors for depression circulate within psychiatry, which can be seen as shaped by familiar medical disease concepts. This can be productive, generating testable hypotheses that shape applied research leading to pharmacological or psychological interventions, or it can be unproductive, leading to seductive models and arguments that are untestable. I have amplified Patten's list by exposing the metaphors that were previously only hinted at:

1   chemical imbalance (metaphorical because there is an assumption about what a normal 'balance' of neurotransmission in the brain might be – balance then becomes a metaphor rather than a measure);
2   degenerative (based on assumed atrophy of specific brain structures – a metaphor of the 'unseen');
3   'toxicological' (assumed exposure to an abstract 'noxious' psychological environment, and not measurable chemical changes such as nitrous oxide levels in the air);
4   assumed material damage to the brain as a result of psychological stress (again based on the unseen);
5   assumed deficiency of neurotransmitters such as serotonin (based on a metaphor of lack without any measurable baseline);
6   lingering use of largely obsolete categories such as 'consumption' (historical metaphors with little contemporary impact);
7   reference to a 'medical mystery' paradigm-shifting breakthrough (a metaphor of pending 'discovery');
8   assumed evolutionary vestiges (once adaptive mechanisms are now maladaptive as environments have changed – the metaphor of 'vestigial function').

Ronald Pies (2015) points to the very real suffering of the mentally ill and the disservice we may do them by assuming that psychiatry's nosology and practices are both rhetorical and metaphorical. However, mental illness 'may be metaphorical in certain contexts', suggests Pies. What does he mean by this? First, critics who say that psychiatry is a metaphor seem to be wielding 'metaphor' as a technical and literal instrument by which psychiatry's ambiguities can be readily exposed and moralized, rather than celebrated. Metaphor teaches us not only to tolerate uncertainty but also to think with uncertainties. We should be pleased to find a medical specialty that trades in metaphors without embarrassment – although, as we have seen, the new wave of reductionism in psychiatry (symptoms will ultimately be explained by brain anatomy, physiology and biochemistry) has perhaps come to hold metaphor at arms' length, even as it employs metaphor with abandon.

We must warm to, or befriend, metaphors – we cannot afford to leave them out in the cold, they cannot simply be applied cold, and they do not drop into our laps as cold calls. Metaphor works only if there is intention and audience reception, suggests Pies. So, 'my husband is a clown' appears to be a metaphor, yet in this case Mrs Jones' husband does in fact put on make-up, a wig, a funny nose and huge feet and apes around entertaining children at parties as a paid professional. Nobody would laugh at Mr Jones' clowning if his intentions and his audience's expectations did not match – all through the medium of metaphor. Mr Jones throws a bucket of confetti 'as if' it were water and the kids duck; he hits himself on the head with a hammer, but everybody knows the hammer is made of rubber; he mimes climbing a ladder and we all agree that the ladder is not there. We then *co-create* metaphors as a common social endeavour – again, they do not simply fall out of the sky, and they do not work solo in front of a mirror. Brains alone do not do this – language and performance, along with the use of artefacts (such as cooking utensils, shelter, spectacles, books, computers and transport), knit brains together.

Yet, it can be argued that the expression and the reception of mental illness do not work in this co-creative way of shared production. In fact, their dynamic may be entirely different. A mentally ill person might indeed stand in front of the mirror and, in misrecognition, circulate metaphors amongst herself and her alter egos. Studies of dissociative identity disorder (DID) suggest that multiple identities, or subpersonalities, are metaphorical in nature. They do not show shifts in underlying physiological functioning or memory. 'Alters', suggest Merckelbach and colleagues (Merckelbach *et al.* 2002), are metaphors for different emotional states.

The eruptions of a schizophrenic episode may be neither expected nor desired by the audience; and the same goes for a depressive episode that was not welcomed by the person suffering from depression, and therefore lacking intention. Rather, it felt more like a visitation – that of the 'black dog', one of the most famous metaphors in psychiatry, with a history that goes back a long way before Winston Churchill (Foley 2005). These are not, says Pies, 'intentional comparisons' (as with a metaphor that works) but literal mis-takes in, or on, the world: slippages.

While not rejecting the real suffering of people with a mental illness, it is common to be perplexed by such symptoms where they are liminal, borderland, a 'thinking otherwise' to logic. Shakespeare wrestled with this in *Macbeth*:

Macbeth:

…

how does your patient doctor?

Doctor:
Not so sick, my lord,
As she is troubled with thick-coming
Fancies
That keep her from her rest.

Macbeth:
Cure her of that.
Canst thou not minister to a mind diseased,
Pluck from the memory a rooted sorrow,
Raze out the written troubles of the brain
And with some sweet oblivious antidote
Cleanse the stuff'd bosom of that perilous stuff
Which weighs upon the heart?

Doctor:
Therein the patient
Must minister to himself …

Macbeth Act 5, Scene 3, page 3

A modern translation might be:

MACBETH: 'How's my wife?'
DOCTOR: 'She's overwhelmed by visions that will not allow her rest.'
MACBETH: 'Can you not treat an ill mind by taking away her memory of sorrow? Can you not use some drug to erase the troubling thoughts from her brain and ease her heart?'
DOCTOR: 'In that respect, the patient must heal herself.'

So, the patient must indeed look in the mirror and ask 'Can I make sense of this – or, in what way might this make sense?' This returns us to Arnhild Lauveng's wolves – neither night nor day dreams, but rather, metaphorical realities offering a kind of logic, a way of 'thinking otherwise', or perhaps of not thinking, 'keeping the wolves from the door' – having just enough resources to keep alive – for 'wolves' (life's predatorial quality) are killing machines.

Macbeth is pleading for his wife's mental health, but is saddened when the doctor claims that he cannot heal the emotionally ill. This leads to Macbeth accusing the doctor of not being a doctor at all, because he is not able to cure psychological illness or point to a drug that will do the job. How contemporary this sounds!

Let's sit down to a Chinese takeaway

As a young biologist, psychologist and budding psychotherapist, like many of my peers, I was caught up in the UK 'anti-psychiatry' movement of the 1970s. The terrible twins of the movement were Ronnie Laing and David Cooper. Many of us warmed more towards Cooper's (1967) work for its fusion of Marx and systems psychology. His *Psychiatry and Anti-Psychiatry* was a constant companion. I do not now subscribe to the radical position Cooper put forward, but it is worth restating: the psychiatrist–patient relationship is a system engaging a double bind and a knot (Cooper takes these metaphors, respectively, from

Gregory Bateson and Jacques Lacan). As a complex, dynamic, adaptive system, the psychiatrist–patient relationship resists simple analysis or reduction to formulae. It is not a form of logic but a series of contradictory double binds/knots such as 'I love you/now go away' or 'give me a hug/but keep your distance', which are familiar to both (especially the patient) as typical ways in which their everyday relationships, including family dynamics, unfold and then create mental binds. Such binds can be suffocating.

Further, a symbiotic relationship – and one of dependency – is built up between psychiatrist and patient, which questions Freud's formulation that the patient is cured when the transference/counter-transference (and resistance/counter-resistance) dynamic is resolved. Cooper suggested that the dependency dynamic between doctor and patient is 'for life', the psychiatrist acting metaphorically as 'hero' to the patient's 'lifetime dependency'. Drawing on a Marxist model, Cooper then suggests that this translates into a 'lifetime of income' for the psychiatrist (whether private or paid by the National Health Service (NHS)), giving both participants no incentive to break out of the dependency cycle, but rather, to deepen it. This is a capitalist strategy of exploitation of labour – the work that the patient puts in to progress to a cure is, in fact, a lifetime of slavery to the psychiatric establishment's strategy of increasing capital. On the one hand, there is no incentive for the patient to get 'better', and on the other hand, there is no incentive for the psychiatrist to seek a 'cure'. When I say that I do not subscribe to this position, what I mean is that I take Cooper's argument seriously but not literally. Rather, it is an argument based on a lacework of metaphor. It is, in fact, a double bind or knot in its own right.

I once went to a talk by David Cooper in which he asked a member of the audience to pop out and buy a Chinese takeaway for one. The person returned with a few steaming aluminium serving-trays and, at Cooper's request, laid them out on the stage. At the end of the talk, Cooper said to the audience, 'Let's sit down to a Chinese takeaway.' He stripped the cardboard tops from the foil trays and proceeded to sit down in each tray in turn. The metaphor of 'sitting down' to a meal was taken literally. 'That', said Cooper, 'is what we call madness.'

Madness, then – in Cooper's case, he was referring to the schizophrenias – is, again, to take the otherwise imaginative and metaphorical world literally. The symptom is, then, one of impoverishment, for metaphors are tasty, rich and nourishing – and so often full of additives – like the Chinese food itself. Paradoxically, the world of metaphor is not the fantastic world of symptom in which the schizophrenic may be entangled, but the cure for the symptom of literalism or the urge to concretize the fabulous: 'there's somebody hiding in the bushes and they want to kill me'. This paranoia – literally a 'parallel knowing' – is not a losing of touch with reality but a literalizing or concretizing of irreality, one of such increased touch that there is a suffocation of metaphorical possibility. The illness then requires a dose of metaphor. Or, the fabulism needs to be made real, not by literalizing but by a form of the literary genre of magical realism.

I am arguing – again paradoxically – that it may be metaphor that gives us a binding and a boundary, illustrated in magical realism. Magical realism works on the basis that we take its fantasies seriously but not literally. Without metaphor, we fall into literalism, or taking things concretely. The world of the literal comes prepackaged with given boundaries, but is suffocating. Imagine having a conversation with somebody who says 'That is just an echo from the past' and becoming completely fixated on attempting to hear that echo, literally. In the Greek myth of the nymph Echo, told in Ovid's *Metamorphoses*, Hera, wife of Zeus, has been slighted by Echo, who is a notorious chatterbox, and punishes her by cursing her conversation. Echo is only able to remember and repeat – verbatim – the very last thing that anybody says to her. Isn't that a good definition of authority structures or hierarchies? And maybe of some forms of psychotherapy and psychiatry!

Echo's extreme form is found in the figure of Narcissus. Echo falls in love with the hunter Narcissus, but he rejects her. Settling down by a pool after hunting deer, Narcissus captures his own reflection in the water and falls in love with himself. He is unable to move, as his gaze is so firmly fixed on the reflection, and gradually wastes away, becoming a narcissus flower. He also gives rise to the name for pathological and extreme self-love – narcissism. Narcissism is being caught in the trap of only ever hearing your own echo. Then, the metaphor is literalized and becomes symptom. Isn't that a good definition of authoritarian figures as heads of hierarchies?

Félix Guattari, a psychotherapist, and Gilles Deleuze, a philosopher, described the 'schizophrenic' state in metaphorical terms as 'smooth' (unbounded) rather than 'striated' (having boundaries), or as a 'body without organs'. This may be back-to-front, as the schizophrenic can be strictly bound by a literal perception, as we have seen. The body-with-organs is a metaphor for the classification systems with which eighteenth-century European Enlightenment thinking was obsessed. Medical education became structured through organ systems, so that a typical curriculum (even today some curricula follow this model) was developed as units studying the vascular system, the nervous system, the reproductive system, and so forth. This obsessive packaging or compartmentalization in no way captures the holistic, dynamic and complex way in which a life in a social context works, let alone an isolated body. It is a form of 'striation' or portioning up the world in order to manage it. Thinking 'organ systems' also reduces the mind to the brain.

A typical striation is longitude and latitude. This system does not appear in nature, but is a convenient way of mapping space and location. The 'body without organs' is a metaphor for a 'smooth' space that remains unmapped and undifferentiated. It also captures anomalies that do not fit striated schemes, such as the platypus and madness. When the skin of a platypus was sent back to a curator at the British Museum in 1798 by the then governor of New South Wales, Australia, the 'flat-footed duck' was thought to be a hoax because it did not fit the current taxonomy conventions. In other words, it remained a metaphor. The curator, George Shaw, summed up this scepticism:

> Of all the Mammalia yet known it seems the most extraordinary in its conformation; exhibiting the perfect resemblance of the beak of a Duck

engrafted on the head of a quadruped. So accurate is the similitude, that, at first view, it naturally excites the idea of some deceptive preparation.

We might say the same thing about madness. It is as real as the platypus, yet remains in the minds of some as a confabulation, undoing the best attempts of rationalists to place limits on human experience and to ignore the liminal and uncanny. What, then, is the best way to tame the unruly beast that is the platypus when it does not fit any of the boxes? Answer: generate ever more complex boxes – taxonomies and classifications. Make a box that the composite and unruly beast fits. In other words, create an infinitely malleable house of metaphors, edition by edition. And so the DSM was born.

One man's metaphors can create an industry

An 1840 census in the USA attempted to record the frequency of 'idiocy/ insanity' across the population. By the 1880 census, seven forms of mental illness classifications were used: mania (heightened passions), melancholia (depression), monomania (obsession), paresis (hysterical paralysis), dementia (memory loss), dipsomania (alcoholism) and epilepsy. This list constituted an idiosyncratic collection of symptoms that may even indicate symptom in those who conceived the classificatory system. Up to 1921, the system was used less as a prospective psychiatric diagnostic symptom and more as a retrospective health statistic. After this date and the formation of the American Psychiatric Association (APA), a system of tally (openly metaphorical) became literalized. The first edition of DSM was published in 1952. A body-without-organs became stratified. Patients could now be carefully located on a latitude and longitude grid, placed rather than dis-placed – pinned as specimens rather than remaining as floating anomalies.

In 1974, an American psychiatrist, Robert Spitzer (1932–2015) was asked by the APA to write a new version of DSM. This was published in 1980. Cynically, the new, more complex, system was adapted to the availability of a new wave of pharmaceuticals developed by a burgeoning drug industry in the late 1950s. Whatever illness classifications were included could be tailored to potential profits for pharmaceutical systems. Spitzer, reputedly authoritarian, had a powerful hatred of psychoanalysis and expunged mention of its influence in psychiatry in subsequent editions of DSM. This, one would imagine, would make DSM less of a metaphor-friendly handbook and more rigid in its approach. The opposite was the case, as new classificatory descriptors were coined that, some argued, appeared to invent the disorders they described, such as 'hyperkinetic reaction of childhood', now termed 'attention deficit hyperactivity disorder' (ADHD), and 'post traumatic stress disorder' (PTSD).

Alan Schwartz (2016) argues powerfully that the profit motive of 'Big Pharma' widened an originally narrow classification band for ADHD, so that once beneficial medication for a small number of people has now become a serious dependency problem for many. Expanding any classification of a supposed mental illness to include a population of the 'worried well' is akin to attempting to treat a metaphor. To his credit, in 1973 Robert Spitzer led a protest against maintaining 'homosexuality' as a disorder.

Here is the entry in DSM-5 for 'Anxiety Disorders':

Separation Anxiety Disorder

Selective Mutism

Specific Phobia

Social Anxiety Disorder (Social Phobia)

Panic Disorder

Panic Attack (Specifier)

Agoraphobia

Generalized Anxiety Disorder

Substance/Medication-Induced Anxiety Disorder

Anxiety Disorder Due to Another Medical Condition

Other Specified Anxiety Disorder

Unspecified Anxiety Disorder

This is an extreme case of English for Medical Purposes (EMP) (see Chapter 3) – naming as reification. Other than 'panic attack', will patients be using this EMP list, or will they be employing richer and more imaginative metaphors? What better than the 'blues' for melancholy and sadness; or the 'black dog', whose origin is in Robert Burton's *The Anatomy of Melancholy* (1621) (Foley 2005)? Isn't 'free-floating' anxiety more evocative – and true – than 'unspecified anxiety disorder'?

Cross-cultural issues and metaphors

The APA has a raft of web pages devoted to explaining and exploring the latest edition of DSM (V) (2013). One page is devoted to 'Cultural Concepts in DSM-V', explaining that the manual now 'incorporates a greater cultural sensitivity'. The rationale for this knowledge is that it will sharpen the diagnostic acumen of the psychiatrist.

Examples are cited: 'uncontrollable crying and headaches are symptoms of panic attacks in some cultures, while difficulty breathing may be the primary symptom in other cultures'. In Japanese culture, 'social anxiety' is described not as a worry that I might not fit into a social group, or that I fear meeting people, but rather, the concern that I might unintentionally upset somebody else. Manners are balanced on the knife-edge of anxiety. The assumption is that there is an underlying condition – such as anxiety – that affords a range of differing cultural expressions. Fine, but does anxiety itself not have an underlying cause? Is there, for example, a common neurological or physiological cause for anxiety, or is such physiology (for example, a fight-flight reaction of the sympathetic nervous system in which adrenaline levels are raised) the correlate of anxiety?

As we think this way, we find ourselves thinking in circles. Surely the particular cultural 'cause' of anxiety – personal embarrassment in one culture, fear of offending others in another culture (the distinction between such 'guilt' and 'honour-shame' cultures, respectively, was drawn in 1940 by the American anthropologist Ruth Benedict) – is the idiosyncratic cultural expression? Such a view, notes Angel Martinez-Hernaez (2013), is to turn a biomedical theory of stress into an ethnographic object, or cultural metaphor. If this is the case, while 'anxiety' is patently deeply felt and real, it is also an embodied metaphor. A good metaphor is felt somatically and emotionally, as we have seen – my earlier example was 'peeing through ground glass' or 'peeing fire' as analogies for the first urinations after a trans-urethral resection of the prostate (TURP). Could all psychological symptoms – anxiety, depression, phobias – be thought of as embodied metaphors? This is not to devalue the symptom – the knee jerk reaction (a fine embodied metaphor) that a metaphor is not 'true' and therefore not worthwhile – but to better understand it.

While, to a psychiatrist, the outward sign of a mental illness (for example, the patient is experiencing tangible delusions) points to a universal condition (possibly schizo-affective disorder), what the patient experiences is a highly contextualized set of symptoms. For example, as noted earlier, 'Things like ants keep on creeping in various parts of my brain', an Igbo (Nigerian African) 'idiom of distress for the somatic manifestations of a mental disorder' (Martinez-Hernaez 2013, p. 1021), is, in other words, a cultural metaphor.

The use of metaphors in psychiatrist–patient communication

Steslow (2010), amongst others, points to the disparities in style and power between the voices of (i) the psychiatric establishment backed by 'Big Pharma', (ii) commentators on mental illness (for example, patients such as Arnhild Lauveng who have 'recovered' and offer articulate accounts of their symptoms, or creative writers/novelists commenting on mental illness 'prescription culture' (Bleakley and Jolly 2012)) and (iii) the general public, as patients or clients, who consume psychiatry and psychotherapy but whose voices are generally peripheral to debate. Patients, of course, find voices in support and pressure groups, such as 'Relate', and in the increasingly powerful phenomenon of posting videos online (YouTube) or comments on social media. The voices of the previously disenfranchised are also represented on television medi-soaps that articulate common mental health issues and provide helpline support.

In the context of this book, crudely, the psychiatric-pharmaceutical industry avoids metaphor for scientific account and plain description (EMP); the artistic communities' representations of mental illness and the psychiatric establishment are largely metaphor based; while the largely disenfranchised public appear clumsy with metaphor, framing their experiences in metaphorical terms, but not consciously, critically or reflexively.

There is certainly a disjunction between psychiatrists' and patients' uses of metaphor that may be readily bridged. Lorna Rhodes (1984) discusses the use of metaphor (such as 'this will clear your mind') for medication, particularly anti-psychotic drugs, in psychiatric settings. Drugs are not passive but active agents in transformations of identity and personality, behaviour and experience. They are artefacts – agents or technological 'actors' networking with persons and concepts. Where patients describe their effects metaphorically, psychiatrists might resort to biochemical descriptions. However, close listening to the metaphors that are used by patients may help psychiatrists in their work.

Rhodes argues that patients do not necessarily engage in cause-and-effect talk about medications, but rather, how medications allow them to take a stance towards their illness or think otherwise about symptoms. This may be expressed as both metaphor (enhanced meaning) and persuasion (rhetoric): 'This stuff fogs my mind, I don't need it all the time.' This may lead to an equally metaphorical and rhetorical response from the psychiatrist, in offering an alternative medication: 'This will clear your mind.' A common metaphorical ground, or agreement, between patient and psychiatrist is that something is contaminating, taking over, smudging or controlling the patient, and the psychiatrist argues that the medication will clear, relieve, dissolve, absorb or displace this irritant, providing some clarity. Do pharmaceuticals cure 'unhelpful', even 'bad', metaphors?

The issue about the relationship between patients' and psychiatrists' language is largely one of power rather than creating mutual understandings. Psychiatrists use language assuming epistemic supremacy, while patients need ontological (meaning) and axiological (values) orientations to their conversations. The patient fails to speak with authority if she resorts to metaphor, whereas the psychiatrist claims authority through EMP – but the language is stilted, even mute. Patients offer – albeit partial and incomplete – narratives, while psychiatrists again employ the rhetoric of DSM-based diagnostic classifications. The patient's narrative is the jumble at the back of the shop of idiosyncratic examples, the doctor's formulaic response the neatly stacked shelves at the front whose stock is based on market research.

Rather than proving a hindrance to a supposedly objective, scientific and reifying psychiatry, metaphors can offer a powerful therapeutic possibility (Wirtztum *et al.* 1988), especially at the level of the 'extended metaphor' that is the story. Metaphors offer specific therapeutic leads: one depressed patient says 'I'm down in the dumps', whereas another says 'I can't see a way out' and a third, as reported earlier, 'my head's in a vice'. The metaphors invite differing therapeutic responses.

An online account tells a story of psychiatric institutionalization and treatment as one in which the patient's metaphors were viewed as illegitimate and she had to learn to engage with the standard metaphors of the psychiatric establishment (www.medscape.com/viewarticle/726590_2).

Does psychiatry actually have a relatively impoverished metaphorical language?

In an Italian study, Alfonso Santarpia and colleagues (Santarpia *et al.* 2010) have written on metaphorical conceptualizations of the body through a corpus analysis of texts from psychiatry, psychotherapy and literature. Their study suggests that the landscape of modern psychiatry is shaped by an overriding didactic metaphor, 'The Body as Container', in which psychiatry textbooks utilize weak or 'fuzzy' metaphors of the body such as 'anorexics want a subtle body without flesh', whereas Italian poetry through the ages draws on highly specific or strong body references, for example zoning in on one organ, such as 'Whose heart burned' and 'a heart of marble' (Petrarca in Santarpia *et al.* 2010). We have seen that 'body as container' is one of the small group of primary metaphor complexes that structure cognition, according to Lakoff and Johnson (1980).

The body as container reinforces the point I made earlier concerning the historical shift from ancient Greek views of the body as porous and subject to attack from external forces such as gods or natural forces (Padel 1992) to the modern view of experience and symptoms as events within the container of the body. Psychiatry has been instrumental in promoting this view when it follows reductionist arguments seeking the origins of symptoms in brain mechanisms. The didactic metaphor then shapes the medical culture. Culture and metaphor are co-conspirators in shaping 'taken-for-granted' worldviews such as an internalized personal identity that is 'owned' as given. However, 'ownership' of identity can be located in trends of modernism, Protestantism and capitalism, and is held in a web of metaphors such as 'don't invade my personal space' (where the martial and individualism meet). Such views themselves might be seen as 'mad' in collectivist cultures.

Perhaps only an Italian study could ask the important question concerning the value of metaphor: 'Can these two worlds of psychiatry and poetry inform each other?' Might there be a metaphorical cluster other than a fuzzy and abstract notion of the 'body as container' that shapes the world of psychiatry quite differently, indeed, explicitly in a poetic rather than a conceptual way? Through a corpus analysis of psychiatric manuals, the body is, again, considered in terms of a didactic metaphor – 'Body Container' – with a great many non-specific attributes. In contrast, a sample of Italian poetry from Dante (fourteenth century) to Pasolini (twentieth century) talks of the body in specific organ terms such as heart, blood, flesh and head. But these organs do not signify separate body systems, or present as imprisoned specimens in jars. Rather, they poetically inflect the psychology and affect of the whole person.

Importantly, both patients and psychiatrists were found to describe symptoms through organ metaphors. A patient with panic attacks says, predictably, 'my heart was racing'. A patient with agoraphobia describes her symptoms more poetically: 'my chest feels as if it was enveloped in a light sheet that protects me from an attack of invaders'. Note that the symptom's origin is in the world, not in the person. The organ provides a landing site or dwelling place for the feeling. Again, for the ancient Greeks (captured particularly in Homer), this is a visitation from a god – but that does not constitute 'madness'. A patient with an eating disorder says, simply, 'My body is empty.' Other common metaphors include, again, 'my head's in a vice', and, more striking, 'my body has disappeared'. In turn, psychiatrists using therapeutic techniques such as guided imagery or Ericksonian relaxation commonly use phrases such as 'imagine your body is melting'.

The authors of the Italian study draw on Ritchie's (2003) Context-Limited Simulation Theory of metaphor. This suggests that metaphors are always generated according to context or a 'field of meaning', so that they are both culturally specific and associated with an idiosyncratic personal history. Primary and secondary perceptual stimulators form 'custom-made' metaphors for an occasion such as a conversation, a therapeutic episode or a memory recall – 'It was like a shark attack, sudden and vicious' (primary metaphor/simile and perceptual stimulator), followed by 'It was like being caught in a scene from *Jaws*' (secondary metaphor/simile and perceptual stimulator).

The body is, then, constructed as a series of abstractions or metaphorical representations that invoke associated feelings – terror, coldness, abject misery, desire and so forth. Following the rule of metaphor, 'ordinary' experiences are transported into the extraordinary, imaginative and unexpected in a shift of ground, like the artist's brushstrokes invoking far more than marks on a canvas. At the same time, it is common for hackneyed or tired metaphors to be employed (again, 'my head's in a vice', 'my heart was racing').

While psychiatric consultations generate a range of such metaphorical and 'fuzzy' body references, the corpus analysis of psychiatric textbooks revealed remarkable consistency in describing the body as 'container'. The authors draw on six Italian psychiatry textbooks and also on the entire DSM-IV for the corpus analysis. While the '*body as container*' represents the superordinate category (in which there is a sense of containment or suffocation), there are subordinate metaphor categories within this:

- The body is a covering – protection, safety, filter, containment or constraint with the possibility of some free movement.
- The body is a building – protection, safety, housing things.

Typically, metaphors here refer to 'losing myself in my body', to inside/outside, closed/open and over/under.

Other superordinate categories revealed by the corpus analysis are:

- *Body-substance*, with subordinate categories:
  - The body as an object (loss of subjectivity, depersonalization).
  - The body as a natural element (water, fire, air, earth).

o   The body as an instrument or tool (lack of leverage: in relationships, 'I find it hard to pick up somebody').

• *Body-divine*

o   The body as divine – from a psychiatry textbook: 'anorexics want a subtle body without flesh'.
o   The body as supernatural.
o   The body as a sacred object.

• *Body abstract*

o   From a psychiatry textbook: 'Every part of the body can become an erogenous zone' is an abstraction. What does this mean in concrete terms?

In contrast to the corpus analysis of psychiatry texts such as DSM, the corpus analysis of poetry texts revealed the use of the following metaphors:

• Body-organism

o   Body as an animal – cat-like, predatorial
o   Body as a plant – vegetating, blossoming

• *Body synaesthesia:* the body as a field of meaning, or mixed sensations.
• *Body metamorphosis:* the body changes and adapts.

The striking finding of the study was that psychiatry – apart from psychoanalytic approaches – utilized metaphors that were abstract and did not relate to specific body parts (psychoanalytic approaches did, as expected, refer to the genitals and the anus and mouth – as genital, anal and oral stages of development). Perhaps, in expunging psychodynamic approaches from psychiatry by privileging short-term, functional approaches such as cognitive-behavioural therapy (CBT), psychiatry has also lost its metaphorical range and compass. In short, metaphors referred to non-specific attributes, dissolving the concrete for concept. In contrast, poetry specifically referred to blood, chest, arms, eyes, breasts, face, head, heart, skin, hands and flesh, curiously absent from the corpus of psychiatry textbooks. But again, these bodily sites were dwelling places for experiences, emotional shifts, insights, pleasures and pains.

The authors imply that psychiatric metaphorical language is anaemic and lacking and could learn from the more concrete focus of poetry as a 'Literary Construction of the Body', where 'poetic thought could serve as an important resource in the conceptualization of the body'. We might ask whether psychiatry is failing to learn from its more florid patients about the value of metaphor as a means of understanding the 'thinking otherwise' of such psychotic patients in particular. Taming the language and thought processes of such patients by adapting them to a chronically anaemic psychiatric language may not be as productive as entering the lion's den of the patient's language and trying to understand his or her thought processes from within, where 'sitting down to a Chinese meal' may be exactly what it says.

This recognizes that the use of metaphor is particularly complex with psychotic patients, primarily because part of their symptom complex is the inability to see the difference between reality and a metaphorical state, so that (paradoxically) florid language is used literally. When a psychotic person says 'somebody is poisoning me', she is experiencing the metaphor literally and concretely. Rather than shifting to the conceptual and classificatory (DSM) language of 'paranoid delusion', the psychiatrist might engage with the patient's metaphor through specifics: 'is there a bitterness in the poison?'

Didactic metaphors in psychiatry

In previous chapters, we have seen how corpus research exposes typical metaphors used in a specialty. Overarching didactic metaphors – medicine as war or violence, the body as a machine, and the patient's account of illness as a journey – trump these. The public imagination rather than the medical landscape, according to Lakoff and Johnson (1980), is shaped by a number of metaphorical clusters commonly used in everyday life – for example, 'life is a journey' ('she seems to have lost her way'; 'I wish he could find a direction'; 'there's light at the end of the tunnel') and 'understanding is seizing' ('she's got a grip on the situation'; 'you must take the opportunity with both hands'; 'I don't know that you fully grasp the seriousness of the situation'). The 'body as container' has emerged from one piece of research as a didactic metaphor, as described above. Are there others in psychiatry?

My argument throughout this book is that where guiding, leading or dominant metaphors – 'didactic' – historically and culturally shape the landscape of medical cultures and its practices, this suggests that, reflexively, we might shift the metaphorical shaping of a cultural landscape. This, of course, is a shift in values, but it presents as a different use of language and performance, for example in consultations with patients, in talk with colleagues and in the ways academic articles and books are written.

Psychiatry, for example, can be seen to have chosen a language of scientific objectivity (over more poetic possibilities, discussed at length in Chapter 9) that distances patients and provides a rational defence against psychiatry itself being diagnosed as an irrational practice. But, again, say critics, this is plainly ideological; for example, it fails to distribute intellectual capital amongst stakeholders in psychiatric work, where psychiatrists retain such capital as a means of exercising power (Taussig 2001). Such scientific objectivity – reflected in the baroque edifice that is the DSM-V – suggests fairness across gender and ethnic mix in diagnosis and treatment, but this fails to address why certain ethnic groups consistently make up the majority of inmates in psychiatric institutions.

I have considered the multiple appearances of metaphors in medicine as this relates to treating symptoms of body and mind. In the following Chapter 8,

I follow the appearances of metaphors in medical education. From Abraham Flexner's influential shaping of medicine curricula and medical schools just over a century ago, to contemporary thinking about distributed cognition and reflexive practice, medical education theory and practice have been shaped by metaphor.

8 Metaphors in medical education

The pedagogic imagination

'Out, damned brain!': the embodiment of metaphor and metaphors of embodiment

Metaphors may cluster, for good reason. An ailing metaphor is attended to, treated or critically addressed by another metaphor. One metaphor becomes an educational lens through which we learn about another metaphor. The values and meanings of metaphors are best appreciated through metaphors themselves, as a layering. For example, brain anatomy ('locations' and 'architecture') and functioning (neuronal 'pathways' and 'firing') might be described in exquisite material detail drawing on metaphors, but we resort to another layer of metaphor when it comes to translating the 'firing' of neuronal networks into explorations of consciousness (Valle and von Eckartsberg 1981), affording experiences such as falling in love, irrational hatreds and fears, and the sublime and terrible ('The miserable have no other medicine,/But only hope' – Shakespeare's *Measure for Measure*, Act III, Sc. I).

Metaphors and similes appear to 'work' because they transpose from a conceptual state to a physical state, or embody a thought. That metaphors afford tangibility is a basic tenet of Lakoff and Johnson's (1980) groundbreaking work – thus, 'as right as rain', 'dig where you stand', 'the sky's the limit' and 'smooth as silk'. This is positive reification or embodiment – the rain and the sky are ideas dressed up as things. As previously noted, Gaston Bachelard provides a masterful phenomenology of such substantial poetic metaphors through his books on the four elements: *The Psychoanalysis of Fire* (1977), *Air and Dreams* (1988), *The Flame of a Candle* (1989), *The Poetics of Space* (1992), *Water and Dreams* (1994) and *Earth and Reveries of Will* (2002).

A poetic metaphor – such as Lady Macbeth's 'Out, damned spot!' – occupies three territories at once: the physical (compulsive wringing of the hands, pacing); the emotional (fear and loathing); and the cognitive (obsessive thoughts). The 'origins' of the metaphor can be sited in two places at once, like the simultaneous wave and particle forms of light – in the world (a socially responsive moral conscience) and in the stuff of the brain.

Functional magnetic resonance imaging (fMRI) allows us to see which parts of the brain control metaphor production and appreciation. Such mapping can be achieved also through studying persons with neurological deficits whereby metaphors cannot be recognized or formed. Metaphor production has been associated with focal activity mainly in left cortical hemisphere regions (the left angular gyrus, the left middle and superior frontal gyri, and the posterior cingulate cortex) (Benedek *et al.* 2014).

Such reduction of language effects to brain locations does not necessarily explain, but sites, metaphor production and use. To better appreciate the relationship between the levels of (i) brain 'architecture', (ii) cognitive 'maps' and 'strategies', and (iii) actual, situated social behaviour, we have to use a metaphor such as 'extended cognition' or 'the extended mind' (Clark and Chalmers 1998; Menary 2010). The thought experiment that underpins the extended cognition thesis is this: imagine a person who has Alzheimer's but is able to keep a diary in which all thoughts are recorded – would that diary not constitute an extension of cognition? Indeed, in the age of advanced computers and mobile phones and of pharmaceutical treatments (whether compensatory or enhancing), surely we cannot confine 'thinking' to what is inside the skull? Also, surely a shared language system that has evolved historically and culturally is not just inside the head but is 'in' social exchanges, activities, performances and non-verbal exchanges?

Metaphors are neither 'in' the brain nor 'in' the culture, but are the means by which we appreciate the relationship between mind and culture. Metaphors are connectors that 'mind the gap'. Again, while Lakoff and Johnson (1980) argue that container metaphors ('in and out of love', 'thinking outside the box', 'she led a sheltered existence', 'it's well within his reach') are one of our most commonly used metaphor clusters, the point of a 'container' metaphor is that it breaks free of containment. Being 'in' love captures the sense of total, exquisite entrapment. 'Out of my head' is the banner metaphor for extended cognition. Inspiration and expiration are first breathing, and second, life and death – 'she was totally inspired', 'he just expired'.

An example of inhabiting both mind and culture simultaneously is provided by Shakespeare and is called by psychologists the 'Lady Macbeth Effect' (Risen 2006). This is again a metaphor employed to explore another metaphor, or metaphor layering. In Shakespeare's *Macbeth*, the guilt-ridden Lady Macbeth tries to clear her conscience through symbolic handwashing – as compulsive handwringing – while sleepwalking: 'A little water clears us of this deed', 'All the perfumes of Arabia will not sweeten this little hand' and the better known 'Out, damned spot!' Those who study metaphor and the brain have asked: 'Are moral purity and physical cleanliness linked?' In the Lady Macbeth Effect, moral and bodily purification converge. Cognition is, indeed, embodied and extended – the gloopy mind does spill over.

In a creatively designed research study, Zhong and Liljenquist (2006) asked participants to recall an ethical or unethical act and then to fill in missing letters of incomplete words such as SH_ _ *ER and W_* _H. Subjects who had recalled ethical acts filled in words such as SHAKER and WISH, while those who recalled unethical acts mainly filled in SHOWER and WASH. In another test, subjects recalling an ethical or unethical act were offered a choice of objects – an antiseptic wipe or a pencil. Three-quarters of those who recalled an unethical act chose antiseptic wipes, while two-thirds of those recalling an ethical act chose a pencil. A third task was to recall an ethical or unethical act and then describe it on a computer. The researchers told the participants that the keyboard was dirty and gave them the opportunity to wash their hands.

They then asked all subjects whether they would help out a researcher who was desperate for volunteers for a study but could not pay them. Those who had washed their hands were 50 per cent less likely to volunteer for this fictional study, suggesting that as they were newly cleansed, they had absolved themselves, and felt less guilty about not participating for the needy researcher. In a further study, Zhong and Liljenquist (2006) found that participants who hand-copied a story about an unethical act subsequently were more likely to rate cleaning products as very desirable in relation to a control group. From the results of these studies, it would appear that physical cleanliness is related to moral purity. The embodiment of metaphor is laid bare.

Innovative researchers have been keen to replicate the Macbeth Effect in differing fields of inquiry. Gollwitzer and Meltzer (2012), for example, showed that novice video game players playing a violent game showed a strong preference for hygiene gift products in comparison with other gifts when prompted to make a choice between options after playing the game. In comparison with experienced gamers, who had developed ways of rationalizing the unethical violent content of some video games, novice gamers reported distress after playing such violent games. Cleansing products symbolically attend to the 'damned spot!' Subsequent attempts to replicate Zhong and Liljenquist's studies have proved to be difficult, however. One objection was that these researchers used relatively small groups of participants. Using much larger groups, Earp and colleagues (Earp *et al.* 2014) from Oxford University failed to replicate Zhong and Liljenquist's second study, finding no evidence of a Macbeth Effect. Further replication of the study seemed to be needed.

Schaefer and colleagues (Schaefer *et al.* 2015) reopened debate about the Macbeth Effect by suggesting that the social phenomenon can be mapped topographically onto the somatosensory cortex – or, there is an embodied metaphor effect at work. This study tested the theory of embodied cognition's suggestion that knowledge is represented in modal brain systems derived from perception – just as the Macbeth Effect suggests, where physical cleansing and moral purity converge. In other words, metaphors have meaning at the historical, cultural, social, behavioural, cognitive, anatomical, physiological and biochemical levels, again as layered effects. The researchers asked participants to enact scenarios where they had to perform moral or immoral acts with the mouth or the hand. After lying in a voice mail (the immoral mouth), participants showed strong preference for mouth wash; and after writing a lie (the immoral hand), strong preference was shown for hand wash products. fMRI results indicated activation in those parts of the sensorimotor cortices (mouth or hand areas) that mirrored the immoral activity. The authors conclude: '[T]he involvement of the sensorimotor cortex for the embodied metaphor of moral-purity is somatotopically organized.'

Movement from the study of metaphor in historical, cultural and social contexts to cortical mapping of metaphor production and use is itself governed by dominant or didactic metaphors leading us to feel a mixture of ease and discomfort with the Cartesian mind–body split. Ease, because all activity and experience has a neurological basis. Discomfort, because we know that this is a reductionist view that does not engage with the fact that ours is the age of cognitive extension beyond writing and language use to computer-assisted and extended activity. 'Hard wired' is an inappropriate metaphor for brain activity, which is all 'software', but a good description of extended cognition in our reliance upon artefacts, especially computers and mobile phones, in a world often described as 'bioinformational', where biology and engineering are bedfellows.

The English language, according to Lakoff and Johnson (1980), utilizes a restricted and readily mapped number of core 'metaphors we live by', as noted earlier with reference to 'container' metaphors. These include space and place metaphors, such as location ('I feel down today so I may take some uppers'), that include containment (inside/outside/contained/loose). Where such containment metaphors are dominant in the culture, in science and in medicine, then we think of brains in heads, of minds in bodies, and of bodies separated from other bodies in space. Again, this is what we commonly refer to as Cartesian dualism and Protestant-capitalist individualism. What, however, if these dominant spatial metaphors were replaced by those of motion or process? What if minds were loosed and bodies (as they technically are) seen as 'open systems'? Here is a multiple shift: from the linear to the complex, and from the 'closed' (a functioning boiler) to the 'open' system (a body, a weather system). The body as open system has an element of unpredictability, described by Deleuze and Guattari (1988a, 1988b) through the metaphor 'lines of flight': 'one day, he woke up and realized that his life was in tatters'.

Such an awakening might make you nearly jump out of your skin. Where discrete bodies are defined by the body's biggest organ, the skin, the body is imagined as a sac containing discrete organs such as the liver, heart, lungs and so forth. The body's system is reduced to a closed one, an engineering problem – a boiler with a thermostat and feedback system. This discrete organ system has become a metaphor for a traditional medicine curriculum, guided by topic-based content arranged as a body-organ-system and based on anatomy as a foundation. The curriculum is hardly precision engineered, but it is designed, and can be fine-tuned through feedback. This content bias ('topics') may be extended somewhat to process ('themes'), to include physiology and biochemistry, where the curriculum is now segmented into the pulmonary-vascular system, the autonomic-and-central-nervous system, and so forth.

What, however, are the implications for a medicine curriculum in which the 'open' system of the body (a dynamic, adaptive, complex system subject to entropy and at maximum complexity at the edge of chaos – hence its predictable tipping into physical symptoms and psychological distress) is tied to the 'open' system of the body's environment, and metaphors are used such as 'extended' cognition (examples of 'lines of flight') and the 'bioinformational post-human' (indicating a human augmented and supplemented by technologies)? What might an open (dynamic, adaptive, complex) curriculum look like? And what metaphors shape such curricula and pedagogies involved in 'delivering' curricula? Indeed, why should a curriculum be 'delivered' at all, implying an efficient and guaranteed parcel service to your front door?

The postman always rings twice: metaphor and medical education

Forgive my rhetoric – I persuaded you into stereotyping medical education with my insistence above that 'delivery' can be likened to a postal delivery. This conjures up a mechanical, teacher-led, information-packaged view of education, better described as 'training'. (I recoil from describing medical education as 'training' or reducing such education to 'competences' and 'skills'. Medical education is much more complex than this. Training also makes me think of instructors and 'trainers', an unfortunate metonymic link, as 'trainers' further make me think of running shoes, so that medical education is now best described through metonyms of track and field competition!)

Returning to the postman's delivery, 'delivery' can mean a birth, and also the style or manner in which something is done, from a formal speech to a bowler's delivery in cricket (for example, with speed and accuracy, venom and rise, or spin and disguise). Medical education is not simply the process of transmission of knowledge and skills, but rather, the creative interpretation of curriculum content and process. This creative element is largely achieved through metaphor comprehension and production within areas of ambiguity such as values conflict and novelty. There are too many compulsive handwringers in medical education, trying to design spotless curricula. This is education by strangulation. The curriculum must breathe and have elements of liquidity: preparing medical students for work has a bottom line – education for tolerance of ambiguity (Bleakley *et al.* 2011).

Getting comfortable with the white space

Again, the single most important trait of a good doctor – in diagnostics, team-based treatment and patient-centred care – may be tolerance of ambiguity. While this trait has been reified in both sociology (adapting to the 'risk society') and psychology ('anti-authoritarianism'), and then opened to measurement (tolerance of ambiguity questionnaire scales) (Furnham and Ribchester 1995; Furnham and Marks 2013), it can be read as a metaphor: or, indeed, as a metaphor for metaphor itself, where metaphor use and appreciation invites tolerance of ambiguity. 'Metaphor making', suggests Cone (2013), is a way of educating for tolerance of ambiguity.

Many people find Minimalist art (especially conceptual art) discomfiting, even stupid or pointless. Minimalism refers to stripping down an object so that it has no reference point but its own matter and positioning in space (usually a 'white cube' gallery space). Conceptual art refers to the 'display' of an idea – such as a light bulb going on and off in an empty room (clearly, a great metaphor for 'ideas' themselves). Minimalism is based not just on instrumentally stripping things down to 'dry essences', but on conceptually facing people with dilemmas and contradictions. Cone (2013) describes this as 'getting comfortable with the white space'.

Let us remind ourselves that, according to Michel Foucault's (1976) *The Birth of the Clinic*, it was medicine and not Modernist art that invented the purifying white space as the 'clinic'. This is echoed in the white cube of the art gallery and Le Corbusier's architecture – the dwelling as a cube painted white, whose interior is saturated in natural light, and which is raised off the ground to avoid muddying and pollution of the whiteness. The clinic is the antiseptic white space (a metaphor: unblemished, signifying purity) within the larger clinic of the hospital that legitimizes otherwise invasive intimate examinations, especially by male doctors with female patients.

Doctors once visited patients in the privacy of the patient's home with the family gathered. This customarily inhibits intimate examination and reduces doctors' power. Foucault argues that the clinic, the doctor's own space, affords power and authority and legitimizes professional intimacies. The subsequent white coat is the embodied metaphor of purity, power and professionalism. Ironic, then, that the doctor's white coat has long since been abandoned in the UK (as a potential source of infection) – where the milk-white coat has turned sour. The clinic, too, is where the sharp end of medical education occurs, as work-based experience. And here, the hierarchies and power structures are most apparent. In the UK, white doctors, too, are three times more likely to be picked for senior posts than those from ethnic minority groups (Cooper 2013).

The clinical white space is echoed in the laboratory, outwardly a place of control but actually a place of messy experimentation. As noted previously, Mangione (2012, p. 546) describes the rise of scientific medicine and its divorce from the arts and humanities as a product of the shift in influence from French to German medicine in the 1870s, when the outcome of the Franco-Prussian War 'shifted the axis from Paris to Berlin, and medicine went the German way'. Where the French way privileged the bedside, the German way privileged the laboratory. Medical education was stripped of its interest in a liberal education, so that the early socialization (and consequent identity construction) of doctors was shaped as anatomists and bench scientists. As noted previously, this was largely due to the influence of Abraham Flexner, the son of German immigrants to the USA, whose 1910 report on medical education shaped the next century of medical practice (Flexner 1910; Cooke *et al.* 2010; Nevins 2010; Bleakley *et al.* 2011). Mangione (ibid.) further notes that use of the arts and humanities in medical education 'may increase our tolerance of ambiguity, a trait sorely lacking in modern medicine'.

Erotic faculties and thinking with mother's milk

I discuss at length in Chapter 4 how the landscape of medicine is shaped histori-cally by dominant or didactic metaphors that are masculine in tone – collec-tively, an industrial–military complex of machine and violence metaphors grounded in the archetype of the hero. Abraham Flexner's 'quality' reforms of medical schools in the wake of his 1910 report led to the closure of poorly resourced schools – the very schools that gave women and black minority stu-dents an opportunity to study medicine (Hodges 2005). Flexner turned medicine into a white, male establishment. This was a kind of violence.

In the context of end-of-life or palliative care, the work of the 'Metaphor in End-of-Life Care' (MELC) group (Demmen *et al.* 2015; Semino *et al.* 2015; Demjen *et al.* 2016; Potts and Semino 2017) offers empirical evidence that health professionals and patients use violence metaphors that are sometimes mis-placed. Paradoxically, persons who are dying may use such metaphors more fre-quently than the healthcare professionals and carers who are caring for them, but this may be a contamination effect in which patients use metaphors borrowed from medicine in an unreflective way. The outcomes of this research study also suggest that 'journey' metaphors are a common alternative to violence meta-phors in end-of-life care. This is echoed in healthcare's increasing use of the metaphor of 'pathway' for integrated, team-based and patient-centred care.

Recording frequencies of use of metaphors from corpus analysis of, say, online forums does carry the danger that we do not get at the contextual nuances of the uses and impact of metaphors. For example, habitual or casual use of a violence metaphor does not necessarily correlate with a person's, or a discourse community's, investment in the power and meaning of that metaphor. On the other hand, habitual use of metaphors should also ring alarm bells, as stubborn, negative or unproductive practices may be shaped by such metaphors, now tech-nically 'dead' or overused. The MELC study does include qualitative inquiry that can get closer to the meanings invested in contextual use of metaphors, such as violence or journey metaphors within discourse communities and across genres (such as speech and online postings), and this data suggests that we cannot make blanket judgements about the uses and meanings of violence meta-phors. First, such metaphors have multiple expressions – from subtle control to outright warfare and battle; and second, they are contextually sensitive, changing meaning and value according to context.

In spite of these two conditions, what might it mean to shift wholesale from a leading or dominant archetypal masculine metaphor complex to a more feminine complex, for example? This is a question my colleagues and I have posed and addressed in previous medical education texts (Bleakley *et al.* 2011; Bleakley 2014, 2015). In order to provoke thinking about the complexity of this problem, let us consider the challenge to dominant masculine metaphors put forward by recent French poststructuralist feminist thinkers, represented by Luce Irigaray (2004) and Hélène Cixous (1991), amongst others. Irigaray is more of a separa-tist feminist than Cixous and bases her feminist metaphors (how to think, or epistemology; how to be, or ontology; and what to value, or axiology) on the woman's body – a position that has been challenged by the emergent transgender movement. Irigaray characterizes a feminist education (how to think ideas and how to form a just society) as challenging the patriarchy in terms of an historical notion of 'loss' based on the genitals. Freud famously characterized women as a 'puzzle' and a 'problem' in terms of the castrated male or lack of the phallus. Irigaray and other feminists turn the tables on this position, first bodily and second linguistically (and both metaphorically).

For Irigaray, the man is lacking what the labia offer, characterized as the constant conversational 'meeting' of the labia, as 'two lips', to speak a fluid, moist, erotic language. The transgender movement challenges this as old-style essentialism, but the 'erotic' can be taken as a guiding metaphor. Joanna Frueh's (1996) *Erotic Faculties* is one of the few contemporary texts – albeit grounded in, and referenced to, radical performance art – that explicitly aim to celebrate eros in pedagogy and the Academy. In sections such as 'Fucking Around', Frueh asks why eroticism and the sensual body are treated as no go areas in pedagogy, and then closeted, rather than being exhibited as part of the learning process.

Hoping that the reader will take her seriously rather than literally, Frueh asks for the eroticization of the curriculum, not, for example, through acting out attractions, but through making pedagogic capital from such attractions. Positive transference might facilitate and inform the transfer of knowledge. Reading Frueh in this way, we can ask: how can medical education become thrilling, pleasurable and satisfying, even multiply orgasmic – based on women's potency? Can learning express generalized romantic aspirations and inspirations? Where is there expressive sensuality in the curriculum, and how might students come to love their learning, engaging more passionately with the curriculum? Can medical education, in Irigaray's term, speak a 'moist' language? What is an erotically charged curriculum that is free from inappropriate sexual content or innuendo, as 'acting out'?

A patriarchal language is characterized as dependent upon an hierarchical power structure expressed as phallic (stiff and unyielding) and through linguistic binaries, such as Male:Female, in which female/woman is the inferior term. This is continued as White:Black (racism and imperialism), Logical:Irrational, and so forth. Such a discourse is famously characterized as 'phallogocentrism' – the term was originally coined by Jacques Derrida – favouring masculinity and logos over femininity and eros; and the 'dry' Western canon of male authors over an alternative succulent and diverse, or 'multiply orgasmic', canon including women writers. Irigaray (2004) also calls for a shift in studies from single metaphors to 'metaphoric networks', especially through mobilizing more radical discourse communities of women and feminists.

Structuralism, with its search for a universal underlying law or logos to consciousness, draws on the masculine/logos oppositionalist model (e.g. Lévi-Strauss' one logic to all myth structures: the Raw vs. the Cooked or Nature vs. Culture). Poststructuralism critiques this view, suggesting that there is no oppositional model that structures language and thought; rather, we should celebrate multiple structures and metaphors. Hélène Cixous introduces the metaphor of 'writing with mother's milk' to characterize poststructuralist feminist thinking. Here, writing is nourishing or succouring, and 'invisible' or does not leave a trace, a metaphor for both a lightness of touch and a lack of the wish to inscribe self upon Other. Masculinist imperialism is characterized as heavy-handed and bent on inscription and ownership through self-serving capitalism and imperialism.

Three case studies

The relationship between metaphor and pedagogy in general is well researched, with a large critical literature. However, the uses and abuses of metaphors in medical education is a field that has not attracted much research and is ripe for development. A starting point for such research would be to consider the importance of analogical reasoning and the specific use of metaphors as vehicles for learning in undergraduate medicine in particular. The basic principle to be considered as an educational process is how one thing may be better appreciated, understood or applied in relation to another thing, or how thinking with metaphor may turn the ordinary into the extraordinary, and the merely 'additive' into the self-generating 'expansive'.

Following Lakoff and Johnson's (1980) influential model, we have seen how embodied metaphors are good to think with. One concept or conceptual cluster can be used to heighten the meaning of another concept or conceptual cluster to improve 'grasp' of knowledge. Through metaphor, the well-known distinction that Jerome Bruner makes between ways of acquiring learning – the enactive (doing), the iconic (images) and the symbolic (language) – can be collapsed and placed under the one heading of 'embodied metaphor'.

It is important to recognize that most medical education consists of *reproduction* of knowledge, skills and values (usually described by the metaphors of 'transmission' and 'training'). This is necessary to form a platform from which 'expansive' learning (Engeström 2008) may occur. Knowledge transmission must be eclipsed by innovation – the *production* of knowledge. This knowledge must then be disseminated – this is the issue of 'transfer' in learning as the expansion of a network. Such innovative expansion turns training into education. By 'knowledge' I mean conceptual capital, emotional capacity, activities (skills, performances), and values that are socially oriented and culturally contextual.

I will illustrate the use of metaphors in medical education through three contrasting examples. The first is based on an article by Fleming *et al.* (2012), entitled 'You Too Can Teach Clinical Reasoning!', outlining the pedagogical structures of an efficient clinical reasoning method in paediatrics. The authors never use the word 'metaphor' in the article, but metaphor is at the heart of the learning process they outline for diagnostic proficiency in paediatric medicine. I use it to illustrate how thinking with embodied metaphor can help medical educators to 'scaffold' the learning of medical students. Briefly, 'scaffolding' is a metaphor for extended cognition and for providing facilitation for learners so that they can move from one level of understanding and practice to a higher or more complex level without failure, aided by the stepwise help of a well-designed learning experience, expertly facilitated.

The second example is a brief analysis of an online text introducing brain synapses from a website – 'Neuroscience for kids' – that was, in the author's words, 'created for all students and teachers who would like to learn about the nervous system'. It is an example of the unreflexive use of metaphor in supposedly introducing 'objective' scientific facts to a largely raw audience. The third example is a largely unsuccessful, misguided or clumsy use of metaphor in attempting to teach medical students elements of pathology – more on this later.

1 Stepwise use of formal metaphors that structure clinical reasoning: 'semantic qualifiers' and 'illness scripts'

Semantic qualifiers and illness scripts are, it is claimed, 'in' the brain. Well, let us free these birds from their cages to carry out some 'in the wild' natural history observation, turning semantic qualifiers and illness scripts into living, embodied metaphors *in vivo*.

In my first example, taken from the medical education literature (Fleming *et al.* 2012), a teenager presenting with acute symptoms is turned into a 'patient' and further framed as a 'problem' to be solved. This is a rhetorical use of metaphor, arguing for efficiency in medical education. I object in principle to such objectification of persons, whereby medicine itself is reduced to 'treating the numbers' rather than encouraging sensitivity to the unique individual. However, as we shall see, such initial instrumentality can serve as a useful heuristic – a problem-solving short cut – in our illustrative example, where the patient is a 16-year-old boy with a history of two ear infections, presenting with three days of fever and abdominal pain, who registered a 10 out of 10 rating on a pain scale when admitted to hospital:

> The pain started as a dull ache in the peri-umbilical region, moving to the right lower quadrant ... [he] had one day of vomiting and two days of decreased food intake. A physical examination revealed abdominal tenderness, rebound tenderness, and guarding ... white blood cell count was 20,000.
>
> (Fleming *et al.* 2012, p. 795)

A narrative- and case-based approach – focusing on the teenager's 'chief concern' rather than medicine's interest in the 'chief complaint' – would enlarge upon this, taking a more detailed history that would almost certainly multiply up the metaphorical count. This approach would also take into account the teenager's distress, rather than putting this on the back burner or rationalizing it as part of the 'presenting symptoms' profile. Focusing on the 'numbers' (population- and evidence-based medicine) invites a Minimalist approach that articulates the 'problem' as one of semantic qualification. Semantic qualifiers are a shorthand way of representing the patient's narrative and capturing symptom presentations as a tight metaphorical group. First, the presenting symptoms can be written out as a series of one-line statements, and this, in turn, is reduced to a small number of semantic qualifiers, usually as metaphorical pairings such as 'acute–chronic'. This is a burning down to dry essences, a conscious process of reduction – not as a depersonalizing tactic but as a mnemonic for diagnostic reasoning.

Here is the restatement of the boy's presenting symptoms that form the semantic qualifiers:

- 'Two ear infections' becomes *otherwise well*
- 'Three days' becomes *acute*
- 'Decreased food intake' becomes *anorexia*

The key findings from the history, physical examination and laboratory tests are synthesized to form the most plausible (differential) diagnosis. The 'dry essences' are, in fact, metaphors. The boy is not anorectic – 'anorexia' serves as a memorable metaphor (also a semantic qualifier) for decreased food intake. 'Acute' serves as a memorable metaphor (and semantic qualifier) for 'just three days of symptoms'. These are metaphors, because one thing (just three days of symptoms) is substituted for another, more memorable and striking, descriptor ('acute'). Acute means intense, sharp, penetrating, severe and potentially dangerous. In medical terms, it means 'sudden onset'. Of course, like 'chronic' – from the Greek god *Chronos* or Time, meaning long period, and constant – acute has lost its metaphorical 'hit' through overuse. In medicine, it is an habitual or 'dead' metaphor. Rather, it is part of tacit knowing. The boy in question buckles under the actual, terrible, sharp, penetrating pain, while 'acute' is an embodied metaphor.

The 'dry essence' statement about the boy is then:

> an *otherwise well* 16-year-old *boy* who presents with *acute* onset of *fever, severe, focalized* abdominal *pain, vomiting* and *anorexia*. The physical examination and laboratories were significant for *right lower* quadrant pain, *guarding, rebound tenderness*, and an elevated white blood cell count. This patient's presentation is most consistent with acute appendicitis.
>
> (Fleming *et al.* 2012, p. 796)

The authors italicize the single keywords at the heart of the already reduced semantic qualifiers. Of the 11 keywords, five are metaphors in context or technical metaphors ('acute', 'severe', 'focalized', 'guarding', 'rebound tenderness'). 'Rebound tenderness' is a wonderful metaphor for unusual sensitivity to *removal* of touch or pressure (although it is not an entirely reliable palpation technique), and an illustrative example of a metaphor as activity. Its alternative name 'Blumberg's sign' – in memory of the German surgeon Jacob Mortiz Blumberg (1873–1955) who first developed the technique – is merely descriptive and honorific, an eponym.

As doctors gain expertise, they develop the ability to make clinical judgements from pattern recognition – again, termed Type 1 reasoning. Familiarity with symptom configuration ('I've seen hundreds of these'; or 'I saw this once before and will never forget it') allows snap judgements. This is discussed at length in Chapters 5 and 6. Prior to gaining expertise, students must use Type 2 or conscious, linear clinical reasoning, such as decision trees, whereby differential diagnoses patiently emerge from summing up the evidence of the presenting symptoms. Experts under conditions of uncertainty also revert to Type 2 reasoning. Pattern recognition may look like the 'blink of an eye judgement', but it requires mobilizing of an unconscious or tacit 'illness script' as a basis for making such a clinical decision.

Illness scripts are hypothesized (and hypostatized) cognitive maps that are clusters of facts based around remembering groups of patients presenting with certain symptoms. Such scripts contain little pathophysiological data, but lots of clinically relevant material. Once the 'chief complaint' is identified, the doctor searches unconsciously for recognition of an encoded illness script that matches the symptoms. 'Chief complaint' is a medically centred metaphor for symptom presentation and can be reconfigured as another metaphor, the patient's 'chief concern' (Schleifer and Vannatta 2013). Indeed, the potential mismatch between the metaphors of the chief complaint and the chief concern is a source of rhetorical conflict in the doctor–patient interaction. Further, the chief complaint is referred to as a 'pathophysiologic insult' – a metaphor for major or minor injury or infection (viral 'invasion' – another war metaphor, local inflammation, perforation and so forth).

Returning to the semantic qualifiers for our 16-year-old boy above, this list unfolds:

1   Acute abdominal pain.
2   Poor oral intake.
3   Pain began around umbilicus but has moved to the right lower quadrant.
4   Febrile to 39.4° centigrade.
5   Has associated nausea, vomiting and anorexia.

Thanks to the presence of tacit 'illness scripts', even by later years in medical school, a differential diagnosis of inflammatory bowel disease, acute gastroenteritis or appendicitis will normally have been readily reached by number 3 in the list above. A diagnosis of appendicitis will normally have been reached by number 4, thanks again to a unique tacit 'illness script'. An 'illness script', also known as 'encapsulated knowledge', is a metaphor for a cognitive event, where the tangible act of interacting with patients and clinical teachers shapes neuronal patterns within the jelly of the brain and its concealed electrochemical work.

2 *Jumping synapses and orgasms*

My second example of the use of metaphor in medical education enters that jelly of the brain with its tangle of neurons, to discuss learning about transmission of 'information' at the synapse. Such transmission is not caught by a 'pipe' conduit metaphor – such as the vascular system's 'pipework' that Lakoff and Johnson (1980) describe as a primary embodied metaphorical frame ('our idea has gone down the tube'), but, traditionally, by wiring metaphors: 'there's a blockage in the flow of information'. Neuronal networks, however, are not continuous, but have gaps (synapses) where one pathway ends and another begins. Further, transmission of nerve impulses is not an all-or-nothing process but depends upon the build-up of 'potential' until a critical point is reached and then firing occurs. This can be compared to an orgasm.

Here is part of an online description of 'the synapse' from the webpage 'Neuroscience for kids' (https://faculty.washington.edu/chudler/synapse.html) – I have highlighted metaphors in italic:

> axons take *information* away from the cell body. *Information ... flows ...* across a synapse.... For *communication* ... to occur, an electrical impulse must *travel down* an axon to the synaptic *terminal*.... When a neurotransmitter *binds* to a receptor ... it changes the postsynaptic cell's *excitability*: ... either more or less likely to *fire*.

Again, a metaphor allows us to understand one thing in terms of another. This bundle of metaphors (eight in 49 words) allows us to picture the workings at the synapse in terms of an 'information transmission' (or bioinformational) model conjuring up physical things like 'hot' electrical wiring, where, paradoxically, 'communication' that 'binds' is achieved through the 'flow' of information (*information travels down or flows in a fiery and excitable way that binds one thing to another as a message*). You get the picture – but in terms of the metaphors provided by the authors. This is, then, a rhetorical use of metaphor aimed at an audience ('Neuroscience for kids', where 'kids' is used tongue in cheek or metaphorically, meaning neuroscience for beginners). A neuroscience for adults might well have explained the incremental build-up – a balance between excitation and inhibition – prior to a synaptic firing, and then the firing itself, again in terms of an orgasm.

3 *Can sports metaphors help in teaching pathology to medical students?*

Kanthan and Mills (2006, no pagination) remind us that

> Although the use of metaphors, analogies, and similes is pervasive in our language, not much has been written about its use as a potential active teaching strategy in medical education to explain complex or abstract concepts.

The authors argue that metaphors, analogies and similes can be used as aids in teaching pathology to medical students. The first example above, of the use of semantic qualifiers and illness scripts, explores an established process of diagnostic reasoning. The second example uses well-worn expressions to conceptualize synapse functioning. This third example is different – it involves the production and employment of novel metaphors for complex curriculum content in pathology teaching. This content is perceived as difficult to teach when it comes straight out of the can and may be indigestible. Learning must be scaffolded in some way, and the authors chose 'sports metaphors' (the study is based in Canada, and the sports chosen are tennis, hockey and American football). The thinking behind the use of metaphors is sound, but the choice of metaphors proves to be rather mundane and does not fully capture the students' interest. The study reported limited success as a result.

Analogies were used across two consecutive years of an undergraduate pathology course for medical and dental students in Canada, first to facilitate understanding of complex concepts, including acute and chronic inflammation, infarction, thrombosis and embolism, and second, to offer students practice in communicating complex medical concepts. In particular, the authors hoped that visual metaphors would help in both of these areas, especially in recall of information. Metaphors did aid teaching and learning in a limited way, and helped students to learn how to better communicate with patients when discussing complex medical issues, but, again, the study fell short in terms of impact.

On the basis that one thing can be taught and learned in terms of another more familiar and perhaps more striking thing, the authors used sports analogies/metaphors to teach pathology. However, the design of the pedagogy always meant that students would not necessarily substitute an ordinary thing for something extraordinary, as an imaginative conceptual leap ('steel yourself'; 'what storms then shook the ocean of my sleep' – from Shelley's 'Epipsychidion'), but rather, substitute the ordinary (a sports strategy metaphor) for the extraordinary (the body in inflammation). This seems rather forced when medical concepts of exudation, transudation, oedema and pus were explored using game strategy plans. For example, inflammation was described in terms of where the sport was played and the make-up of teams (hardly a gripping notion), so that

> the vascularized connective tissue became the playing field; the teams were Team A (the circulating cells in vessels – neutrophils, eosiniphils, basophils, and platelets) and Team B (the connective tissue cells – mast cells, resident macrophages, and lymphocytes); and the extracellular matrix … became the 'reserves' on the 'bench'.

Further, the 'quick kill' of acute inflammation was likened to a 'blow out' (an easy or one-sided victory) in hockey or sport in general, while chronic inflammation was likened to 'repeated overtimes'. Chronic inflammations, such as persistent infections and autoimmune diseases, were also described as resembling a five sets tennis match with alternating deuce/match points, while acute inflammation was likened to winning in three straight sets. Thrombus/infarction was compared to the toilet getting blocked by a tennis ball caught in the S-bend. As the ball absorbs water, flushing becomes erratic. Eventually, the system breaks down with a messy, stinking flood. The fate of a thrombus offers possibilities from no effect, to intermittent blockage, to full-blown infarction with complete breakdown of normal structure and function.

Students were also asked to generate their own metaphors for acute inflammation. These included relationships and sex, and war, conflict and violence. Students also generated visual metaphors for thrombosis, embolism and infarction: these included gardening, plumbing and construction analogies. Students showed insight into how such metaphors might be used to succinctly explain what was perceived as difficult medical information to patients. The researchers and students noted that poor or ill-fitting metaphors (like some of the more forced sports metaphors) could disengage learners and produce misunderstanding.

High ground and swampy lowland

Many years ago, I ran a medical education course on which the majority of the participants were senior consultant doctors and surgeons. On the very first session, I introduced Donald Schön's (1983, 1990) model of reflective practice. Schön describes the technical-rational knowing and practice with large amounts of certainty as a 'high ground', and 'indeterminate zones of practice' that carry large amounts of uncertainty as 'the swampy lowlands'. The latter includes the unique, the unexpected and value conflicts – everyday concerns for doctors, as Schön himself points out. While the participants seemed to enjoy the session, the following week, I was met with several questions demanding clarification.

Many of the doctors, and especially the surgeons, were perplexed about the use of the metaphors 'high ground' and 'swampy lowlands'. They could not quite cope with the slippage between the conceptual and the tangible that is the hallmark of an embodied metaphor. I asked them to read an extract from the American surgeon and writer Richard Selzer's (1996) *Mortal Lessons: Notes on the Art of Surgery*, where I had highlighted this description:

> With trust the surgeon approaches the operating table.... With a blend of arrogance and innocence the surgeon makes his incision, expecting an organ to be exactly where he knows it to be.... But this morning, as the surgeon parts the edges of the wound with his retractor, he feels uncertain.... Blood is shed into the well of the wound. It puddles upon the banks of scar, concealing the way inward.... It is an alien land. Now all is forestial, swampy.

The 'high ground' and 'swampy lowland' are examples of the 'spatial' grouping of embodied metaphors described by Lakoff and Johnson (1980) such as 'up there', 'upbeat', and 'down here', 'down in the dumps'. The confusion rested with the link between these spatial metaphors and levels of uncertainty. These doctors and surgeons could not accept that they were dealing with high degrees of ambiguity in their work, or that tolerance of ambiguity was an essential value for that work and something that should be educated in medical students. Rather, they resisted and deflected this argument by refusing ambiguity, saying that their patients expected clear and concise diagnoses just as they sought such clarity themselves. They were shaped by the didactic metaphor of the doctor as heroic dragonslayer (medicine as war, doctors as warriors) 'saving' patients, and this put them in denial about the pervasive nature of uncertainty and ambiguity in their work. Such uncertainty was both the elephant in the consulting room and the skeleton in the mortuary cupboard – or, like medical slang, brushed under the carpet. Such institutional blinkering occluded an appreciation of the value of the newly introduced pedagogical metaphors of a technical-rational 'high ground' in conflict with a 'swampy lowland' of uncertain practice – again, the complex of values conflict, the unexpected and the unique.

From terra firma *to* terra incognita: *bread and butter content metaphors are displaced by a new breed of process metaphors*

As noted previously, Kathryn Montgomery Hunter (1997, p. 167) sees medical education through a series of 'alimentary metaphors', or learning as ingestion and digestion of facts. Here, 'students are spoonfed, forcefed; they cram, digest, and metabolize information; and they regurgitate it on tests'; however, this leaves them 'metaphorically starving'. Bleakley and Bligh (2006) use a food metaphor in describing the limitations of learning by simulation, where they see 'hungry learners' being fed 'menus' rather than food – learning by simulation becoming simulation of learning. Hunter playfully notes that medical teachers must not overcook their teaching, but maintain good taste – information must not be allowed to go stale, so you must 'periodically check that information for freshness'.

Medical education, however, has changed since Hunter's astute observation. Individuals are no longer force fed in order to go through bulimic cycles of regurgitation of facts. Learning and assessment in medical education are rapidly focusing on what medical students and junior doctors need to know to work well in interprofessional, team-based and patient-centred practice. Learning is not just about individuals accruing knowledge capital (much of which is archaic or surplus to practice concerns), but also about identity formation and legitimate entry into communities of practice. Learning is about social participation and collaboration.

This is a paradigm shift in medical education – away from reliance on individualistic to social learning theories (Bleakley 2014). This, again, can be seen as an important part of the shift from heroic, masculine, competitive medical culture to a more team-based, collaborative and feminine approach. This shift has spawned a number of key metaphors. The 'spiral curriculum', mentioned earlier, describes topics being revisited in greater depth throughout a course of study ('curriculum' itself is derived from the Latin *currere*, describing Roman chariot races around a 'course') (Pinar 1975).

'Scaffolding', also mentioned previously, describes helping learners by setting tasks that are just out of their reach, but providing the means by which they can be successful in the task. Jerome Bruner introduced the term 'scaffolding' in the 1960s, based on the Russian Lev Vygotsky's model of assisted learning. Vygotsky developed his theories of learning soon after the 1917 Russian Revolutions, and so it was not surprising that he used collectivist metaphors as rhetorical, even ideological, devices. Vygotsky described a 'zone of proximal development' (ZPD) as what a learner can achieve beyond current limits with assistance (again, emphasis on collective support).

Social learning theories (Bleakley 2014) such as Cultural-Historical Activity Theory (CHAT), Actor-Network Theory (ANT) and Communities of Practice (CoP), employ a number of neologisms that act as metaphors. CoP approaches describe 'legitimate' entry into a community of practice (such as medicine and then medical specialties) through an apprenticeship that invites knowledge of codes and an emergent identity. CHAT approaches describe developments in teamwork participation and understanding through 'teeming' (a pun as well as a metaphor) and 'knotworking' (an alternative to 'networking' in which health professionals come together temporarily for specified tasks, creating 'knots' that hold only as long as they need to and are then undone). 'Wildfire' activities describe the constant management of uncertainty in clinical practice, where spontaneous incidents flare up that have to be attended to as an emergency (Engeström 2008).

ANT (Latour 2010) describes how 'nets' can be made through 'work' ('worknets' rather than networks) in the process of translating practices, information and ideas that 'expand' a network rather than allow it to crystallize or collapse. While their component parts are tangible (people, artefacts), networks are often not visible per se; we can only get the 'trace' or 'smoking gun' – that is, whatever the networking achieves in the way of product.

Yrjö Engeström (2008) describes learning in terms of the metaphor of 'expansion' of 'activity systems'. An activity system 'expands' as its members innovate through collaborative learning. Much learning becomes tacit, especially in expertise (recall the use of 'illness scripts' in clinical judgement), and is held as a network that Engeström compares with mycorrhizae – underground fungi that are symbiotic with tree roots and grow over vast areas. Engeström (2009, 2010) suggests that education has outgrown the 'acquisition' metaphor to explore the 'participation' metaphor (Sfard 1998). This led to interest in 'communities of practice', referred to above. However, in CoP theory, the leading metaphor to describe communities of practice was 'binding' ('legitimate' entry; clear processes of socialization; bounded identity constructions).

Times have changed – for example, contemporary healthcare is characterized not by stable teams with centripetal characteristics, but by ad hoc, fluid teams with centrifugal characteristics, loosening rather than binding, while still maintaining a sense of collectivity such as a common goal, or respecting other colleagues. 'Liquidity' is a chief metaphor to describe this postmodern landscape (Bauman 2000). In terms of Sfard's distinction between acquisition and participation metaphors for learning, Engeström says we must move beyond 'participation' to be more specific about kinds of participation. 'Binding' participation is not a helpful metaphor in a world of shifting grounds (helpfully returning us to swampy lowlands of practice).

The shift from bounded to fluid teams needs new descriptive and explanatory metaphors. Centrifugality chimes with the 'expansive' activity systems noted above. Rather than tighten associations through centripetal activities such as 'team identification', networking and translucency, new, looser and more dynamic healthcare teams attract metaphors of centrifugality such as 'negotiated knotworking', deliberate transparency and 'whistleblowing'. These are looser, more ethically conscious, deliberate attempts at widening participation and inclusivity rather than the exclusivity shown by traditional 'tight' teams. Negotiated knotworking invites loose but attentive associations and temporary bonds. Meanwhile, the curriculum, through time, spirals and frays.

How, then, is a sense of 'binding' nevertheless achieved in these new clinical work structures? Crises or emergencies necessarily produce 'amoeba-like' 'wildfire activities' involving 'runaway objects' (such as protocols so heavily adapted for context that they are unrecognizable), where cogency is key because people have clear roles (such as a resuscitation team). Co-ordination of such teams is not achieved through old-style hierarchy and authority power structures, but through negotiation. Power is distributed through recognized expertise or ability to innovate, so that these new order team members learn what Engeström calls 'swarming' and 'multi-directional pulsating' – metaphors of engagement and collaboration based on shared ethical concerns and mutuality.

The 'patient' was once fixed in a bed on a ward as a stable object for treatment. As patient-centredness developed, the patient became problematic as his or her status changed, and so multiple 'pathways' of care were developed to tether the patient, or keep him or her visible. The patient is also what Engeström (2009) calls a 'runaway object' – hard to pin down (like a displayed specimen) other than through objectification, treated in multiple spaces across multiple, fluid teams (for example, seeing a different doctor on each visit to a general practice surgery).

Engeström's key metaphor in describing this new era of clinical teamwork is, then, the 'horizontal' over the 'vertical'. The vertical, with its metaphor of the tree, symbolizes tight hierarchies and centripetal activity around a stable trunk of practice, knowing and values. The embodied metaphor that Engeström chooses to best describe horizontal, democratic associations is 'mycorrhizae-like' activities. Mycorrhizae are symbiotic associations between fungi and the roots or rhizoids of a plant. Growing centrifugally, the fungal underground web can cover a massive area, and many plants depend upon such a web to receive adequate nutrients and water. In return, the plant feeds sugars back to the fungi. Such fungal webs reproduce through their visible structures – mushrooms. This is another often-used metaphor to describe the development of ideas, associations and practices ('the team's practice ability just mushroomed'). Mycorrhizal structures are not 'tight' like nets, but invite loose associations through knotworking. Although this brings vulnerability, it also brings flexibility. Cussins

(1992) describes a similar metaphor in the theory of 'cognitive trails', and Knorr-Cetina (2003) in the paradoxical term 'flow architecture'.

These are, then, metaphors with which to think a new, more open and fluid clinical teamwork practice in which collective improvisation is key – a model for which is the communication between members of a jazz group (Haidet 2007). The group needs some vertical structure (collective statement of theme or melody, chorus), but is largely characterized by improvised solos (although these, too, will have some vertical backbone, such as chord progressions). 'Expansive swarming engagement' and 'multi-directional pulsation' are star-like patterns of activity around the patient, or around a central model of care, or a care dilemma such as that introduced by the UK government, which led to the spate of English junior doctors' strikes during 2016. Here, a radically politicized workforce displayed focused swarming and pulsation, advertising 'flow architecture' in which the house/yurt was built, dismantled, built again, and so forth, in nomadic fashion. Doctors would set up cognitive trails by moving away from set patterns of activity to rethink them and improvise, and then move back to a collective activity through directional swarming, as they tried to make sense of the government's NHS workforce planning through acts of resistance rather than capitulation (BBC News Channel 2016).

Such liquid metaphors are unlikely to become common currency anytime soon in medical education, but thinking with such metaphors invites a paradigm shift. Glenn Regehr (2010) notes that health professions education research is not 'rocket science'. The latter has become a metaphor for simplicity over complexity: 'It's not rocket science.' But, literally rather than figuratively, rocket science is based on strict physical laws that are linear (albeit complicated), but not complex. Hence, 'rocket science' is not a good metaphor for medical education research, which is messy, full of uncertainty and ambiguity. The distinction between 'hard' scientific research (testing hypotheses, seeking facts, the 'imperative for proof' – summarized as an 'imperative for generalizable simplicity') and 'soft' social science and humanities research is not helpful. Researching medical education demands high tolerance of ambiguity, as the subject matter is often complex, to do with social interactions, highly contextualized and messy. Regehr describes this as:

> Reorienting education research from its alignment with the imperative of proof to one with an imperative of understanding, and from the imperative of simplicity to an imperative of representing complexity well.
>
> (Regehr 2010, p. 31)

Such an approach may deflect researchers' interests away from 'search for proofs of simple generalizable solutions' towards 'the generation of rich understandings of the complex environments in which our collective problems are uniquely embedded'.

Mobilizing Engeström's brave new world of metaphoric imagination for applied medical education is an exciting prospect. It might directly address

Regehr's plea for a future medical education research programme. Such a vision is not pie-in-the-sky. A common medical aphorism is 'splint 'em where they lay' – real-life problems require rapid responses in the moment; also, moving the person may create further unnecessary injury. Medical education, for some, is a broken limb (the person met the lumbering lorries of the 'competence' movement driven by incompetent educationalists with limited vision) that must be fixed *in situ* – in the workplace. Engeström (2009, 2010) suggests that if technologies were more efficient and dependable, general practitioners working with patients could readily network online in real time to share their diagnostic and treatment dilemmas, confirming Marshall McLuhan's infamous catchphrase (and metaphor) that 'the medium is the message' – from 1967. This would be an example of what is known as 'open source knowledge production', actually a realization of 'sharing and caring'.

Back to the brain

Many of the structures of the brain, such as the limbic system that controls our emotional states, do not look like the diagrams in anatomy textbooks when the brain is dissected. A solid and defined block of colour with a shape in the text turns out to be a squidgy mess on first sight. For example, without the map (the anatomy textbook) in front of you, it is hard to recognize within the human limbic system the hippocampus (the seat of memory) as looking like the 'sea horse' after which it is named. While the 'sea horse'/hippocampus may seem to be merely a linguistic descriptor and nominalistic, it evokes much more. There is fragility, a sense of something floating in a medium, a sense of the ancient – an embodied metaphor acting as teacher. Metaphors in medical education are our greatest resource, but we treat them with light disdain.

Finishing this chapter on a metaphor and image instead of a literal reading of a brain location (lulling us into a false sense of security as we imagine we have discovered the source of the river) is deliberate. It is an invitation into the poetics of medicine and medical education that is the subject of my next chapter. Poetics offers the fundamental ground for metaphor as content and process (Lakoff and Turner 1989). Without developing a poetic imagination, all this talk of metaphor will seem like camouflage, or deflection from the real problems that medicine faces as an applied science. I believe that to get the best out of thinking medicine and medical education with metaphors, we need a metaphorical imagination, or a 'poetic diction' (Barfield 2010). An education into the poetic imagination introduces ways of 'thinking otherwise'.

9   Poetry, metaphor and the medical imagination

Part of this chapter was developed from dialogue with a medical student – Komal Parmanand – at Peninsula Medical School, UK, for whom I was a tutor while she was in her fourth year in 2015–2016. Komal has graciously allowed me to draw on that dialogue and to use two of her poems to illustrate points made in the chapter.

A literary construction of the body

Studying and writing poetry in medical school, suggests Rafael Campo (undated) – doctor, medical educator and poet – can make medical students (and their tutors) better listeners. You have to listen to, into and through a poem in order to get at its juice – same thing with patients, and with colleagues. The flesh of a poem is like the flesh of a person – it captures and displays symptoms. It is not just the writing of poems that educates the kind of sensibilities needed for both clinical acumen and caring communication, but also the reading of poems. Just as doctors tend bodies forensically, so poems are bodies made by humans that are tended by readers, whose forensic work we call 'criticism'.

When symptoms appear in bodies and minds – a skin rash, an abdominal pain, shortness of breath, anxiety, obsessive thoughts, depression with suicidal ideation, anorexia – we can think of these as embodied metaphors. This poetic framing immediately gives a richness and depth to observation of symptoms that is lacking in the reductive formal language of medicine, even of psychiatry, and in the deeply impoverished language of the pedagogy that informs mainstream medical education, with its reduction to the mechanics of 'skills', 'objectives' and 'competences'. The poetic approach allows us to more readily 'think otherwise'.

Thus, depression: leaden, heavy, stuck; anorexia: stripping back the flesh to a bare minimum for existence, floating above anything that might anchor, stain or stink, like menstrual blood or shit. While depression is a chronic weight and burden, anorexia is a series of acute episodes of unburdening through starving, stripping back almost to disappearance. When metaphors appear in poems, as the flesh of those poems, they, too, must be read as symptoms – of the embodied imagination, necessarily out on a limb because poetry is essentially deranged, but positively abnormal (*surhumaine*).

The symptoms of the imagination that poetry catalogues also offer a cure for culture's ailments – chronic lack of innovation, entrenched habits and petty-mindedness. Done well, poetry is an elevation of language and of the human spirit that is emotionally and intellectually challenging. As positive derangement, poetry affords a treatment for repression, sourness, underperformance and mundanity in culture. Not many people do it, and few read it, however. The body and mind fruitfully derailed is Walt Whitman's 'the body electric', a generator of light and heat, and a battery of metaphors.

We have seen that a metaphor is a term or phrase that does not make literal or ordinary sense, but raises the meaning through curious comparisons ('he had egg on his face', 'she forced the issue', 'a tissue of lies'). The ordinary can then become extraordinary, raising mundane understanding to imaginative insight. A symptom, too, does not make ordinary sense but shifts a bodily or mental state into the territory of the extraordinary – fractures, rashes, hives, boils, sudden pains, blinding headaches, bleeding, swelling, vomiting, discharges, strings of expletives, memory loss, hallucinations, assumptions of godhead and invincibility, plain but unmoveable greyscale sadness day after day. Metaphors again appear in the flesh and psyche as symptoms, and are repeated in the bodies of poems as descriptions of anxiety, swellings, rashes, narcissism, phobias, boils, pains, discharges and flatlining. We are all Job, under the thumb of Nature.

'Good listening makes physicians better diagnosticians and promotes better patient satisfaction', claim Ronald Schleifer and Jerry Vannatta (2013). Where do these big claims come from? Well, there is plenty of evidence to correlate active listening with both diagnostic acumen and patient satisfaction (Bleakley 2014). It is harder to provide evidence that embedding oneself in poetry necessarily leads to better listening, and we must be satisfied with assumptions that have a ring of authenticity. Danielle Ofri (undated), like Rafael Campo a doctor and writer, unconditionally celebrates poetry's value for medicine, when it moves us beyond 'good listening' to 'interpreting metaphors': 'poetry is important … because interpreting metaphors is a critical clinical skill in diagnosis; patients' symptoms often present in metaphorical manners and we doctors need to know how to interpret our patients' metaphors'. What constitutes good poetry (and effective handling of metaphor) is another matter, and is dealt with at length later in this chapter.

Prior to interpreting metaphors, we respond to them. We must first learn to appreciate them, since appreciation precedes explanation. Writing, reading and critically engaging with poetry is like taking a bath in metaphor, soaking in its goodness. But, just as the bath can scald if it is too hot, and then in time gets cold and unpleasant, so metaphors can turn nasty. They can be too hot to handle (over-metaphorizing, mixed metaphors). Here is a headline from the daily paper that I read today at the beginning of the Rio de Janeiro 2016 Olympics about the Brazilian football team's initial underperformance: 'Brazil's caravan of angst totters under the burden of obsession.' (Ironically, Brazil went on to win Olympic gold.) Or, they can become 'dead' and cold metaphors through overuse and overfamiliarity ('a piece of cake'); worse, they can become malignant (again, sorry to beat the drum, but do exhausted people with terminal illness really want to know that they are 'battling' cancer?).

This chapter presents a case study of one medical student (Komal Parmanand) – aided by feedback from a small group of her peers – working with one medical school professor (myself) and using poetry as a medium to explore 'listening' to patients. By 'listening', I do not just mean taking in and responding to what another person says. I have a broader view of listening that encompasses 'thinking' medicine with metaphors. We can call this a 'deep listening', not just an informational listening. It is a full appreciation and acknowledgement of another's presence, and also of his or her suffering, that refuses to filter out what Schleifer and Vannatta (2013) call the 'chief concern' of the patient rather than just the 'chief complaint' (presenting symptom).

The patient's 'chief concern' is his or her overall condition in relationship to presenting symptoms, such as emotional anxieties, worries about co-morbidities, concerns about side effects of treatments, and so forth, presented as a complex of metaphors. Such patterns of symptoms can include mental health issues and medically unexplained symptoms ('I'm worried to death about this constant ache that I have in my side and the woolly feelings that go with it, like I'm sapped of all my energy, and then there's the stomach churning too …').

Poetry and prognostic consciousness: ahead of its time

Conversation with another demands constant movement or positioning within a backwards and forwards flow of listening and speaking (to the other and to one's inner thoughts and feelings, spiked with memories, imaginative leaps, speculation and fantasy), co-ordinating the verbal and the non-verbal, presenting and creating identities while moving in and out of roles with set scripts and potential for improvisation around those scripts. This complex of factors has been described as a web of 'affordances' (Clark 2008). The latest neuroscience suggests that consciousness is already prognostic – we are always in the process of detection, slightly ahead of ourselves, predictive, not reactive. Andy Clark (2016) compares this to surfing, where the fastest part of the wave – the 'pocket' – is just ahead of the breaking curl in the most critical section.

Our minds, or consciousness – the primary emergent property of the complex adaptive system that is the central nervous system, the autonomic nervous system and the enteric system of the gut – surf just ahead of the curl, not because of some inner urge but because of adaptation to environmental flux, that is, a fundamentally uncertain world of embodied metaphors. Metaphors offer links between one experience and another that afford development or innovation. Hence, we always have one foot in the known and another in the unknown. This may be why the most common mental condition suffered by humanity is free-floating anxiety or existential angst.

Complex environmental cues can become clues to the perceptive doctor, as she has her antennae up for key information from her patient's talk and demeanour in recounting a history. Close listening requires a certain kind of sensibility, the sort that appreciates poetry for its rich, embodied language, compression and rhythms. This kind of perceptual awareness is best expressed again in the psychologist James Gibson's (1979) notion of 'affordance'. Gibson turned perception theory on its head by suggesting that it is not individuals who orient to stimuli in the environment, but rather, the environment affords, or gives off, patterns of events that educate attention, shaping interests and embedding us in a complex process of environmental flux. This flux shapes us; we do not shape it (other than by the fact that we are part of this flux for another). I do not hear the birdsong; the birdsong attracts my attention and educates it so that I might better orient on another occasion.

As individuals, we offer affordances for others and are embedded in a flux of affordances. In this way, doctors learn how to diagnose through pattern recognition. Repeated exposure to certain patterns creates affordance – the pattern 'grabs' your attention and educates it for the future. This is commonly called 'gaining expertise'. We saw in Chapters 5 and 6 how resemblances help to educate such expert, or Type 1, reasoning.

Malcolm Gladwell (2009) suggests that we need a minimum of 10,000 hours of dedicated, reflective practice to gain expertise in fields such as music and sport. Apply this to relationships, and Gladwell's theory is squashed. Many of us have 10,000 hours of dedicated practice in intimacy, lovemaking, child rearing, small talk, speculation and duplicity, but we still get it horribly wrong on so many occasions. Perhaps we read relationships literally rather than metaphorically; or relationships are lived through either hot and impossibly potent, or tired and dead, metaphors. A relationship, of course, is the best illustration of a metaphor – two things coming together in a way that suggests a transformation to a more intense expression. But often, the metaphors are mixed or over-egged, causing nausea, or they become dead through habit and repetition. A relationship is not a skilled conjunction (as if doctor–patient relationships could be 'taught' as 'communication skills' and 'professionalism'), but an imaginary conjunction – again, a metaphor: 'it'll be alright on the night' and 'like two peas in a pod'.

Amongst the richest kinds of environmental affordances are spoken and written languages as we compose sentences – not just the language of others, but also listening to one's own voice(s). Such language varies in its density and intensity. Cultural artefacts such as medical diagnoses and poems – bound by rules and historical conventions – are metaphor-dense and -intense. The metaphors educate our attention, and we come to appreciate them through repeated exposures. The Elizabethan English that frightened us at school when we first studied Shakespeare now affords pleasure in recognition and new insights. The patient – an embodied poem – demands the total listening that poems demand of us, where the patient's symptom presentation, embedded in his or her self-presentation, is a complex and layered poem demanding multiple readings and educated responses.

Schleifer and Vannatta (2013) suggest that 'poetry, especially the encounters with metaphors that poetry almost always occasions' can educate for a listening that takes the doctor beyond the 'chief complaint' to the patient's 'chief concern'. Rafael Campo (undated) argues passionately for the value of poetry from a structural perspective: 'poetry is a pulsing, organized imagining of what once was, or is to be'. Poetry is simultaneously diagnostic and prognostic, both memory and foretelling made flesh or fleshed out.

Poets love the fizzing body electric – Campo's 'pulsing, organized imagining' – just as doctors tend to it when the skin erupts in boils, the heart races abnormally, or everyday social interaction habitually spills over into threatening behaviour. While poets sing the body (Homer's epics were song cycles long before they were written down), doctors' work is tending the body – not just instrumentally fixing and maintaining it, but also educating patients into how to balance risk with regulation: 'safe' sex, 'balanced' diet, UV 'protection', 'mindfulness' as an anxiety prophylactic. See how those metaphor vehicles – 'safe', 'balanced', 'protection', 'mindful' – seem so bland on first hearing in comparison with their tenors: 'sex', 'food', 'sun', 'anxiety' (sounds like a young couple's typical summer holiday), and yet how those vehicles can come to howl, given time. The vehicles normally carry the unexpected image and then the weight of surprise ('my head is a jungle'). But in the examples above ('safe', 'balanced', and so forth), the vehicles are tonally greyscale rather than hot primary colours. Metaphors can work this way, too, through greyscale intensities.

Consider Sylvia Plath's (1960) poem written when she was in the third trimester, nine months into her pregnancy, aptly titled 'Metaphors' (available at http://genius.com/Sylvia-plath-metaphors-annotated). In the poem, Platt comes to see her pregnant body not in colour and blooming, but tonally greyscale as 'a ponderous house', and elephantine. She unfolds her confession that the potentially exotic feeling of pregnancy ('a melon strolling on two tendrils', a big loaf with its 'yeasty rising', 'new-minted' money in a 'fat purse') has become not only functional ('a means', 'a stage', 'a cow in calf'), but also bitter ('I've eaten a bag of green apples') and without hope ('Boarded the train there's no getting off'). Medical students, GPs and psychiatrists in particular could benefit from studying Plath's metaphors; many women suffer from hopelessness rather than hope during pregnancy and postpartum. Postnatal depression may occupy the greyscale spectrum – cold ashes, low and threatening skies, an immobile pewter sea.

The work of poets such as Plath captures the complex experience of being embodied, but experiencing life as something that transcends the physical moment. Good poets capture ordinary experiences through strong physical descriptions and make them extraordinary. Physicality is displaced, as it is in both anorexia (rising away from the disgusting earth) and depression (sinking into the engulfing earth). Poetry can echo the rhythms of the body (iambic pentameter is based on the heartbeat: lub-dup/lub-dup/lub-dup/lub-dup/lub-dup: 'Now is the winter of our discontent/Made glorious summer by this sun of York'); in Plath's poem, as the opening line tells us, each line has nine syllables, the poem is nine lines long, and 'metaphors' has nine letters, echoing the round nine months of pregnancy. Or, the language can capture the round bodily shape, as Plath's does, such as the dome of the belly inside and out – melon-like, a purse, a red fruit.

But, in Plath's confession, her body is just a vehicle in which she has been imprisoned. Plath had two children before she committed suicide at the age of 31. Her last poem, 'Edge', begins: 'The woman is perfected./Her dead/Body wears the smile of accomplishment.' This is not the healthy 'red fruit' of the pregnant woman; rather, it is greyscale sadness come full circle.

Poems employing embodied metaphors are gestural. They resemble 'speech acts' and are performative. Michael Rosen (2014) says:

> You have to live the poem with your whole mind and body.... You pass a poem to the audience through the words as embodied.... And the people listening and watching come back at you in an equally embodied way.

Poetry is not just performed when read aloud, but performs on and off the page when read to oneself. David MacNeill (1985) introduced the notion of 'metaphoric gestures' that are on a continuum from 'expected' to 'unexpected' (a metaphorical dislocation). An expected metaphoric gesture is a common cultural action that is readily understood, such as a 'conduit' metaphor, discussed earlier (Reddy 1993) – the cardiologist says to the patient in the process of an angiogram:

> We are going to give you a local anaesthetic and intravenous sedation. I will insert a small catheter into an artery in the crook of your arm and thread that towards your heart. We will then put in an iodine contrast dye for the X-ray. After a while, you will feel a warm sensation flooding your body, like a fluid running through you.

As he says this, he gently sweeps his arm across your body as if tracing the course of the contrast dye. An unexpected metaphorical gesture is the warm, flooding feeling of the dye, something unique in your experience. It is surprisingly pleasant – warm and moist – in amongst the cold and forbidding 'angio' paraphernalia surrounding you.

Poems that work are like this extensive, warm, flooding feeling. There is no prior cultural image or model that prepares you for this unique feeling. It is an utterance that is simultaneously a fracture of the known and a snapshot of the future, both diagnosis and prognosis. You, the patient, have the sensation of the coursing dye, while the cardiologist presents you with the evidence of the symptom – the extent of your furred artery, the damage and its limitation. The speech act (verbal or gestural) offered by the doctor is, in intention, illocutionary – it aims to explain what is going on. However, it may be received by the listener/viewer as perlocutionary or ambiguous in meaning. A poem is a speech act and a gesture that is intentionally perlocutionary (Platt's 'A melon strolling on two tendrils').

The cardiologist says to the patient recovering after the angiogram:

> Good news! We found some narrowing of a distal cardiac artery caused by a build-up of plaque, but the constriction is not severe enough to warrant an intervention like putting in a stent, so you can manage this on a drug and lifestyle regime: statin, beta-blocker, ACE inhibitor, low dose aspirin and exercise with a good diet. OK?

What the cardiologist found plain, straightforward and stripped of metaphor (an illocutionary gesture), the patient found ambiguous and metaphorical (a perlocutionary gesture), for it is the patient who must live with the uncertainty of the prognosis while the doctor champions the certainty and literalism of the diagnosis, the revealed symptoms. From the patient's perspective, however, the cardiologist was, paradoxically, speaking poetry and metaphor: 'narrowing' and 'furring' of the artery; 'management' of symptoms; and 'drug regime'.

The rhythms and images that shape the dynamic cognitive architecture necessary for medical diagnostic work can mirror the pulses and shapes of poems, but with a key difference – as William Empson (1930) famously said in *Seven Types of Ambiguity*, poems aim to create ambiguity for literary effect. As noted, diagnoses and treatments, on the other hand, aim to reduce ambiguity. As noted in Chapters 5 and 6, a radiologist looks at an X-ray showing an 'apple core lesion' in the colon. (For more on the radiological imagination and metaphor, see the conclusion to chapter 11.) His diagnosis is swift, based on pattern recognition (he has seen this shape many times before): 'There is an area of narrowing in the sigmoid. The undercut edges give an apple core appearance. This is colonic carcinoma.' This could be rendered as a Minimalist poem:

> There is an area
> of narrowing
> in the sigmoid.
>
> The undercut
> edges give
> an apple core appearance.
>
> This is colonic carcinoma.

The Minimalist poet William Carlos Williams (also a doctor) famously described a red wheelbarrow (in a poem simply called 'XXII' from the collection *Spring and All*, first published in 1923 and reprinted in 2015, which begins in uncertainty). The first stanza says that 'so much depends/upon' a red wheelbarrow, and then the wheelbarrow is plainly described as 'glazed' with rain water and standing beside some white chickens. Williams had simply observed the scene in a friend's farmyard, but turned an observation into a conundrum.

Again, the key difference between the two tangible observations is that the radiologist shows certainty ('There is' and 'This is'), where Williams shows uncertainty ('so much depends upon'). Of course the radiologist's account is also of pathology and suffering, raising deep feelings of concern, while Williams' account is purposefully on the surface, one of plain description raising nostalgia at best. In Minimalism, depth is found in surfaces. Doctors know this from their collective socialization into presenting 'cases' as succinctly as possible. Both the radiologist and Williams as poet work their way into the body of things – on the one hand, a human gut, and on the other, the guts of a backyard. Both are limned with bright metaphor and images: 'narrowing', 'undercut edges', 'apple core appearance' from the medical diagnosis; and 'so much depends', and 'glazed' from the poet and doctor, diagnosing human existence, a state of being that is about relationships with things around us – our con-texts.

The major metaphor underlying both sets of words is 'juxtaposition' – one thing set against another that surprises, excites or signals disease or being ill-at-ease: healthy colon set against cancerous colon; an inanimate but brightly col-oured wheelbarrow set against animate but white chickens. Setting one thing against another in this way is how to construct a metaphor: 'Life is a fiddler and we all must dance.' Life fiddles with your body, and the music is not sweet but sour – boils, bruises, discharges, damage, broken parts, dark weather in the psyche, a clogged artery, a sliding hiatus hernia, violin string adhesions in pelvic inflammatory disease.

Metaphor is the vital spark that turns ordinary, loose and watery language into the oils and earths of poetry as a radical but creative reduction – the alchemy of distilling to liquid densities and of burning down to dry essences. Cognitive psychologists call this reduced matter 'tacit knowledge' (Polanyi 1983) and a 'cognitive unconscious' (Reber 1996), stored as metaphors and made explicit as expert diagnostic acumen. Poetry, read silently from the page or spilling from the mouth, echoes the making explicit of schemas of narrative knowledge that doctors use in diagnosis. Schemas are tacit narratives – 'illness scripts' (discussed in Chapter 8) – absorbed from patients' histories and stored as cognitive architecture (Custers 2015).

Poetry at the bedside

How many medical students currently studying worldwide will *formally* be introduced to poetry and/or metaphor as a part of their education into diagnostic acumen, including close attention to patients' stories? Students will learn communication skills, but when will the words 'metaphor' or 'poem' be uttered? If they are lucky, they will hear about something called 'narrative based medicine', along with the tip from the archives of the great physician and aphorist William Osler that the diagnosis is in the patient's story (if you listen). Osler, in col-lapsing medical sleuthing to pithy maxims, was a Minimalist artist before Minimalism.

As Danielle Ofri (http://danielleofri.com/poetry-in-medicine/) insists, medical students can benefit from learning about metaphor in medicine, and there is no better place to start than poetry, the metaphor cauldron:

1   Medical language, particularly specialty-based lingo, is saturated in metaphor and often used (and abused) in diagnoses. Doctors need to be reflexive about the language they use with both patients and colleagues. Communication with patients can be improved through understanding their uses of metaphor and how medical metaphors can confuse patients if misused by doctors. Medical culture sees most illnesses as everyday or mundane (except for rare or unexplained symptoms, which are always fascinating for doctors), while for patients, illness is not everyday but something out of the ordinary. Medical language – especially scientific descriptions – often objectifies and dehumanizes patients, as it turns persons into symptoms and refuses everyday or lay descriptions: 'Mrs K presented with a hematoma' (Mrs K thought she had bruised herself in a fall – actually, the doctor will argue that a bruise is not quite the same as a hematoma, but Mrs K does not need to know that). What is commonplace and commonly understood by a shared term – a bruise – is not made extraordinary by a scientific description.

2   The landscape of medicine – its values and practices – has been shaped by two dominant metaphors for nearly 500 years, as discussed throughout this book. These are 'the body as machine' and 'medicine as war'. We need to understand why this cultural shaping has occurred, what it means for patient care and safety, and how new metaphorical landscapes are emerging.

3   Medicine outwardly refuses metaphor in the same way that it refuses ambiguity. Intolerance of ambiguity is a mark of fixity. Contemporary team-based and patient-centred medicine needs adaptable doctors.

Dog-tired and disaffected: case study and context

Peninsula Medical School in the UK was formed from a union of Exeter and Plymouth Universities and had its first intake of students in 2002. With the addition of a dental school, the medical school expanded to become Peninsula College of Medicine and Dentistry (PCMD). In 2012, Peninsula was dissolved to create two separate medical schools within the two universities, Exeter and Plymouth. Medical students from the 2012 intake continued under the old name of Peninsula Medical School, and the final cohort graduated in 2017.

Peninsula has a reputation for an innovative curriculum, including a high profile for the medical humanities, which are both core and integrated. In the fourth year, all students study for an assessed longitudinal Special Study Unit (SSU) in medical humanities, choosing from a long menu of topics, from life drawing to stand-up comedy. This runs over an academic year, with three two-day sessions (one per term) of six hours per day with one or more academic tutors, who may be clinicians, social scientists, humanities scholars or artists (or a mix of these, and many SSUs are co-facilitated; for example, doctors pair up with artists). The students curate their own one-day, end of SSU conference to present work. This work is written up and assessed, and there are formal awards for the best work. Typically, then, students complete a creative piece of work such as a film, a piece of creative writing or a performance; write a reflective account of producing this piece of work that puts it in the context of their clinical learning, adding both relevance and meaningfulness or depth of insight; and present the work at the student-led conference, which has an organizing committee, a conference brochure and a guest speaker. Work is archived and often presented at subsequent exhibitions or conference presentations.

At the time of writing, I run the SSU 'Touch/Don't Touch: The Art of Communication'. Students are encouraged to both see communication – particularly with patients – as an art or a development of style, and to represent communication issues they see as problematic or complex through an art form, such as creative writing. They are then left to evaluate whether or not the medium of representation – such as poetry – enhances their appreciation and understanding of patient care and safety, or of the human condition.

As a student on my SSU, Komal Parmanand chose to study three leading metaphors in medicine – 'medicine as war', 'the body as machine' and 'illness as a journey', to see how these shaped styles of communication and whether these were helpful or unhelpful for patients. She looked at the historical roots of the metaphors; how pervasive the metaphors are in contemporary medicine; and how they affect doctor–patient communication. This involved talking with patients and senior doctors on rotations including end-of-life care. While she wrote a formal, reflective account about the place of leading or didactic metaphors in medicine, she also wanted to represent the power of metaphor through a metaphor-rich medium, and chose poetry to do this. As her tutor, I gave formal feedback on her work, but also wanted to respond to her poems in kind, and so gave feedback on the poems by both suggesting edits and rewrites, and writing 'mirror' poems in response. This poetic dialogue replaced the usual academic monologue provided by tutors, and resulted in Komal entirely rewriting the poems. Two of the poems were entered for the Peninsula Students' annual poetry competition, one winning second prize.

As an illustrative example of the process of dialogue, below is one of the poems that Komal first drafted to break the skin of the medium, to get underneath that skin and to feel the way that a poem might better capture a strong experience than a formal, reflective account of the sort that is encouraged for students in their reflective portfolio work. Komal's poems vividly describe her experiences with patients, and engage issues around the three metaphors of medicine as war, the body as a machine and illness as a journey. Again, these metaphors are especially prominent in medical talk in end-of-life care.

As previously noted, Elena Semino and colleagues (Semino *et al.* 2015) have studied what they call the 'violence' and 'journey' metaphors in end-of-life care by patients and healthcare professionals in online forums for cancer patients, in the light of a current drive by the NHS to replace descriptive 'war' metaphors with 'journey' metaphors for cancer patients. Semino and colleagues found that patients themselves employ war and journey metaphors in both productive (empowering) and unproductive (disempowering) ways. War metaphors are not, then, by default negative and journey metaphors by default positive. However, they can be used inappropriately – a dog-tired and disaffected person suffering from a terminal illness may not want to be told that he or she must 'fight' that illness.

On the palliative, or end-of-life, care rotation, as KP considered dominant metaphors such as illness as a journey and medicine as battleground, she made the critical move of suspending knowing, to ask the existential question: 'how do any of us know?' about end of life. This highlighted a key metaphor – that of 'mystery'. In engaging with mystery, Komal wrote the following poem (one of three that she first submitted to me for comment), beginning with a rhetorical question:

How do you know?

You live your life a certain way,
Whatever that may be.
And then one day, they tell you softly,
That it's time to let things be.
They say, they're sorry but there is no more.
The end of the road is now ahead.
From now on, your days are short and few,
And there's nothing more to be done or said.
What road is it that you're on? I wonder,
Is it a peaceful country lane?
Or is it a chaotic road filled with dismay,
And grief, and suffering and pain?
How do they know what lies ahead? I wonder,
Or how much time you have left?
What if they've miscalculated your future,
And left you feeling empty and void and bereft?
Will there be the white light of heaven,
Waiting for you with open arms?
Will you be at peace and loved and joyful,
Or filled with dread and worry and qualms?
Is there anything you would want to do,
Before it all comes to an end.
How would you want to be remembered?
What messages to the world would you want to send?
The worry of what lies ahead,
Is an ongoing thought as you prepare.
For the worst, or the best of it all,
Questions you cannot spare.
And once it's all over and you are gone,
Life continues on, and still
These questions we all have about what lies ahead,
Remain gaps we cannot fill.

(Reproduced with permission of the author)

As I pointed out to Komal, this is less a poem and more a prose piece cut up into lines. There are some very good lines ('the worry of what lies ahead'), but there is also inconsistency and 'clunky' listing of words in obvious metonymic chains ('And left you feeling empty and void and bereft?', 'Or filled with dread and worry and qualms?'). Simplicity might be better here: 'And left you feeling empty'; 'Or filled with dread'. The opening stanza could be improved by deleting one line:

Original:
You live your life a certain way,
Whatever that may be.
And then one day, they tell you softly,
That it's time to let things be.

Suggested revision:
You live your life a certain way
And then one day they tell you softly
That it's time to let things be.

Why do 'they tell you softly'? In sharp contrast, the poet Dylan Thomas, in 'Do Not Go Gentle into That Good Night', urged us not to go gently at death but to 'burn and rave' as we get to the 'close of day', so that we 'rage' against the failing light. A simple solution for Komal's poem is to just drop the 'softly': 'And then one day they tell you.' And so forth.

Komal was open to constructive criticism, because the thinking she was using to construct the poem is part and parcel of the thinking she uses for diagnostic and caring tasks when adapting intelligently to webs of affordances in medical work. As noted above, I suggested that I would write a poem in response to 'How do you know?' and that Komal should write another poem in response to mine. The ground-rules were: no 'line pinching' and no obvious 'lifting' of ideas. The poem must emerge as a felt response to what my poem afforded and not as an intellectual exercise in trying to work out what a poem is, or what a metaphor should be.

Below is my poem and its justification. The poem is elliptical, hence the title 'Taking the curves'. It follows a heartbeat in its traditional metre (iambic pentameter), again the basic rhythm of the body based on the heartbeat's 'lub-dup, lub-dup'. It draws on metaphors of the heart and then returns to itself, excited by its own process – the main circuit of the body electric. The heart's configuration as a muscle and engine in the chest is undone, but at the end of the day we have to recognize that the heart has a lifespan, a sell-by date. The poem is deliberately brief to offset the stereotype that end of life is a drawn-out affair, and deliberately upsets the notion of loss by framing death as a prospect that makes the heart race.

Taking the curves

> The heart may be a glistening muscle
> Blistered by pressures or a tired pump,
>
> A fat-covered engine in the chest
> Running down under a damp bone grille;
>
> But it is also a language peppered
> With stinking cusses and crosswise diction
>
> As cursed as Job in its tireless strain
> To make the next landing, or navigate
>
> The next blind bend, a curve so perilous
> That the heart itself races at its prospect.

So, I set Komal the task of rethinking the personal link with her end-of-life patients and their dilemmas using a totally impersonal poem, but a poem that is wholly tangible, grounded in body and replete with well-known ('blind bend') and original ('stinking cusses') embodied metaphors – some taking anatomic liberties ('fat-covered engine'). Komal's original poem has too much metaphysical musing for me. She did not entirely shake this off in her rewrite, but her metaphors had a lot more physical presence (sunlight 'pouring', the heart is 'heavy', ink 'flowing', 'agitation' in the breath; 'pump' of the heart). Many of these are common metaphors, such as 'heavy heart' and sunlight 'pouring' through an open window – but why not? If there are weeds to be removed, use a hoe, the right tool for the job.

Here's what KP came back with. She decided on the genre of a love letter written from the patient's perspective:

> *What lies ahead*
> To my love,
> The sunlight pours
> Through an open window
> As I write to you with a heavy heart.
> The ink that flows
> Is black with burden
> And writes with affliction.
> For our future
> Is only alluded to
> And riddled with mystery.
> And so I cannot answer your questions
> About what lies ahead.
> They told me months ago

That this was it
And yet I live on with fear
And agitation in each breath,
Each pump of my tired heart
As if it were my last.
Friends have come and gone,
And left only pieces of a puzzle
That will never be complete.
Some devour from tall trees of aching fruit,
That couldn't be controlled
By the sweet juice of relief.
Others strolled through meadows of bliss
And danced with glee
As their minds clouded but bodies found liberation.
Every friend, a solitary portrait
Of what lies ahead.
I write to you, my love,
As the light caresses my face
With the promise of heaven.
I pray you do not suffer
From uncertainty
As I have, for it helps no man
Find liberation.
It offers nothing but insecurity
Masked only by the unfaltering beauty
Of what we wish our lives to be.
            (Reproduced with permission of the author)

This draft offers a marked transformation from the first poem. The poem now demands close, critical reading. While a scan of the body of metaphors shows some predictability (sunlight 'pours', the heart is 'heavy' and 'tired') and sugar coating ('meadows of bliss'), there is exciting innovation ('black with burden' – a nice alliteration too; 'aching fruit', 'sweet juice of relief'). Some of the images are powerful: ink is not only black but, again, 'burdened' with its blackness, and 'afflicted'. So, the body of the ink itself – the voice of the dying person – shows symptom; the embodied metaphor is sick and asking for care. Actually, it demands attention. Just as the ink runs out of the pen and then the pen runs out of ink, so the writer's life is running away (as is the life of the person to whom he or she is writing).

'Some devour from tall trees of aching fruit' may seem a little forced at first, but the metaphors are apt. Fruit does ache to fall from the tree when heavy or ripe. Making the tree tall increases the tension of the 'aching fruit', which will now drop from a great height. There is an element of surprise hidden amid the tension of the aching fruit. And the tall tree means that the fruit cannot be readily plucked as low hanging.

The first big shift from the original poem is that the patient is now the subject and not the object of the poem. The reader is invited into his or her world by sharing an intimacy – a love letter written to a partner. Suddenly, the poem is no longer a case study objectifying the patient, but a bedside encounter listening to the dying person's story. The second big shift from the original poem is that the metaphysical now gets physical: the future is 'riddled' with mystery (now a double mystery, for who is doing the riddling? We riddle fires, but we also set riddles or mysteries). While the line below might benefit from a simple edit – 'Some devour from trees of aching fruit' – it is a relief that 'relief' is embodied as a 'sweet juice' rather than floating away as an abstraction:

> Some devour from tall trees of aching fruit,
> That couldn't be controlled
> By the sweet juice of relief.

Conclusion: poems, like suffering people, may be bruised black and blue

KP and AB then had a conversation about the relationship of poetry to medicine, anatomizing that relationship – where convergence takes place, where there are parallel meanings, and where there is plain divergence and mismatch. Here are the descriptions of the meetings of the territories of medical and poetic labour (both unpaid work for medical students!).

We aligned guidelines for poetry style with medical practice's verve:

1 A poem has a rhythm like life has rhythm – for example, and as already noted, iambic pentameter, Shakespeare's diction, is like the beating of the heart (lub-dup, lub-dup, lub-dup, lub-dup, lub-dup). Medical work, too, must have rhythm, especially on long shifts, and these rhythms are easily interrupted. Finding and keeping this bodily rhythm stops you from tiring easily and making mistakes.

2 Alliteration (repetition of the same sound – 'the wild weather weakens') in poetry is like emphasis in music. While it creates insistence, alliteration can easily be overdone and decline into a cheap trick, a poor imitation of Anglo-Saxon and Medieval verse, and so should be used sparingly. Alliteration, again, should be like hammering on the anvil, or the pounding of the chest in resuscitation; but alliteration can be subtle too, like a drummer playing with wire brushes rather than sticks, or a doctor palpating a patient's abdomen, or percussing the chest.

Saeed Jones (2014) is a young, black and queer American poet whose debut collection *Prelude to Bruise* has been received with critical acclaim. In the poem 'Prelude to Bruise' (available online, read by Jones: www. buzzfeed.com/juliafurlan/5-poems-from-prelude-to-bruise-read-by-saeed-jones?utm_term=.kuyXZz4yn#.ppMajmw92), an imagined white, racist man in Birmingham, Alabama talks to a black man unsparingly about how he likes to 'break in' young blacks like horses, brutally, with queer sexual overtones. Jones says that he wrote the poem 'very quickly while saying it out loud', fearing that 'it would fall apart in my hands' if thought about for too long. So, Jones works like a doctor percussing the body, rapping us rhythmically with his provocations.

The poem is choreographed alliteratively: black, blue, broke, bootblacks, with 'bruising' and 'Birmingham' in the background. B & B = bed and breakfast, or bread and butter. Bread and butter pericarditis, where adhesions occur. The rub of the heart in pericarditis is heard as a grating sound through a stethoscope. There is so much scope for poetry in this, where symptom patterns, to the keen senses of the doctor, are alliterative too. They may be foregrounded as signal against noise, like the crack of a joint, or a rasp like the fine crackles of rales in inhalation for a patient with respiratory disease. Or the alliteration may be an insistent, recurring symptom, like tinnitus or thumping headaches that suggest further investigation. Like Saeed Jones' bruised bodies, we can suffer the blues as melancholy until they turn black and a depression grips. The doctor must be able to track and anticipate the colours of moods.

3   Finish lines on a strong word. There is nothing worse in a poem than finishing a line with a weak or trailing word – this is usually the easiest symptom to spot in a novice writer. Good poets often finish lines with emphasis, or plain recognition of what in nature is a startling phenomenon. The first stanza of a poem by Matthew Francis (2013) called 'Sea at Low Tide' describes how the sea has 'frittered' away in rockpools to create not just a 'mist', but – the final word – a 'sandshine'. While the sea has receded, the poem keeps the sea in our vision through nouns – things – 'rockpools', 'mist' and a wonderful neologism, 'sandshine', finishing each line strongly, keeping the receding sea present, not just in the mind but in the senses. You can smell the rockpool, feel the mist and see the sandshine. This is the presence of absence. Similarly, in medicine, do not let the diagnostic clues recede like the falling tide, but keep investigating the rockpools and the traces (mist and sandshine). In conversing with patients, do not trail off, but keep the conversation going with strong, positive response.

4   Finish the poem strongly, or with a puzzle. Just as lines should finish on a strong word, so the poem itself should finish strongly. This does not necessarily mean coming to a conclusion; it may mean setting a conundrum or a puzzle. Consultations may finish with unknowns, uncertainties, but finish conversations with patients on a strong word. Doctors may think that patients want certainty in the diagnosis, whereas there may be a high level of ambiguity and uncertainty. Actually, what patients want is a good relationship with their doctors underpinning and informing excellent medical acumen. Where this trust is established, ambiguities are better tolerated. We do not read poems for answers, but to ask better questions.

5   Talk with, not about. Poetry, of course, is descriptive, but stronger writing talks *with* things rather than *about* them: 'A screaming comes across the

sky' (the opening line of Thomas Pynchon's *Gravity's Rainbow*). When Herman Melville begins *Moby Dick* with 'Call me Ishmael', Ishmael does not want to describe himself to you; he wants you to sit down next to him and join, or enter, his voice. Similarly, you need to talk with your patients and colleagues, not about them. Enter their worlds. Talk with their symptoms, not about them. KP's turnaround in her poem above was to switch voices from hers to the dying person's.

6   Do not preach, but do send a message. There is nothing worse than a poem that finger wags or subsists on the thin gruel of piety. Similarly, in medicine, do not tell people what to do, but be clear and firm with guidance.

7   Write a poem, not a piece of prose cut up into lines. This was a criticism I made above of Komal's first poem. A piece of prose cut up does not have an internal rhythm, and usually lines finish on weak words. Make every clinical interaction a rounded poem, not a series of cut-up sentences or interactions.

8   What does the poem 'weigh'? Is it 'lite' or profound? Poems, of course, can be light and elegant, but avoid 'lite' – poems that are too abstract and have no ballast (or are not based in tangible experience). Is your medical intervention weighty or 'lite'?

9   Where do you mostly feel the poem? Poems gain gravity by carrying ideas that have substance, and these should be felt in the gut and heart as much as they are understood or turned over in the mind. Similarly, you should feel your patients' symptoms and suffering in your gut and heart as you calculate diagnoses and treatments in the head.

10   Does the poem bring new insight or understanding, or surprise? A poem can be a conundrum and might take some time to unwind. Similarly, every encounter with a patient should bring insight. Each patient is unique.

11   The poem is a concentrated experience – poems punch far above their weight. Similarly, clinical interventions should have gravity and purpose.

12   Every word counts – make sure that you are using the right words; use the right tools. The best way to learn to write poetry is to read lots of poetry, to immerse yourself in the field. By your side, have a dictionary and a thesaurus. Bathe in words and befriend them. Use the right words at the right time. Similarly, in medicine you get to know your best tools – textbooks, protocols, formularies. Most tools are now portable apps. Poetry-to-go is also a good idea. Medical students should not just immerse themselves in clinical texts but also in medical biographies and autobiographies, in medical history and in medical fiction. Reading Chekhov may give greater insight into bedside practice than reading formal texts on communication in medicine.

13   Rewrite often – polish and polish. Scrap the poem and retain the idea, then rebuild. Practise – scrap and rebuild expertise. Unlearn and relearn. Medicine or poetry – both are arts and crafts that require lifelong learning.

Coda

I have brought clinical practice and poetry into complex conversation to show how the conventional arts and science divide is a sham. Medical education can benefit from the use of poetry, and the poet, in turn, can become what Gilles Deleuze (1998), after Nietzsche, calls a 'diagnostician of culture': a person who treats culture's symptoms – lassitude, mania, social injustice, inequality, consumption – with metaphor. Gaining expertise is not just down to hours of practice, but hours of practice with active, ongoing reflection.

Writers often persuade themselves that they work in solitary ways – sitting in front of a computer screen and churning out the first drafts, then refining and refining. Instrumentally, this may be the case, but the reality is that writers carry over what they learn and hear in social interaction, or in research through reading other writers. Every piece of writing is in some sense collaborative, resulting initially from interaction – dialogue, overheard conversation, and so forth. I am interested in forefronting this collaborative aspect of writing.

The chapters (5 and 6) on resemblances in medicine were shaped through dialogue with a colleague, Robert Marshall, who is a senior consultant pathologist and medical educator. This chapter benefitted from my conversations with a senior medical student, Komal Parmanand. The following two chapters expand collaboration through bringing together in a symposium setting a group of doctors, medical educators, artists and humanities scholars, all of whom in some way are engaged with the topic of metaphors in medicine, to discuss the state of the art of 'thinking with metaphors' in medicine. The results led me to scrap two chapters from an earlier draft of this book and replace them with two new chapters that capture cutting edge thinking about metaphors in medicine, and represent the range of thinking and the intensity of ferment in the field. I have also benefitted from correspondence with a number of other clinicians and scholars in the field who could not attend the symposium and are now part of an expanding network focused on the website www.medicalmetaphors.com, set up with generous funding from the British Academy/Leverhulme Trust. I am grateful to them all for sharing their collective wisdom.

10 'Thinking with metaphors in medicine: the state of the art'

Part I: the odyssey

Welcome to the drinking party

In order to sound out current thinking about metaphors in medicine, what better way than to invite a bunch of artists, scholars and clinicians with a passion for the study of metaphor to a symposium to share perspectives? And what better place to meet than Dartington Hall, set in the heart of the Devon countryside, with its mixture of historic buildings, formal gardens and rolling landscape – the composite metaphor that is 'Englishness'? Dartington Hall was first developed as a great country house in 1384 by King Richard II's half-brother John Holand, and its original gardens included a practice jousting arena and a bear pit – both excellent metaphors for academic spats. In 1925, Dorothy and Leonard Elmhirst bought the estate and developed an innovative arts and education centre that has continued to the present day.

While the symposium was held over just three days, it felt more like the Odyssey – a returning home extended to 10 years of adventure and unforeseen circumstance. The following two chapters capture the best of the ideas that flowed from the meeting. I witnessed no academic spats, but rather, a ferment and proliferation of new ideas conducted with grace and good feeling. I wish universities and medical schools were more like this.

This chapter was, then, written as the aftermath of collaboration with 18 other people, and I would like to acknowledge the important contributions of the participants: Tess Jones, Arno Kumagai, Sue Bleakley, Stella Bolaki, Gianna Bouchard, Julie Bligh, Giskin Day, Bella Eacott, Martina Ann Kelly, Teo Manea, Mick Mangan, Robert Marshall, Martin O'Brien, Nicole Piemonte, Steve Reid, Caroline Wellbery, Tom Nutting and Victoria Bates.

The group was international and cosmopolitan: three from North America, two working in Canada (one Irish doctor, and one Japanese-American doctor who has recently moved to Toronto), one doctor from South Africa, and 13 mixed professions from the UK. There were six medical doctors in total, one visual artist, four performance artists/performance and theatre academics, and eight academics in medical and healthcare education, medical humanities, applied ethics and philosophy. These labels offer a crude summary – many are experts in interdisciplinary praxis: a performance artist whose provocative work is politically sophisticated and who is a theorist and teacher in his field; a doctor who first studied Classics at Oxford University; a professor of family medicine who has specialized in rural general practice and plays in a string quartet; a diabetes specialist who is a medical educator drawing on current critical theory; a Theatre Arts, Literature and Gender scholar who works in healthcare education with a specialism in disability studies, and is a long-serving editor of the primary North American journal of medical humanities and a co-editor of the leading international text on health humanities; and so forth.

The symposium was entitled 'Thinking with Metaphors in Medicine: The State of the Art' and convened at Dartington Hall between 24 and 26 June 2016, generously funded by The Wellcome Trust and the British Academy/Leverhulme Trust. On the back of this funding, a parallel, purpose-built website was set up (www.medicalmetaphors.com). The aims of the symposium were:

1   to gather intelligence on the state of the art of thinking with metaphors in medicine;
2   to form a network for future collaborations;
3   to add content to the website;
4   to collectively shape a final chapter or chapters in this book.

A 'symposium', defined as 'a conference or meeting to discuss a particular subject', follows the model of Plato's *Symposium* (385–370 BC), in which a drinking party is described where the topic of discussion is the many faces of 'love' (eros). The metaphor 'Platonic love' has its origin in this account. The Romans developed the symposium into the convivium, describing both a banquet and a conscious separating off from everyday life to provide a space for deeper discussion. The participants in Plato's symposium discuss sexual attraction, beauty, and Socrates' account of the love (*philia*) of knowledge, wisdom and learning as the vocation of philosophy. Erixymachus' speech notes that love is an important component of medicine, reminding us not just of the love of medicine as a vocation, but also that medicine requires love – something that we have crassly reduced to the instrumental, as 'communication skills', 'empathy' and 'patient-centredness', boxed up to be 'delivered' to students. Love itself is medicinal, says Erixymachus, because it fosters 'association', and this heals. As medicine, love then acts as a 'master' metaphor (forgive the gendering), lifting people from the ordinary mutuality of recognition to the extraordinary plane of care, affection and desire.

Being or falling (an apt metaphor) in love surely represents the most extreme form of uncertainty, occupying a place, as Socrates notes in his *Symposium* speech, between the gods and humanity, between imagination and bodily desire. Socrates concludes with the metaphor that beauty is truth, famously restated in John Keats' 'Ode on a Grecian Urn' from 1819, in which the poet describes the contemplated Urn as a 'still unravish'd bride of quietness'. Take away the questionable 'still unravish'd', and 'bride of quietness' remains as one of the most beautiful metaphors in literature. Medicine was our 'bride of quietness', the subject of our contemplation, and, like Socrates and Keats, we hoped to address both the truths and the beauties of medicine's metaphors, and perhaps to expose some ugliness too. What, then, were the fruits of our drinking party discussions?

Let's begin at the end: the polyphonic wonder of the drinking party

As I started to shape the multiple contributions to the symposium into some kind of order, the order that emerged was metonymic: a chain of associations in which one 'take' on metaphor on medicine was replaced by another 'take'. I am grateful to Caroline Wellbery, one of the participants, for pointing out that this reading re-creates the cultural hegemony of the individual voice, the solo artist, at the expense of the polyphony of voices that you would hear at carnival rather than Socratic symposium. This latter format regulates, relegates and even silences, in Caroline's words, 'all the interruptions, digressions, objections and ponderings' that happened at the Dartington symposium and in any carnivalesque setting. Here is Caroline's response in full, as a welcome antidote to the formulaic 'procession of speakers' so loved in particular by British audiences:

> Perhaps we would want to elaborate on the concept of 'symposium', and given its drinking party origins, add to it notions of frenzy, ecstasy or carnival. Not that we were anything but orderly and polite, outwardly anyway, at Dartington. Yet in writing up our discussion, the opportunity presents itself to move away from the hegemony of the single author. Rather than amalgamate or appropriate the presentations by describing and then riffing off of them, though Alan does so amusingly, brilliantly, and above all metaphorically, wouldn't this be a place to represent the carnival, to present the 'world turned inside out and upside down'? And isn't there a way in which by summarizing and interpreting the formal presentations a decision is made not only about how speech is assembled but who gets to speak? What happened to all the interruptions, digressions, objections and ponderings from the group? I could have imagined a more cacophonous performance of voices, or at least something like Jane Cardiff's amazing sound installation '40-part motet.' As SF Moma's website describes it: 'Individually recorded parts are projected through forty speakers arranged inward in an oval formation, allowing visitors to walk throughout the installation, listening to individual voices along with the whole.' Or the artist Ragnar Kjartansson's 'The Visitors', shown most recently (I believe) in Montreal, where listeners can go from virtual room to room to hear each musician's contributions to the songs while enjoying their idiosyncrasies, including Kjartansson's own as he plays naked in a bathtub. The arts offer ample metaphors for a collective in which each plays a contributing part. In the words of Martin Buber, 'Even as a melody is not composed of tones, nor a verse of words, nor a statue of lines – one must pull and tear to turn a unity into a multiplicity.' As dialogic madness, the form of these summary chapters could have commented in its

own way on the destabilizing, ec-centric redistribution of sensibility, carnivalesquely chopping the authorial, authoritative voices of the official speakers into conversational confetti.

(Reproduced with permission of the author)

I love Caroline's intervention – it reminds me of Bruno Latour's (2002) distinction between 'iconoclasm' and 'iconoclash'. The former is the destruction of cherished images, beliefs and institutions (only to replace them with others), while the latter is the ringing cacophony of a meeting of images, beliefs and institutions. Dominant metaphors run the course of addiction: they begin on a high, and fade as tolerance sets in; when they no longer serve a purpose, they can become irritants and then potentially destructive. Iconoclasts of various persuasions help with the demise of dominant metaphors, only to replace them with the single voice of authority. What Caroline's plea and Latour's 'iconoclash' ask for are, of course, radically different. Given the constraints on finishing this book to the publisher's deadlines, there is simply not enough time to explore how polyvocalism might have played out in reporting the Dartington symposium from quite another angle than the one that I have adopted. The way of carnival certainly chimes with my suggestion in previous chapters that the current dominant metaphors shaping medicine ('machine', 'war', 'journey') may be replaced not with other dominant metaphors or didactic frames, but rather, with a spray of 'small narratives', localized and contextualized, but listening to each other despite the cacophony.

Ethically murky metaphors

Tess Jones opened the symposium with a 'future shock' scenario in which she reminded us, through three medico-ethical case studies, that the future is already with us. In 'near future' science fiction, such as that of J.G. Ballard, we are often faced with bodily, medical and epidemiological metaphors describing ethically sensitive practices such as cloning, transplantation, genomics and theranostic nanomedicine (the development of individualized therapies through nanoplatforms that combine diagnostic and therapeutic capabilities within a single treatment agent (Xie *et al.* 2010; Lammers *et al.* 2011)).

Your body is a purse: unzip it and donate

Tess framed her talk through Kazuo Ishiguro's (2005) dystopian science fiction novel *Never Let Me Go*, describing an English boarding school – Hailsham – in which clones are raised as organ donors, and 'harvested' several times until they are literally exhausted of their crops. This is their purpose in life. The novel is a meditation on mortality and an awakening to the uses and abuses of the body, and to what constitutes 'humanity' in an era of 'organ trafficking'. As Tess explained, Ishiguro employs a number of novel biomedical metaphors, such as excision as 'donation', surgical procedures as 'unzipping your body', surgical sites as 'recovery centres', living as 'deferral' and dying as 'completion'. Of course, the use of terms such as 'harvesting' and 'banking' of organs (and this extends to 'transplantation tourism' and 'organ trafficking') already provides a range of 'productivity' and 'economic' metaphors that, in forefronting functional activities, mask the human concerns.

Pillow angels

Tess then described three case studies, each ripe for discussion of ethical dilemmas in medical treatment, where a metaphor is used as a kind of encryption and 'gift wrapping' of the 'case' – behind which, of course, is a suffering person. Ashley X was born with static encephalopathy, a severe brain disorder. While alert to her environment and breathing, sleeping and awakening independently, Ashley is tube fed, cannot lift her head or sit up, and cannot talk. Like other children with severe brain disorders, Ashley developed puberty very early, at six and a half years. This raises issues such as how parents and carers might deal with menstruation in a child who has to wear nappies, and with body weight gain that would make mobility and repositioning increasingly more difficult. The parents 'resolved' some of these issues by consenting to Ashley undergoing a hysterectomy, appendectomy and removal of early breast buds, performed at a hospital in Seattle in 2004. In 2006, Ashley also received oestrogen therapy so that her future growth in size and weight would be inhibited. This became known as the 'Ashley Treatment' (Pilkington 2012).

In a blog set up in 2007, Ashley's parents explained why they had consented to these treatments – known as 'growth attenuation' – as they continued to care for her at home: such as preventing possible bedsores, menstrual pain, appendicitis, discomfort from the predicted growth of large breasts, and the risk of breast cancer that runs in Ashley's family. An article published in 2010 offered testament from two bioethicists that the 'Ashley Treatment' is in the interests of the recipient (Diekema and Fost 2010). Disability rights activists, however, heavily criticized the treatment as a violation.

Ashley's parents nicknamed her 'Pillow Angel' (pillowangel.org) because she always has her head on a pillow. Ashley has become an example of a new category of 'permanently unable' children made possible through advancements in medical interventions. Ashley's parents' blog (pillowangel.org) in time created the new category of 'pillow angel' children and includes the stories of 'Charley', 'Erica' and 'Tom' – three of an estimated six 'pillow angel' children globally. the metaphor 'pillow angel' already deflects from some thorny ethical issues raised by disability activists in particular, especially critical of ableist perspectives, although Ashley's parents have posted that they are not concerned with the ethical debate but just want to get on with caring for their child.

Destination therapy and bridges to recovery

Tess's second metaphor example was 'destination therapy'. This refers to medical interventions that are in themselves end-points or destinations and not bridges or transitional stages to another intervention or therapy. This metaphor sits neatly under the master metaphor of 'illness as journey'. Destination therapies usually refer to interventions for patients with severe heart failure who are not candidates for transplants. Instead, a left ventricular assist device (LVAD), a mechanical support that aids circulation, serves them. The complex of metaphors around heart functioning is already problematic – such as heart 'failure' in the context of inevitable death for us all. An LVAD may be implanted in a person waiting for a heart transplant or a person with temporary heart failure. These are called, respectively, a 'bridge to transplant' and a 'bridge to recovery'.

Innovative treatment/care

Tess's third metaphor example was 'innovative treatment/innovative care'. This is where unusual, idiosyncratic or innovative medical or surgical interventions and/or acts of healthcare are not carried out as part of systematic data collection or formal 'research'. This means, of course, that the 'innovation' does not need formal ethics approval as part of a systematic research study, although informed consent would be gained from the patient. It does not mean that there are no ethical implications for the intervention or act of care. 'Innovative' acts as a gloss; 'new' or 'improvised' does not necessarily equate with 'safe'.

Metaphors inhabit medical ethics as rhetorical ploys

While there are lively debates about 'pillow angels', 'destination therapies' and 'innovative treatment' in the medical and healthcare ethics literature, what is often excluded from such debate is the power of the metaphor to persuade, dissuade, clarify or obscure, and this is what Tess brought to the table. Metaphors act rhetorically and are not simply signposts or labels. They are ethically sensitive phenomena in their own right.

Medical and healthcare ethics arguments used to be dominated by the application of principles such as autonomy and beneficence (Beauchamp and Childress 2013), but principlist approaches have recently lost currency, replaced by casuistry, or argument based on the single case and context. 'Casuistry' is an unfortunate descriptor, as it also means sophistry, or specious but clever reasoning. Tod Chamber's (1999) penetrating analysis of seminal ethics cases based on literary exposition, or taking ethics cases as narratives, reads quasi-scientific and quasi-logical claims as 'fictions', in which rhetoric and metaphor are used for effect.

In fact, the term 'narrative bioethics' may have its origin in a metaphor. Helmut Dubiel (2009, 2011) suffered from Parkinson's disease and underwent 'deep brain stimulation' therapy, subsequently entitling his autobiographical account *Deep in the Brain*. 'Deep brain' is a powerful metaphor. Relatively and literally, there is little depth to the brain, as compared with, say, 'deep ocean' or 'deep space'. However, 'deep brain' conjures up an unfathomable and hidden process, paired with deep attention by deep neurosurgeons in the deepest recesses of the hospital – the operating theatre. 'Deep brain' accrues power from contrast with what Dubiel himself calls 'high-risk technologies' (deep brain stimulation achieved from a risky high 'above' perspective, both surgically and morally). Lakoff and Johnson (1980) remind us that key and commonly used metaphors – such as 'container' metaphors – are structured in space (e.g. above–below).

Dubiel describes how he came across a 2007 'dissertation' (presumably doctoral) written by a 'young theologian', Katrin Bentele, that drew heavily on Dubiel's own account of Parkinson's. She uses the term 'narrative bioethics' (although the term 'narrative ethics' had been used since at least 1997 (Jones 1999)). Dubiel notes the shift in bioethics from 'overgeneralized' universal Kantian principles (moral imperatives) – such as justice and truthfulness – to 'second order principles' such as respect for self-determination of individuals. Engaging with these second order principles, for Dubiel, is a narrative process – people engage in conversation, make judgements and tell further stories about those judgements. In her work, Bentele argues that facing illness produces an identity crisis, which, in turn, generates 'reflexive efforts' to maintain integrity in the face of potential dissolution, where such 'reflexive efforts' amount to telling stories. Describing ethics as 'narrative', in a climate in which medical ethics craved scientific respectability, also metaphorized medical ethics as an imaginative approach to medical conundrums. In each of the three case studies of ethical dilemmas and their metaphorical wrapping or couching raised by Tess Jones above, reflexive effort or storytelling is paramount, and embodies rhetoric or persuasion.

Dubiel notes the classic distinction made by philosophers between 'having a body' and 'being in a body'. The latter is a body with an identity. The former is the body treated by medicine that suspends the patient's 'chief concern' to focus only upon the 'chief complaint' (Schleifer and Vannatta 2013). Suffering and identity collide in 'being in a body', but, paradoxically, suffering can drive out self-recognition and fragment identity so that a person is separated from his or her body and merely 'has a body'. Where the body is restored as 'text' (Kamps 1999; Bleakley *et al.* 2011), and is co-operatively 'read' by patient and doctor, being in the body is also restored. The ongoing 'production' of the medical body can be seen as that of sharing stories about symptoms.

Embodied metaphors, again, act as the binding agents that give these stories presence – the flesh made word and the word made flesh. The key metaphor in this process may be 'rupture'. Time and again, as the body's perceived wholeness and integrity are ruptured through the eruption or the slow simmer of symptoms, so identity can be ruptured in the emergence of vulnerability. In this scenario, therapies that are 'innovative' and have 'destinations' are comforting. Even the fallout from medical intervention is softened metaphorically as a 'side effect'. Side effects can be sharper than this, even fatal. A 'side effect' of poor teamwork communication in surgery, for example, can be the demise of the patient.

Metaphors and metamorphosis: power plays in medical education

Arno Kumagai's symposium presentation argued for the value of a metaphorical imagination in medicine that is best introduced through medical education. Experts in metaphor mostly work in humanities departments, and medical education must embrace this expertise through the incorporation of the medical humanities in medical education, doctors collaborating with scholars in humanities and pedagogy. Beyond the moral imagination, both Tess and Arno remind us that a political imagination (grappling with issues of power, inequality and social justice) is central to medical practice and the shaping of medical culture. The political imagination, too, is shaped metaphorically through a series of metaphor translations.

Arno is a specialist in Type 1 diabetes. The descriptor 'diabetes' itself is a metaphor, derived from the Greek *diabainein*, meaning a 'siphon', referring to frequent urination as a key symptom. Following the derivation of 'metaphor' from the Greek *metaphora* – literally to 'transfer' – what is more unsettling than the inauguration of a chronic illness such as diabetes? It is the embodiment of metaphor, as the tenor/source of 'health' is transferred across to a vehicle/target of 'illness' demanding a new imagination of life. As Arno pointed out, it is a metamorphosis. Just as metaphors can be discomfiting, so patients usually do not see the arrival of this bodily shift into illness as an opportunity, but as a threat. The shift is from relative stability into instability, and the doctor's work, in diagnosis, treatment, management and prognosis, is to help the patient to recover some stability through exploring the 'life metaphor' of the illness, or the nature of the shift, again, from the tenor/source ('health') to the vehicle/target ('chronic illness') that now shapes the patient's being.

Central to this process of metamorphosis is education – for both doctors and patients, often in collaboration – and central to such education is identity formation. The doctor inhabits a culture with a history of established process for bringing about an identity construction in which the education of the 'healer' occurs through a kind of ordination into a techno-medical priesthood. As Arno explained, this stacking up of identity metaphors is described by the sociologist Pierre Bourdieu as forming an 'habitus' (a circumscribed identity) within a 'field' of practice and social relations. 'Fields' introduce potential barriers through privilege and difference – for example, the exercise of power, where the doctor typically has authority over the patient's 'medical condition' in terms of its visibility and management, most importantly through a set of metaphors.

As the diabetic patient plays out his or her 'body-as-siphon' (neatly fitting the 'body as machine' master metaphor), so he or she becomes more transparent to the endocrinologist/diabetologist. At the same moment, the diabetologist remains opaque to the patient, communicating in scientific language supposedly cleansed of metaphor. The habitus of the doctor and the habitus of the patient barely overlap as professional distance is maintained.

'Patient' literally means 'one who suffers', while 'doctor' means 'learned person' and 'teacher'. But the Bourdieuian Field is also a place of contestation and struggle. Metaphor machinations characterize the Field as a site for the playing out in particular of didactic metaphors shaping both medical and patient cultures, discussed at length in Chapter 4 – the body as machine, medicine as conflict, illness as a journey. Again, will the forces in the Field play out historically to produce a new master metaphor, possibly about a feminine 'holding' rather than a masculine 'violence'; or will the master metaphors dissipate as a complex of collaborating metaphors emerges? Even by talking about 'forces' in a Field, we play into the conflict metaphor. What if we follow Wallace Stevens' (1954) advice in the poem 'St John and the Back-Ache' – that the world is 'presence' and not 'force'?

Redistributing metaphor capital through the dialogical imagination

Arno reminded us that Bourdieu's work is complemented by that of Jacques Rancière, who describes a distribution of cultural capital as a distribution of 'sensibility'. Privileged pockets of culture decide how and what the rest of us shall notice, or how we use our senses: a notion developed by Rancière from the work of the German philosopher and social commentator Walter Benjamin, drawing, in turn, from Marx. The political, then, intersects with the ethical and aesthetic. The implication of this distribution, not merely of 'taste' but of basic sensory experience, is that the use of metaphor is subject to structures of power and privilege. This is most obvious in doctor–patient encounters, when patient metaphors for illness are discounted in favour of doctors' (or medicine's) metaphors for disease. But such privileged use of metaphor is structured by the hierarchies of healthcare – doctors over medical students, doctors over nurses and other healthcare workers, and even across specialties, when surgeons cheekily stereotype, say, dermatology as 'dermaholiday'. Again, metaphors are key to political machinations whereby hospital managers can – within the master economic metaphors of healthcare as machine and commodity, and the essence of human life as 'productivity' – see even senior doctors as 'expendable' or 'surplus to requirement'. Such metaphors leach out into medical education, where 'standardization' is a master trope, turning pedagogy into a production line with a master trope of 'linearity'. 'It's the economy, stupid!' stains healthcare.

Arno continued with the observation that the composite master metaphor for medical education has been to reproduce the 'doctor as hero' identity, although this is being challenged by new 'softer' metaphors of collaboration – patient-centredness and interprofessional teamwork. Arguing that the doctor as hero ('I don't need no stinkin' advice') is counterproductive – offering an obstructive identity in postmodern times – Arno suggests that alternative embodied metaphors are developing in medical culture and should be encouraged to root and flower through medical education.

Since medical education can be seen as a moral education as much as an intellectual and pragmatic one, the education of 'virtue' must embody dimensions of social justice, collaboration and critical consciousness, moving from dogma to dialogue. To follow dogma is to shape practice through a set of inviolable principles laid down by an authority – the metaphor of the 'ruler' as both sovereign person and baseline measuring device, and the fount of wisdom in linear pedagogy. Dialogue is sensitive and sensible conversational narrative, returning us to case-based, situational or context-defined ethics (casuistry), where, if principles arise, they are common to a string of cases, and so are not faceless. There is no dialogue without recognition of the value of the face of the Other, along with sacrifice of 'selfsame' identity and self-biased certainties. Emmanuel Levinas' 'Other', which we must face, or give a face to, becomes both emblem and leading metaphor for this new conversational, narrative medicine, which is both ethical and political, but above all is aesthetic, for we must appreciate the face of the Other before we evaluate.

In the consultation and the clinical team, the doctor moves from chairperson for discussion to interlocutor, promoting what Mikhail Bakhtin (1982) calls 'dialogism' and the 'dialogic imagination'. Key to dialogism is to counter mere 'reproduction' with 'production' of insights and innovations, moving us on into new territory. In Jeffery Donaldson's (2015) term, as metaphor can be described as A = B, so the dialogical imagination is a metaphor producing process as A = B, B = C and so forth. Arno reminds us that the doctor's role in this, as a producer of identity, is to bear witness to the mystery of the Other. In dialogue with patients, this does not mean the outright suspension of medical metaphors in order to allow breathing space for the patient's metaphors. Rather, it involves a redistribution of sensibility capital in which metaphor claims bear equal weight as a new, 'blended' metaphoric space is developed (Fauconnier and Turner 2002).

This is necessarily a liminal space for both patients and doctors, and, as such, invites high tolerance of ambiguity. As Arno suggests, this is not the same as the familiar notion of 'reflection' (which can readily become navel-gazing). Rather, it is best described through a range of metaphors: as a freeing of sensibility, a waiting for and waiting upon (again, bearing witness), the doctor as contemplative beggar, and entry into what Heidegger referred to as a 'Clearing' in which Being is disclosed. Paulo Freire (1973) equated this metaphor complex with education as the 'practice of freedom'.

Here is a simple yet important example. Patients discussing level of pain are commonly asked: 'how strong is the pain?' on a 1–10 scale. Deborah Padfield, as discussed previously, as both visual artist and chronic pain sufferer, has developed a set of visual images that can be used to better describe both the experience and the meaning of pain, often in combination. Each of these visual images affords a metaphor for pain. Sensibility capital is immediately and positively redistributed. The doctor does not teach the patient, but facilitates his or her learning, as a form of empowerment.

Both Tess and Arno brought an enviable light touch, elegance and intellectual rigour to their presentations, framing subsequent discussions.

Murky metaphors and medical slang

Metaphors and resemblances are vital to effective medical work, but they can also mislead and confuse. I have already argued that master metaphors such as 'medicine as war' and 'the body as machine' can be misleading for contemporary medicine entering an era of patient-centred and team-based work. These metaphors may be outmoded, not shared by patients and even destructive, as Susan Sontag argued so vociferously, where they stigmatize.

'Smiling assassin' is a metaphor for insincerity, or worse, somebody who on the outside is agreeable and pleasant, but who harbours negative thoughts or feelings. In psychoanalysis, this is referred to as a 'passive aggressive' personality or 'smiling demolition', while Homi Bhabha (2004), writing on postcolonialism, refers to 'sly civility' – the oppressed 'slave' of the colonialist 'master' outwardly showing civility, servility and humility, but inwardly spitting venom. In medicine and healthcare, as Tess Jones showed, the rhetorical work of metaphors – outwardly positive (even gentle), or neutral – can disguise ethical conundrums and paradoxes, such as 'pillow angel', 'destination therapies', and 'innovative treatment/innovative care'.

We have seen again and again that metaphors are not all 'motherhood and apple pie'. While early in this book I placed emphasis upon the role of metaphor as turning the ordinary into the extraordinary, this movement can go into either the light or the dark, the uplifting or the troubling. Of course, language and life are both. However, dark metaphors in medicine can be troubling because they often lead us into ethically tortuous territory. Originally stimulating metaphors can become 'dead' or 'the walking dead' (the zombie, discussed in the following Chapter 11, which has a creative face too) as euphemism, as idiom, or as overused. Bland metaphors, in turn, can become murky, and murky metaphors can become malignant. Chapter 4 traces how didactic metaphors can follow this now tarnished, once Yellow, Brick Road.

Nicole Piemonte, a scholar in medical humanities and applied ethics working at Arizona State University, presented a talk at the symposium entitled 'Caustic Creativity: Why Backstage Gallows Humor and Medical Slang Die Hard'. I drew on Nicole's (Piemonte 2015) article 'Last Laughs: Gallows Humor and Medical Education' in the section on medical slang in Chapter 3. I have talked to many doctors who politely dismiss the notion that much, if any, medical slang is used any more in their work setting. I wonder what they make of the website http://messybeast.com/dragonqueen/medical-acronyms.htm, where a raft of medical (and veterinary) slang from around the world has been gathered by an anonymous author, showing a disturbing, metaphor-rich underbelly to medical culture. This further confirms that what is repressed or denied in the culture returns in a distorted form.

Nicole noted how visual metaphors could be used positively as a postmodern 'Art of Memory' (Yates 1966) through Picnomics for Medicine (www.picmonic. com/pathways/medicine). This covers body systems or topics such as anatomy and epidemiology. For example, Vitamin B deficiency is illustrated as a multi-metaphoric mnemonic. An image 'stands in' for a piece of information as a mnemonic, such as a stomach with stitches = a gastric bypass; a prune-throwing anemone = pernicious anaemia; or 12 Viking bees = B12. The images then work on visual puns, lively associations. Anyway, you get the picture. If you don't, then please look at this image on the website, as it could not be reproduced here.

Many medical students and junior doctors, hard-pressed to find time to revise for tests and examinations, would, I am sure, swap this wordy book you are now reading on metaphors in medicine for the Picnomics for Medicine website, the latter pragmatic rather than gnomic! They will mostly be unaware that they are joining a well-trodden historical tradition of mnemonics used in Medieval and Renaissance periods in particular to educate the memory, brilliantly described by the historian Frances Yates (1966).

But look, for example, at the 'Cardiovascular Basics: Cardiac Cycle – Systole' (www.picmonic.com/pathways/medicine/courses/standard/physiology-184/cardiovascular-basics-287) – all pipes and hard edges; in other words, the body as machine. Please, reader, go back to one of the classic texts, such as Samuel Osherson and Lorna AmaraSingham's (1981) chapter 'The machine metaphor in medicine', to remind yourself of the historical origins of this metaphor and why it matters that we reconsider the metaphor's value. Picnomics, too, as Nicole noted, fails to foster critique, reflection or invention. It does nothing to educate for tolerance of ambiguity in the workplace once knowledge has been acquired in the marketplace of Picnomic inquiry. While Picnomics outwardly draws on metaphor (as likeness), it does not educate for thinking with metaphors, but follows the common epistemic route of rational scientific knowledge acquisition that denies the value of thinking with metaphor (and then 'thinking' at all).

Such denial, or repression, of metaphor, as already explored, has consequences, as the metaphorical stain is admitted in the backstage rather than the frontstage of medicine – as backroom dark, or 'gallows', humour mainly directed at patients, and negative stereotyping directed at both patients and colleagues. Nicole reminds us that this is not just a coping mechanism (for example in intensive care, where gallows humour is common) but also involves the blunt exercise of 'rapid-truthing', or the leaping over political correctness for the acid truth (sensitively discussing the condition of a neurologically devastated newborn in a clinical team meeting, 'Bill' gets tired of beating about the bush, as he sees it, suggesting that the baby 'is more likely to *be* second base than playing second base').

Psychoanalytically (I can feel the rush of wind as those medical students and juniors run back to their first base of Picnomics at the very mention of 'psychoanalysis'!), the inability to cope with their own distress (or medicine's collective distress) may lead to an attitude of hardening to their patients' distress, disguised as 'professional veneer'. This reinforces the dominant epistemology of scientific objectivity (people are patients and patients are symptoms) and ontology (a focus on your own distress or emotional condition will cloud your rational judgement).

In this way, not only can doctors treat symptoms objectively through the medical gaze, but also they can enjoy symptoms and suffering in a paradoxical embrace, with even a relish for the abject ('Wow – I've never seen a blueberry muffin baby, can I have a closer look?').

Let us rehearse the symptoms of the blueberry muffin baby (the resemblance resonates with the 'pillow angel' as a mollification) as described by Nicole: 'congenital blindness and deafness, jaundice, low birthweight, mineral deposits on the brain, enlarged spleen and liver, seizures'. Once considered the baby's body's road map for rubella (German measles, now rare), 'blueberry muffin' symptoms now indicate a differential diagnosis, including metastatic neuroblastoma (extracranial solid cancer tumours) and cytomegalovirus. Usually, technical language acts as filter and defence, distancing patient from doctor, but here the shield against the glare of terrible suffering is a metaphor, a likeness to a delicious cake. This 'food for thought' is an ethical provocation discussed at length in Chapters 5 and 6.

Metaphors and slang are, again, shields against truth or the exercise of inauthenticity. Nicole reminded us that Heidegger, in *Being and Time*, notes that inauthenticity is characterized by a turning away from the terrible face of Being, as Truth: 'For the most part, [a human being] covers up its ownmost Being-towards-death, fleeing in the face of it.' Characteristically, as already noted, and as Julie Bligh pointed out so clearly at the symposium, we resort to euphemisms in the face of the sublime or the terrible unknown: 'she passed away yesterday', 'he's gone to a better place', 'the baby looks poorly'.

Backstage gallows humour can be seen as part of the constellation of defence mechanisms that medical students acquire through socialization, including objectivity and professional detachment, and dark metaphors offer the glue that keeps this constellation of invulnerability intact. It is, suggests Nicole, a form of 'calculative thinking' that is 'seductive because it works'. In the face of this, medicine needs new formative metaphors and narratives, such as 'slower', 'intentional' and 'open to wonder' thinking and being, which are common currency amongst poets. Cultivating a 'slow medical education' demands an education of the moral imagination, requiring maieutic, not didactic, education, an education of exposure rather than telling, based on the metaphor of 'indirection' and not that of 'direction'.

I can see many objecting that surely, undergraduate medical education is already too prolonged and could be shortened. But this would be missing the point of using 'slow' as a metaphor for 'intense' and 'deep'. To push the metaphor to its limits, and without literalizing, slow medical education could be like slow sex. It does not have to be prolonged, but rather, deepened in quality. It is important, too, that such education is in itself authentic and not duplicitous, to encourage authenticity and not duplicity. Medicine must not speak out of the side of its mouth, but must be straight talking while sensitive. For example, Picnomics works with visual sideways associations, and is basically a form of telling and not a door into debate – as Nicole notes, we are otherwise back to those pernicious prunes! In short, again, we need a 'slow' medical education and to recruit to medical schools the particularly gifted educators who understand what this means.

Returning to Heidegger, the person who suffers requires a doctor who sees him or her not as a 'what' but as a 'who' (Being); who, especially in chronic illness, cannot be summed up or grasped in a restricted consultation, but must be experienced as a person projecting towards a horizon of cumulative knowing (Time). Medicine's epistemological frame (let's wrap this up with a clear diagnosis and treatment plan) works against such ontological unfolding (treat the person, not just the symptom).

Dissolving metaphors: lost in translation

Metaphors are the means by which productive translations are made between the known and the as yet unknown. At the time of writing, meetings are taking place at the highest level between American and Russian diplomats to find a way to solve the complex political crisis in Syria and thus end the war. In one round of talks in November 2015 in Vienna, the Russians accused the Americans that their bombing of so-called Islamic State troops was yielding 'no concrete results'. Metaphorically, so far, so good – nobody is thinking in terms of real concrete blocks, but of tangible outcomes. Later, speaking on Russian television, the Foreign Minister Sergey Lavrov suggested that Washington was 'pulling its punches' against the Islamic State. Lavrov, however, did not use that precise boxing metaphor but an idiosyncratic Russian one, in which the USA 'looks like a cat that wants to eat a fish but doesn't want to wet its feet' (http://foreignpolicy.com/2015/11/18/russia-insults-u-s-war-strategy-with-weird-cat-metaphor/). This is new to my ear, and actually, nothing is lost in translation (see the section below). All the elements are known, but their combination is striking.

Colleagues at Maastricht University medical school told me that, in Dutch, the desire to produce 'concrete results' of the kind the Russians alluded to above is summed up in the metaphor 'to give hands and feet' (*handen en voeten geven*) – the idea that only physical work translates proposals into concrete realities (Van Nes *et al.* 2010). This metaphor can be 'understood' logically in English, but it does not have the same impact: for example, 'it was hands-down the best proposal'.

What metaphor conundrums and solutions present themselves in medical translation, when, for example, a non-English-speaking patient presents at a hospital where none of the medical or healthcare staff speak his or her language? A medical interpreter is then needed. This may seem like a straightforward act of 'making concrete' and 'making transparent' what the doctor and the patient say and do. However, 'translation' itself is a metaphor, and the waters of translation are already murky. Literary scholars call for creative and poetic translations, not simply a crude and literal mirroring, while poststructuralist philosophers call for 'hospitality' in reception of the 'Other' language, whereby mutual existence is possible (Farquhar and Fitzsimons 2011). Was hospitality shown on the American side when Sergey Lavrov said that the USA 'looks like a cat that wants to eat a fish but doesn't want to wet its feet'? Or did this merely raise a combination of wry smiles and knitted brows?

One symposium participant, Teodora Manea, is a philosopher and medical ethicist who also works as a medical translator across three languages – English (her adopted language), Romanian (her first language) and German. Imagine, again, a non-English-speaking patient arriving at an Accident and Emergency department with acute abdominal pain, at a loss as to how to describe the onset, location and severity of the pain. The doctor is unable to explain that he suspects that this is a gallstone that has migrated from the gallbladder and is lodging in the bile duct. How might 'gallstone' translate into terms a layperson might understand? This is not big enough to be a stone, or even a pebble, and 'grit' does not do the job. The conversation, with the patient in increasing pain, reaches an impasse. The work of the translator is to explain to the patient whatever the doctor says, with clarity. This is achieved largely through metaphor, but the terrain is slippery.

It's between your legs

Following Lakoff and Johnson, Teo reminded us that metaphors are embedded in specific languages and are not universal; and to attempt to literally translate a metaphor from one language to another is a compound error (Martinez-Hernaez 2013 describes 'cultural' metaphors, or culture-specific metaphors; Ahmed *et al.* 1992 repeat the warning about culture specificity for food resemblances, as noted in Chapters 5 and 6; and Taussig 2001, amongst other anthropologists and ethnographers, warns of the dangers of universalizing metaphors). Teo gave three specific examples from her own experience: one regarding bodily parts (the groin); one regarding biological entities (blood platelets); and a third regarding specific diseases (clubfoot).

While medical interpreting assumes bridging between the host's and the patient's languages, and positions the interpreter as invisible, the reality is that interpretation happens in a live context, where the interpreter is an agent and not just a facilitator, and 'bridging' is disrupted by issues of what is lost in translation. Illustrative examples quickly bring this alive. The 'groin' discussed involved a male patient in cardiology undergoing an angiogram, in which a catheter is introduced into an artery in the groin area. 'Groin' is derived from the Old English *grynde*, meaning an 'abyss', 'hollow' or 'depression' – this is some way from the actual 'fold' between the thigh and the abdomen. 'Groin' is already a troublesome word. Doctors refer to the 'inguinal' area – which is of no help to the patient's understanding – but describing the groin as 'between the legs' muddies the waters even more!

In languages other than English, the equivalent to 'groin' can refer to architectural features such as the edge between intersecting vaults. Teo informed us that in German, the nearest equivalent is *leiste*, which literally means a 'thin, long piece of wood' or a 'strip'. A metaphor in German for the inguinal region is, then, a 'narrow bar' – literally fine, but in English this could mean a tight passageway in a pub, or a thin piece of metal; and now we are miles away from the groin. In Romanian, there is no common language-specific term for groin, and the next usual approximation will be 'between legs'. Along with the unspecificity of the language, the interaction between the (older) male patient and the (younger) female interpreter complicated the dialogue even further.

If you don't have enough of these you will bleed

Teo presented a case study: very young parents who do not speak English have a child with a genetic condition leading to thrombocytopenia, a dramatically reduced platelet count. Treatment involves repeated transfusions with a danger of internal and cerebral bleeding. How should the interpreter explain 'platelets' to the parents? 'Platelet' means 'small plate', and platelets are unusual in having no cell nucleus. They are invisible entities, and only someone with enough biological knowledge knows exactly what they are. Should the interpreter translate 'platelets' from the source language with the equivalent name of an artefact? In a fraction of a second, the interpreter should *catch* the medical metaphor and find an equivalent medical metaphor in the other language. The nearest equivalent is 'plaques'. Further, is it important that the interpreter does not necessarily have medical knowledge? Direct translation of technical terms into another language does not help, just as doctors' unreflective use of medical jargon with most patients will simply fall on deaf ears.

How much medical knowledge should the interpreter have? Should an interpreter know that platelets (which help your blood clot) are different from red blood cells (which carry oxygen) and white blood cells (which fight infections)? What can an interpreter do with terms like *thrombocytopenia*? How does she find, in the rapid flux of a dialogue, the perfect equivalent for complicated Latin or Greek names? For this case, Teo's knowledge of classical languages was helpful, but this was a happy coincidence, and not something that is required of a medical interpreter. The interpreter's own experience of her cat having had, in the past, *panleukopenia* (which derives from a low white blood cell count) was useful to similarly transform and adapt *thrombocytopenia* to her maternal language. Teo noted in her presentation that 'knowledge is situated, incidental, the construction and flow of it is hard to control'. Metaphors can both help and hinder with the construction and flow of knowledge in these pressured situations of translation.

A foot like a horse

Finally, a non-English-speaking woman, pregnant, has a diagnosis after a scan of congenital *talipes equinovarus* (CTEV) or 'club foot'. Equinovarus – 'like a horse' – is already a poor metaphor for club foot, in which ground contact is made on the outer forward edge of the foot. Entering this territory of explanation offers a potential minefield. 'Club' has many associations in English beyond the club as a blunt(ed) instrument. The young woman may only have heard 'club' in the context of 'clubbing' or dancing. Teo resorted to non-verbal expressions in explaining 'club foot', 'using the hands to metaphorize the feet', as she puts it.

Here are Teo's four conclusions from her thought-provoking presentation:

1   For medical interpreting, metaphors may complicate more than clarify things.
2   Some dead metaphors still contain culturally specific representations of body and illness.
3   The dead metaphors have to be revived and re-tailored for a different language.
4   Mastering a language presupposes awareness of its metaphors!

Historically 'dead' metaphors that still walk, and haunt

Mick Mangan is Professor of Drama at Loughborough University. He has a spar-kling CV as theatre director, dramaturge, literary manager, reviewer and play-wright as well as educator and academic. Through a collaborative reading of Andrew Marvell's poem 'A Dialogue between the Soul and the Body' (*c*.1650), Mick reminded us that historically 'dead' metaphors walk amongst us and can still provoke. In his now classic text *The Philosophy of Rhetoric*, I.A. Richards (1965, p. 101) insisted that 'This favorite old distinction between dead and living metaphors (itself a two-fold metaphor) ... needs a drastic re-examination'. Mar-vell's poem makes 'metaphor' redundant, in the sense that all the language in the poem is metaphoric – every plain description is immediately moved to another plane of understanding and provocation as the soul and the body, in turns, deride each other's limitations.

Mick asked us in what sense the 'soul', as Marvell describes it, makes any sense to us in a materialist age, in which the medical body is the master meta-phor for existence. This is a product, in turn, of scientific empiricism and ration-alism, in which only the literal and material, or that which can be exposed to sense-based and instrument-based experimental manipulation, matters. Mick reminded us of the philosopher Gilbert Ryle's description of 'the ghost in the machine' for the relationship between the corporeal and the incorporeal (soul, mind, consciousness, spirit, self). Ryle then reproduces medicine's master meta-phor of body as machine. I became acutely aware that 'metaphor' was replacing Marvell's 'soul' in our discourse, as a catch-all. The more we defined, dissected, analysed and appreciated 'metaphor', the less precise the term became, and the easier it was to mercilessly expand its territory rather than set limits on its defini-tion. This problem is redoubled when we use the term 'embodied' metaphor, so that we not only persuade ourselves of the absolute pervasiveness of metaphors but also imagine that we can tangibly account for their sensuous presences or multiplicities. So, the 'tree' becomes a metaphor for aspiration, the thorn bush a metaphor for 'entanglement', and the 'bog' a metaphor for despair.

Returning to science's literalism, quantum physics has already introduced uncertainties into such materialist assumptions, yet medicine proceeds without recognition of 'alter-bodies' or embodied soul, which acquires the status of a dead metaphor. Yet, it ghosts around as talk turns to death or to 'meaning'. 'Soul' still haunts. Indeed, psychology, or the logos (logic, meaning) of psyche (soul), has spent the last century trying to shake off the psyche from the psychological, reducing soul to brain, thus halving Descartes' vision. Contemporary post-Jungian Archetypal Psychology has rescued 'soul' and renamed it as 'imagination' (another bogey metaphor for scientific psychology and psychiatry) (Hillman 1977).

Marvell describes the body as a prison for the 'soul enslav'd', 'With bolts of bone' 'hung up ... in chains/Of nerves, and arteries, and veins'. Yet, the head is 'vain' and the heart 'double', suggesting that body and soul are conjoined, but reason refuses this condition while the heart accepts it. The body replies that the soul 'Has made me live to let me die', implying that the body is temporary, while the soul is eternal. The soul, in its alliance with death, asks the body why it is so interested in preserving that 'which me destroys'; the body is paradoxically 'constrained' to 'endure/Diseases, but, what's worse, the cure' as it is 'shipwreck'd into health again'. Marvell seems to be asking: what meaning can we give the suffering body? This will be the subject of the concluding part of the following Chapter 11, where I discuss the work of another symposium participant, the performance artist and academic Martin O'Brien.

Marvell's last stanza in this dialogue between soul and body suggests that one does not exist without the other, while the soul brings an imagination of suffering to the body. In other words, we must make meaning of our suffering and symptoms. This is a basic tenet of archetypal psychology (Hillman 1977). The soul brings 'maladies' of a psychological and emotional variety too: 'the cramp of hope', 'the palsy shakes of fear', 'The pestilence of love', 'hatred's hidden ulcer', 'Joy's cheerful madness' and 'sorrow's other madness'. The architecture of the body and the mind, says Marvell, are unnatural, or work against nature; the poem concludes: 'So architects do square and hew/Green trees that in the forest grew.'

Music as a metaphor for the medical consultation

Steve Reid is Professor of Primary Healthcare at the University of Cape Town, Faculty of Health Sciences, but has worked for many years as a rural doctor. He is passionate about music, playing second violin in a string quartet, and argues that music can act as a metaphor for the medical consultation. Paul Haidet (2007) had argued that the consultation resembles jazz, in the sense that much of it is improvisational – unscripted and developed in the moment. There must also be harmony between the patient's expression and the doctor's response. Steve develops Paul Haidet's model through focus on patterns – first, a rhythm (the 'groove') and second, a chord progression (the 'head'). Once this is established, soloists have a base from which to improvise.

There are standard templates for setting up the groove and the head, classically taught in family medicine as a set of communication capabilities: 'deep', attentive listening; necessary interruptions, because the consultation time is limited; extracting key information, perhaps supplemented by a physical or psychiatric examination; absorbing the patient's chief concern – rather than just focusing on the chief complaint – extracted from the patient's necessarily fragmentary narrative; and placing the individual in the context of the population while considering an evidence-based intervention. Key to this is an appreciation of metaphor, used on both sides of the consultation-as-conversation, but not just in the verbal register, as Steve notes. The non-verbal flow of the consultation is key, too.

Much as the individual patient is unique, most patients will fit a smaller number of template patterns: patients seen on a frequent basis; formulaic illness scripts readily applicable to presenting symptoms; typical symptom patterns for a coherent social group (by ethnicity, gender, age). 'Pattern recognition', after all, is the key diagnostic method for experienced clinicians, as detailed in Chapters 5 and 6. 'Solos' here are typically based on predictable chord progressions. But what if a patient comes in with a wild solo that catches the doctor off-guard? Musicians who love improvisation cherish these moments as the music is invented, but this is still against a dependable matrix – notes may be bent or flattened ('blue notes'); the patient may wail atonally and his or her symptoms seem to follow suit (an unexpected pattern), but tonality provides a tether, a point of comparison from which to work.

Taking classical music as a template rather than jazz, Steve reminds us that 'improvisation' here really means 'interpretation' of the composer's original score. This makes sense in medicine – templates exist as evidence-based guidelines, but the consultation is about the individual patient and his or her unique context, and how this is interpreted through the tacit knowledge of the doctor, described by Gabbay and Le May (2010) as 'clinical mindlines' and 'practice-based evidence' rather than evidence-based practice. Disease histories follow classic scores, but unfold as unique illnesses, because every person experiences the disease differently. But patterns, too – familiar scores – can induce boredom and habitual response, both dangerous qualities in medicine. Music as a metaphor for medicine can, then, teach doctors to be experts in both patterns and the breaking of patterns.

The same musical metaphorical eye and ear can be applied to clinical or management meetings. A clinician might metaphorize such meetings in terms of symptoms: the meeting developed a small bowel obstruction; its focus was interrupted by excessive pressure behind the eye, and the meeting became glaucomic; a fracture occurred that will be difficult to mend. A psychoanalyst might see repression, displacement, denial and other defence mechanisms at play in a meeting full of tension; and in another meeting, anal retentives retain control by sitting on information that they refuse to share, while anal expulsives explode without much provocation and behave in a thoroughly shitty manner. Freud has left us with a host of powerful metaphors that are both embodied and create a 'felt sense' just by their use in language. Steve asks us to look at the ebb and flow of meetings in terms of orchestration of talk and silences, noises and gaps:

What is spoken – words, phrases, arguments, proposals, decisions.
What is thought – mutterings, ideas, arguments, reflections.
What is assumed – whispers, meanings, motivations, power.
What is unconscious – feelings, intuition, forgotten things.
What is absent – distractions, silences, gaps, lack of presence.

(Used with permission of the author)

The metaphor of the orchestra for the meeting also brings an overall aesthetic value to bear on the meeting: could we bear the music made? How was the meeting orchestrated and conducted, and by whom? Did the music inspire, soothe or grate? What was the overall tone? Steve concludes:

> Ultimately one can navigate through an experience to make it musical or visual even though it seems not to be; the metaphor allows us to shift our perception of the experience, which can stimulate new and different actions. If music is able to take us out of our sets of assumptions into a different state of being then we need to re-negotiate our role as we re-integrate into the original environment.

(Used with permission of the author)

Martin O'Brien's film excerpts of recent work, discussed at the close of the following Chapter 11, and Steve's emphasis upon the importance of music as a metaphor for the medical consultation and the medical meeting brought home to me the central importance of the performative and non-verbal in the field of medical metaphors. There is far too much emphasis upon the verbal in the literature on metaphors, even though Lakoff and Johnson have popularized the notion that essentially all 'linguistic' metaphors are embodied, and the 'performance poetry' movement (with its origins in Dartington College of Arts) has claimed that writing is not cerebral recirculation of words and phrases, but an activity of placement of marks (inscriptions) in time and space (Hall 2013).

More attention needs to be focused on the historical and cultural circulation of medical metaphors as performed activities and not merely linguistic descriptions and abstractions. The research implications of this are enormous – corpus analysis of written texts and transcriptions of dialogue would give way to analysis of videotape examples, for instance. This book merely scratches the surface of this relatively unexplored field. However, let us open the door to this world of metaphor in medicine as performed, and embrace its radical wing as performed by 'sick patients' with something important to say about the status of 'sickness' – the subject of the final part of the following chapter.

11 'Thinking with metaphors in medicine: the state of the art'

Part II: the tournament joust

Sailing to a land called 'Metaphor'

To recap: 19 of us exchanged ideas on 'thinking with metaphors in medicine' at a symposium staged at Dartington Hall, Devon. The day before the symposium, Britain had voted to leave the European Union, a tragic decision based on the hapless metaphor of 'closing our borders' to immigrants and making a bad joke out of our deliberately cosmopolitan gathering deep in the archetypally English Devon countryside. I thought of printing T-shirts in favour of migrants: 'Migrants are Skilling Britain' (to oppose the crass slogan 'migrants are killing Britain').

At the opening of the conference, tongue firmly in cheek, I projected a cartoon that appeared as a cover to the Archetypal Psychology journal *Spring*, 1980. The cartoon shows a man with a wry smile wandering through a hilly landscape with trees. The man is looking at a tree that has a sign on it: 'Metaphor for Aspiration'. A bird sits on a branch in the tree with the label: 'Metaphor for Lyricism'. The earth underfoot has a sign: 'Metaphor for Stability'. The path the man is on is signed: 'Metaphor for the Possible'. A gate by the side of the path has: 'Metaphor for Limits'. And so on. I showed it as a warning. Once in the land of metaphor, the temptation is to see everything as a metaphor, or to habitually metaphorize the literal. I call this 'bad poetry' and have already discussed such a mindset in Chapter 7 as a form of madness; indeed, a central symptom of psychosis.

I hoped, then, that we would not metaphorize everything in sight. I need not have worried. Steve Reid, a doctor and musician from South Africa, had sent this wry message just prior to the symposium:

A LAND CALLED METAPHOR

In June, 19 of us will assemble at Totnes harbour to board an old vessel, the Dartington. She is untested with this crew, but built on a long tradition of process and reflection, camaraderie and laughter. Captain Bleakley has stated his intention of leaving the country of Medicine, and crossing the sea of Humanities to reach an intriguing and exotic land called Metaphor, which we have all read about and are keen to explore. An ancient civilization, they apparently communicate mostly through gesture (shoulders) and innuendo (eyebrows) rather than words. The rest is up to you. The navigators Arno and Tess know more or less where it is, and will set our course. But none of us have actually been there before, and the crew is new to one another. There are some hardy veterans of lengthy dangerous voyages, who are lucky to have returned alive. These are the sailors who know the ropes of Process, and will ensure our safe passage through the narrows. And there are some newcomers to this journeying on the sea, who are accustomed to life on land, to more certainty and less fluidity. While they will lend a hand at the ropes, they will probably try to avoid getting seasick by keeping their eyes peeled on the horizon for the destination, the more solid shores of Clinical Medicine, Teaching and Publications. The drunkards of course will use any excuse for a party, and keep us laughing, reminding us of why we allowed ourselves to be press-ganged into joining this expedition in the first place. It promises to be an interesting journey.

(Reproduced with permission of the author)

We talked of Dartington's origins as a grand country house in the fourteenth century and of the possibility that jousting was practiced, as was common amongst the nobility of the time. How would our jousting with metaphors proceed? What would be the fallout? We came up with several themes, discussed below. Retaining a focus on metaphors in medicine, we agreed that:

1   *Metaphors are best appreciated through other metaphors.* This is a refor-mulation of what has widely become known as 'critical reflexivity' (Bleak-ley 1999), a development of 'reflective practice'. Critical reflexivity is a reformulation of Nietzsche's form of philosophical relativism as the 'trans-valuation of values'. This does not mean that 'anything goes' – rather, it requires, as Arno Kumagai was at pains to point out in his presentation, that one's assumptions and biases must be tested against other perspectives in dialogue. It is important to examine what values drive your assumptions and whether these values need to be re-examined. Of course, throughout the symposium, this is precisely what we were doing in terms of medicine's framing or master metaphors.

2   *Metaphors are on a spectrum from the sublime and imaginative, to the benign (on the way out, as overused), to the downright misleading or malign.* As Shane Neilson (2015) shows in his work on pain, the appropria-tion of engineering metaphors to map and explain pain is of little use to patients and clinicians and should be rethought. Metaphors can mislead, cloud or close down thinking. Hence, again, we need critical reflexivity in the face of metaphors – why this metaphor, now? Metaphors have life histo-ries like those of minor celebrities – once peaking, popular and game chang-ing, now on the decline or clichéd, and now dead and forgotten.

3   *Dominant, didactic or master metaphors that have shaped medicine histori-cally need not be replaced by new dominant master metaphors but by a*

multiplicity of metaphors fit for purpose, or context specific. The question is: can we tolerate this fan, or spray? Will it be unbearable cacophony rather than the excitement of the carnival?

4   *A new master metaphor may be emerging in medicine – that of 'transparency'.* But beware – this may be a misleading metaphor that disguises greater opacity, working against its supposed intentions.

Each of these four points moves current debates about metaphor in medicine forward. The symposium developed both plumb lines (sounding out ideas) and fault lines (ideas cracking open to reveal pitfalls). While celebrating the power and beauty of metaphors, we were particularly interested in fault lines, such as ageing metaphors turning bad, even rotting and stinking within the body of medical culture. Perhaps such metaphors can act as manure for the growth of new forms.

1 Metaphors are best appreciated through the lens of metaphor

We agreed that metaphors could not be talked about in any depth without using metaphors (the medium is the message, to use Marshall McLuhan's metaphor, and to risk the rapids of alliteration). This does not mean mixing metaphors. For example, metaphor can be grasped through another metaphor as an immersive medium – such as standing in the river of metaphor, or taking metaphor as the air we breathe. Metaphors are layered, aggregated or sedimented.

To illustrate that metaphors are best appreciated through the lens of metaphor, Tess Jones used Renée Magritte's 1937 painting *Not to Be Reproduced*, in which a figure looks into a mirror but sees the reflection of his back rather than the expected front (https://en.wikipedia.org/wiki/Not_to_be_Reproduced). The painting offers a metaphor, the title a pun. This illustrates a blended metaphor. The tenor/source and vehicle/target are one and the same person, but strikingly different because of their gazes, and are interchangeable. The metaphor works because what the person sees is not a mirror image but what is never usually revealed to the viewer. A metaphor does not mirror back a direct meaning, but raises other, surprising, meanings.

Whereas *Not to Be Reproduced* gives another layer to metaphor as the revelation of the always hidden, Magritte's earlier 1928/1929 *The Treachery of Images (This is not a pipe)* works by a different method – that of negation and pun (https://en.wikipedia.org/wiki/The_Treachery_of_Images). Here is a painting of a pipe, but the caption says, in stark denial, 'This is not a pipe.' If this is not a pipe, what is it? An image of a pipe? A smokescreen? A sign? Certainly, again, to appreciate the pun, we must think metaphorically. The image is indeed treacherous, undercutting our expectations not by an act of poverty but a sleight of hand.

Medical educators might ask why contemplating the conundrums of Magritte's *Not to Be Reproduced* and *The Treachery of Images (This is not a pipe)* is of any use to medical students. First, they open the door to considering the value of metaphors. But second, and most importantly, in educating for critical reflexivity, they educate for tolerance of ambiguity. Returning to Arno Kumagai's presentation, the key component of social justice in medicine is the education of a critical consciousness that shapes the self or identity of the doctor – not in the mould of his or her pattern of socialization, but in terms of respect for patients as the Other. The doctor looks into the mirror and sees the back of his (in Magritte's painting) own head, but is warned not to mistake this for himself. Do not reproduce yourself in the mirror of the Other, suggests Magritte. Rather, ask yourself what it is to 'face', or 'give a face to', the unseen aspects of the patient as Other. 'This is not a pipe' reinforces this lesson. Do not make rapid assumptions about what you see, even in pattern recognition, but allow yourself to be surprised. Education for tolerance of ambiguity through critical reflexivity is the formula for a complex model that has been reduced to instrumental 'empathy' (Marshall and Bleakley 2009).

To return to reflexive capacity, or metaphor-in-action, Hegel famously set out a method for knowing – an epistemology of dialectics – that focused not on how we gain knowledge of the world's objects, but on the process of inquiry or knowing itself. In other words, how does the mind work? Hegel saw an ever-present movement of inquiry between thesis (asking a question), antithesis (challenging the basis upon which the question is asked) and synthesis (shifting the question). This gives rise to what we once called 'reflection' in pedagogy (how and why did I do what I have just done?) and to critical reflexivity (what ideas or values drive and shape my assumptions and thinking process?). This is surely the pedagogy of thinking with and through metaphors, described in Chapter 9. As Jeffery Donaldson (2015) insists, metaphor is the evolutionary spark and process through which all biological transformation occurs, in life (bios) and mind (logos). Critical reflexivity, like Hegel's 'synthesis', one might assume, produces a kind of 'ambiguous clarity'. And critical reflexivity is, again, metaphor-in-action.

As Donald Schön (1990) points out, reflection is invoked not under situations of clarity and transparency, but under conditions of values conflict, uniqueness, innovation or newness, and uncertainty: ambiguity and conflict. As one of the symposium small groups concluded through discussion, 'Basically, there is a constant tension between the power push towards transparent language and messy, problematic and ambiguous language.' Metaphors emerge as an evolutionary impulse in the primordial soup or nourishing mud. Consequently, as participants in the symposium noted, 'metaphor actually can confuse, obscure and connect us with ambiguity'. In this sense, metaphor may be seen as an act of resistance to the 'technical-rational high ground' of logical judgement or the mind in certainty, clarity and the politics of transparency.

Metaphor wants us to return for a moment to the life of the stinking mudhopper emerging in the primal swamp – not to get a breathing space, but to suffocate upon our own cherished ideas. Metaphors may not seek clarity or wisdom, but bind, pull us down, confuse, and make us sick. Metaphors are potential pathogens, and our colourless and odourless (transparent) defence mechanisms of literalism and objectivity are flimsy in their presence, open to productive contamination. Metaphors are, properly, error traps – causing and not preventing productive error. 'You are wrong', says the body to the soul in Marvell's poem, discussed in the previous chapter, and the soul answers back 'you are wrong'. We are both wrong; both wrong-footed and sinister. Metaphors can mislead, but understanding how they may mislead is potentially productive.

2 Metaphors can mislead, while doctors and 'medicine watchers' may inhabit differing metaphorical territories

Metaphor can mislead, and be misunderstood or misconstrued, as an overlayering, a distorting mirror or a multiple echo. Looking into the mirror, there is a danger that we do not see the metaphor we embody or exclaim, but rather, another metaphor looking back at us (or, in Magritte's painting, the metaphor forever looking away, ignoring us, escaping, eternally frustrating Emmanuel Levinas' imperative that we give a face to the Other).

An example of misleading metaphors in public health is measures of alcohol consumption. Many countries refer to a 'standard drink', but this is not standard across countries (for example, it is 10 grams of alcohol in Australia, 14 in the USA and 20 in Japan). The UK changed descriptors from 'standard drink' to 'units' of alcohol some while ago, but 'unit' also acts as a metaphor, perceived as an instrument of governance and a confusing measuring device. 'Unit', too, sounds punitive – a prison from which you must escape, another of Lakoff and Johnson's 'container' metaphors – and so patients regularly lie to their doctors about how many units they consume in a week, already irritated by the fog of technical talk.

Research evidence (for example, Carter 1989; Macbeck and Olesen 1997; Arroliga *et al.* 2002) over 20 years suggests that patients to some extent resist the metaphors used by doctors to explain and explore patients' symptoms and prognoses, preferring to filter the doctors' metaphors through their own metaphoric lenses. For example, Macbeck and Olesen (1997) describe patients' 'ethnomechanics' – idiosyncratic ways of explaining bodily anatomy and process in the absence of technical knowledge. The authors describe patients' 'imaginative projections' as a fictional and metaphorical anatomy and physiology that nevertheless serves as a ground through which they can better adjust to and comprehend their symptoms, again adapting the doctors' medical metaphors to their idiosyncratic knowledge and values landscapes. In some sense, this is a narcissistic process of ownership of metaphors, refusing to let go to embrace the 'other' metaphor.

But medicine's metaphors, too, may be grounded in a kind of narcissism – certainties, knowing best, blind faith in science, arrogance. We may hear multiple echoes from medicine's metaphors that create eerie distortions, disguising medicine's original signal with noise. Here, we rehearse the myth of Echo and Narcissus. Medicine can be thought of as Narcissus, fond of his own voice and reflection, perhaps at the expense of others (patients and colleagues). 'Medicine watchers' – such as non-clinician medical educators, sociologists, anthropologists, psychologists, artists and humanities scholars – might be fascinated by medicine, but find that they are unable to initiate a conversation or get their voice in first, and only hear the continuous echoes of their own (critical) responses, characteristically ignored by medicine but echoing around in journals and conferences inhabited largely by the medicine watchers themselves.

Perhaps medicine has the first word and medicine watchers have the last word – but we are concerned with the in-between words, the metaphors that transform first and last words. '*Ceci n'est pas une métaphore*' – it is a pipe. The tree is a tree, not a 'metaphor for growth and change'; the hills are hills, not a 'metaphor for aspiration'; the bird is a bird, not a 'metaphor for lyricism'. Anti-sensual Neoplatonism continues to bug us. Just as medicine watchers may have itchy trigger fingers when it comes to debating the value of metaphors in medicine, doctors may need to refine their understanding of the fabric of metaphor that holds their work together; otherwise, patients – especially those presenting with mental health issues – may stitch them up with their narratives. As one small group discussion summary from the symposium said,

> Listening for the original metaphors that people or patients use – as expressions of difference or uniqueness – some people choose their own metaphors for specific reasons. Unusual use of metaphor is significant, and use of redundant metaphors can be a deliberate expression of conformity.
>
> (Reproduced with permission of the symposium participants)

3 The demise of the master metaphor: first past the 'post-'

In discussing the question 'What are the historical conditions of possibility under which new master metaphors for medicine might appear?', we heard multiple echoes, and this led us to a conclusion that, in a post-postmodern era (there is the echo), there are no master metaphors, just as there are no master discourses of the kind that characterized modernism (such as logos masculinity, oppositionalism, colonialism). We are, perhaps, beyond the imperialism of the master metaphor. Rather, where Jean-François Lyotard (1979) describes the 'postmodern condition' in terms of the emergence of multiple 'small' and 'local' narratives in the wake of the collapse of the master or 'grand' narratives of Imperialism, Fascism and State Communism, so the collapse of the grand metaphors shaping medicine will give rise to a number of local, contextualized metaphors. These will not be the recently emergent master (and both potentially patronizing and infantilizing) metaphors such as 'pathways of care' (maintained and repaired by your local health authority?) and 'personalized medicine' (gift wrapped?).

Nevertheless, as we discussed this emergent landscape of the 'post/post', we could not help but return regularly to the default position of the (masculinized) 'master' metaphor (nobody proposed the term 'mistress metaphors', although this would have been politically correct), asking which new metaphors will be first past the post. Our favourite was the replacement of irritable martial metaphors with those of 'stillness' – chronic disease was described as both 'sleeping with illness' and 'slow death' (see the section later on Martin O'Brien's work).

4 The emerging master metaphor of 'transparency' may lead to greater opacity

Modern medicine's overlooked master metaphor may be 'transparency'. Michel Foucault (1976) certainly thinks so. His masterwork on the establishment of the modern medical discourse, *The Birth of the Clinic*, describes how the medical gaze metaphorically makes the body transparent. The body is revealed through dissection and anatomical learning, and the doctor turns the fruits of this learning back onto the patient's body. This is further amplified through the physical examination employing auscultation, palpation and percussion, and then more and more sophisticated imaging, in which radiology comes to play a vital role. Radiology replaces pathology as the specialty of transparency, imaging trumping autopsy; and radiology also claims the prize for the largest canon of 'metaphoric sign naming' across the specialties over a century (Baker *et al.* 2013; Wikipedia's 'Radiopaedia: https://en.wikipedia.org/wiki/Radiopaedia), again pipping pathology.

Language follows the medical gaze. The 'patient-centred' and 'patient safety' movements in medicine promise transparency, despite the fact that the descriptors 'patient-centredness' and 'patient safety' themselves are lumbering, contested and opaque (Bleakley 2014) – 'god-terms', to borrow from Kenneth Burke. 'Patient-centredness' and 'patient safety' are metaphors for systems-based vigilant care. The patient is not literally at the 'centre' of anything, although he or she may be an attractor in a complex, adaptive system, and is never 'safe' in a world in which risk is relished. Metaphors can, then, bring opacity or even translucency – and we can never look a god-term in the eye, for this is an act of hubris, but forever live in its shadows, somewhat excluded and chilly.

Caroline Wellbery, a symposium participant, is a doctor with a PhD in Comparative Literature. She is also a longstanding, key voice in medical humanities in North America and a passionate supporter of the international spread of the medical/health humanities. She wrote long ago about medical metaphors in her graduate studies, pre-dating the interests of most, if not all, members of the Dartington symposium. In particular, she writes about the metaphoric meanings of the medical gaze in making the patient's body transparent to the doctor. I am grateful to Caroline for drawing attention to the metaphor of 'transparency' in medicine.

Yet, as Caroline notes, medicine refuses metaphor, showing a metaphor-phobia, as a result of its alliance with science's literalism and objectivity. This returns us to a discussion already raised in Chapter 1. However, doctors must grapple with metaphor every day as they grapple with the body's presentation of symptoms, make sense of patients' metaphor-laden explanations, and gaze upon the body 'as if' making it transparent. As Foucault (1976) noted, the medical gaze and a parallel highly structured language combine to manufacture transparency. The body cannot be understood without language, and language use includes metaphor; further, the body's expression or non-verbal language is always a situated performance involving metaphor.

If you doubt this, think, on your own, of a really embarrassing moment in your life and see if you blush. Chances are that you will not, as the memory is forced. However, when the memory comes upon you spontaneously, you probably will blush – but nobody is looking. Your body immediately becomes transparent to yourself. Just as we blush as if we were embarrassed in company, so, claimed the philosopher Hans Vaihinger (1924), much of our collective lives is lived according to 'guiding fictions' or metaphors such as metaphysical doctrines, religious beliefs and moral codes. We 'see through' these 'fictions' in the sense that they provide a filter or lens, but we can also learn to 'see through' such guiding fictions in the second sense of relativizing them through critical reflexivity. 'Guiding fictions' should also not be seen as truth claims, but as heuristics, rules of thumb or ways to gain purchase. The movement from relative health to an acute episode of illness, or the establishment of a chronic pattern, is an historical shift from the familiar to the unfamiliar, a metaphorical shift – a 'falling' ill, or 'becoming' ill; a 'decline' and a 'disability'. We may live our sicknesses, including ageing, 'as if' we were well, our narratives never fully adjusted to our symptoms. This sickness inhabits the everyday social world. Narcissists and tyrants govern countries, crippling their economies and artistic and creative endeavours, but are mal-adjusted to their psychological profiles, imagining themselves as benevolent and loved. Some surgeons, too, suffer from this stain but present fresh as daisies and seem oblivious to their 'as if' narrative presences. It is part of clinical folklore that dysfunctional surgeons can be perfectly charming (Shen 2014).

The body has a language, and this is laced with metaphor: odours, an expressive skin, and depths that are plumbed through dissection, autopsy, physical examination (auscultation, palpation and percussion) and a variety of imaging techniques. Medicine's task is wholly metaphoric in the sense that it must, again, make the pathologies of the body 'transparent' to its gaze and match this with an associated language of classification, diagnosis and treatment. It is a work against opacity. However, while the patient's body is made transparent, the doctor works just as hard to make his or her presence to the patient opaque under the guise of professionalism or duplicitous charm. The metaphoric work of transparency and opacity is the dance of medicine, to which the patient is the passive audience. But recently, patients have begun to want to be active critics in this performative arena, so that 'transparency' takes on a double meaning – that of the medical gaze upon the patient (mysterious to the patient) and that of the patient's (and public's) ethical gaze upon the doctor in a prompt for disclosure and openness (a plea for clarity and transparency).

Caroline Wellbery notes the paradox that while scientific language achieves its own form of transparency through stripping back to highly stylized essentials (including the rejection of metaphor), the varieties of the medical gaze that 'open up' the body (seeking the site of the lesion, the physical examination, imaging, the probing questioning within the consultation) also further texture the body, revealing its complexities – or its metaphorical layering. Grasping this complexity and texture requires textured language, or the use of metaphors. This layering can be illustrated through an example of diagnostic work with pregnant women, where compromised oxygen supply *in utero* can lead to decreased foetal heart rate and then 'foetal distress'. So, we make mother and then baby transparent in the diagnostic investigation, only to arrive back at an opaque metaphor: 'foetal distress', also known (compounding the metaphor) as 'non-reassuring foetal status'. Indeed, the term 'foetal distress' is avoided by many obstetricians for being too fuzzy (or metaphoric?), that is, not precise enough.

Transparency, apparency and radiology (the specialty of transparencies)

In medicine, there is a constant tension between the push towards transparent language and the presence of ambiguous, messy and problematic language. In the search for transparent and logical description, perhaps repressed metaphor returns in a distorted form, resulting in a kind of medical stutter and a muttering under the breath. Certainly, it would do medical education little harm to think about encouraging use of a more poetic and expressive language rather than banging on about 'clarity' as a 'communication skill'. Robert Marshall, a consultant pathologist and attendee at the symposium, has often reminded me that pathologists' reports were once opportunities to write inventive and crafted essays, but now have to be written according to a formula in a literal style whose model is the 'tickbox', reinforcing the English for Medical Purposes (EMP) taxis of reduction and anti-metaphorical 'clarity', discussed in Chapter 3. What was once an appreciative essay on the dead is now an instrumental assay in which language is professionally smothered and the move to 'clarity' and 'brevity' paradoxically acts against transparency. This is because good prose is so often revelatory, opening up the body of concern to inspection, while brevity may obscure clarity or transparency.

By 'transparency', I now mean at least three things, and these are conflicting 'lines of flight', to borrow a metaphor from Gilles Deleuze and Felix Guattari. There is (i) the body made transparent through the medical gaze (including, as above, writing reports about patients and bodies); (ii) the doctor in consultation with the patient; and (iii) medicine in relationship to the general public. The latter includes 'transparency' about, for example, patient safety data, performance outcomes for consultants, and management of resources.

Paradoxically, the more we attempt to 'cleanse' medical thinking of its perceived metaphorical taints, or encourage metaphor to absent itself from medical discourse, the more we encourage metaphor's presence. This can be explored, and perhaps explained, as an effect of resistance to sovereign power. Medical students instructed to write scientific papers are told, implicitly, that metaphor can be replaced through 'organization' of ideas and 'transparency', which, in turn, requires 'cleansing' of affect, anecdote and personal opinion. But, of course, this is a metaphor in its own right. Here, transparency becomes a key issue in medical education.

'Transparency' – introduced earlier – is now a leading metaphor in science, medicine, politics, and the politics of health or public engagement with medicine and healthcare. But it is a relatively modern word, with origins in the late fourteenth century. Mark Fenster (2010) notes that 'transparency' is now the primary descriptive term for an aspect of public administration in which the government discloses information as a measure of that government's accountability. However, at the same time, transparency also acts as a metaphor, as it describes the distance or disjunction between the state and the public that affords an image of the level of democracy. As a metaphor, 'transparency' can be equated with 'open'/'closed' and 'visible'/'invisible' political contexts, where the state is never fully visible or accountable, just as doctors are never fully visible or accountable to their patients, who are not privy to the 'backstage' of medicine. There is always a surplus to such visibility and accountability, and this surplus is what feeds and maintains the metaphor of 'transparency' where the state is fluid, complex and dispersed; the same descriptors can be used for the postmodern roles of doctors.

Armando Menéndez-Viso (2009) notes that the term 'transparency' has been misappropriated. What the public wants is not a lens or a medium to see through, but to look directly at something so that it becomes *apparent*. We can see a gradual 'clearing' from the opaque to the transparent to the apparent, where transparency still has a lingering sense of something not being disclosed (again, there is always a remainder or surplus to transparency that remains unexplored). Thus, transparency acts as a metaphor for apparency, where direct experience is always mediated. In the case of politics, the public never grasps the activity in itself, such as the process of producing legislation, but only as this is reported through the media, where opacity is already conditional upon the political affiliations of such media.

Patients want medicine to be apparent in the sense of being easy to 'see' and to understand or grasp. Apparency is high visibility. What medicine often presents to patients is opacity or low apparency. Medicine's 'transparency' as public or patient accountability, for example in a doctor–patient consultation, can be driven by medicine's own stock of metaphors and not those of the patient. The medium that the doctor hands to the patient, as the metaphoric lens through which his or her symptoms can be understood and responded to, is already opaque. Let us turn to Radiology, the primary medical specialty of transparency and apparency, as a case study.

In medicine, metaphors are stereotyped as tropes that obscure, paralleling the work of poetry. But the opposite is the case. Metaphors surely clarify by generating insight at a higher level of meaning. Radiologists carry out work at a finer level of meaning, being relied upon to clarify what multiple layers of tissue obscure, penetrating those layers through imaging and ultrasound. In this archaeological work, a handy reference, as we have seen from Chapters 5 and 6, is an archive of resemblances such as an 'apple core lesion' (Figure 5.1) and a 'bamboo spine' (Figure 6.2). The radiological 'line of flight' or impulse to transparency strips out the texture of the body, which Caroline Wellbery refers to, in order to clarify the body and organize its otherwise messy structure. From this base, it is easier to diagnose fault lines and folds in this organizational plan. We can think of these aberrations from the 'normal' baseline as metaphorical impulses towards what Martin O'Brien described as 'slow death', discussed at length at the close of this chapter.

While the dermatologist reads the cover of the body, the skin, as book, and the pathologist reads the footnotes as micro-texts, the radiologist reads the leaves of the book, characteristically through multiple imaging of organs. As other physicians rely on the radiologist for clarity, so the metaphors through which the body is read radiologically promise clarity. To patients, however, these images remain 'as clear as mud', a layered metaphor that works through both contrast and irony. How will the radiologist, or, indeed, should the radiologist, discuss test results with patients, when the layperson might describe the radiologist's explanation as 'clear as mud'?

Just before discussing these issues, we should note that a common metaphor circulating in hospitals is that the radiology department is 'error proof' and that the 'proof is in the pudding' of radiologists' self-reported accuracy. However, puddings differ even when sharing a common recipe. Through meta-analysis of studies, a benchmark for accuracy of radiology diagnoses has been established at an average of 4.4 per cent error rate, which is relatively low (Radiology Quality Institute 2012). Everyday X-rays, mammograms and ultrasound come in at a very low 3.48 per cent error rate, while extremely complex computed tomography (CT) abdominal and pelvis interpretations have a very high disagreement rate between radiologists and consulting physicians of 32 per cent (Radiology Quality Institute 2012).

In a *British Medical Journal* (*BMJ*) article from over 25 years ago (Vallely and Mills 1990), the question was asked: 'should radiologists talk to patients?' (the title itself is interesting – why 'talk to' and not 'talk with'?). The authors suggest that although radiologists may be reluctant to talk 'to' patients, as they see their job not as front-line consultation but as backroom diagnostics, while the referring consultant and GP afford the front line, patients may want to get the results of tests immediately from radiologists. In a survey, patients wished to receive news of tests straight away from the radiologist (transparency in testing leading to transparency in communicating results, even if this means breaking bad news).

Radiologists, however, felt they should not give bad news to patients; rather, patients should hear this from their consultant doctor, albeit as soon as possible. The recommendation in such cases, when '[m]alignancy is diagnosed or strongly suspected', is for radiologists 'when talking to patients to use euphemisms such as bowel obstruction or large ulcer'. The medical metaphor for the malignancy is then used to bewilder and buy time. Opacity trumps transparency, and the normally benign euphemism becomes barbed. In the symposium, Julie Bligh, a medical educator with a background in English Literature, again noted that medical metaphors used in practice in medicine, such as the language of the consultation, are often euphemistic rather than metaphorical. Euphemisms are common currency in palliative care ('passed away' rather than 'died') and in medical management ('rationalization' rather than 'cutting resources').

Twenty years on from Vallely and Mills' 1990 article, the mood concerning direct communication between patients and radiologists had not changed radically, despite the fact that many survey studies during that time showed that most patients would prefer to hear the results of radiology interventions directly from the radiologist, even if the results offered 'bad news' (again, another euphemism, often for the presence of cancer). Radiologists perhaps see talking to patients as a little like looking at a stick plunged into water – it refracts. Their primary job of clarification is refracted in the medium of conversation with patients, and this is not a comfortable line of flight.

Smith and Gunderman (2010) discussed the various conditions under which radiologists would give patients outcome results, and the majority of radiologists surveyed reported that they would prefer not to inform patients of poor outcomes, but to leave this to the consultant physician (other than in the case of mammograms, where, in North America, radiologists are bound by law to give results to women on the spot). The authors ask a rhetorical question: what do radiologists feel about giving immediate feedback under these two circumstances: a pregnant woman with a history of vaginal bleeding has (i) normal findings at examination, or (ii) vaginal bleeding 'consistent with fetal demise'? 'Foetal demise' – another euphemism to partner 'foetal distress'? Would the authors dream of using such language with patients?

Radiologists are stereotyped, unfairly says Patrick Malone (2014), as almost patient-phobic, choosing to sit in darkened rooms and deal with circulating images (metaphors?) of bodies rather than sitting face-to-face with patients and discussing those images in person. Of course, the radiologist has not previously taken a history or made an examination or put the patient in a social context, and does not know about drugs or surgery; and it may be unfair on the consultant physician for the radiologist to discuss results with a patient before that consultant physician has even seen the results. Further, while other doctors look to the radiologist to provide the certainty in diagnosis that they cannot provide, radiologists, too, deal with having to manage uncertainty.

We are left with the conundrum that (returning to Chapters 5 and 6) while radiologists may be experts in, and comfortable with, metaphors as likenesses (resemblances) such as 'apple core lesion', they are not comfortable with conveying a poor prognosis, resorting to euphemisms ('there's an obstruction in the bowel, the consultant will tell you more' for 'I'm afraid it's bad news: you have advanced bowel cancer and operating would be too risky'). Metaphors in medicine inhabit two parallel universes that may or may not converge: first, diagnostic, treatment and prognostic clinical work; and second, consultations with patients and colleagues about diagnoses and subsequent clinical interventions.

The above discussion about radiology was not initiated at the Dartington symposium. It is one of many afterthoughts and footnotes that arose as I contemplated the outcomes of that event. It is a mark of respect to the participants that, now they have ploughed the field, further crops will flourish there. I thank them again for their labour, insights and generosity.

Must metaphor work normally be associated with the verbal and with the written text?

Search online for 'performance in medicine', and you will be directed to sites on the medical enhancement of performance (for example, for athletes under 'sports medicine'), or the performance of doctors or hospitals in terms of meeting clinical outcomes. Change your keywords to 'performing medicine' and you will be directed to <performingmedicine.com/>, linking you to the work of the theatre company Clod Ensemble.

Suzy Willson founded Clod Ensemble to set up an educational programme to improve clinical practice and healthcare through arts interventions with medical students, doctors and healthcare practitioners, further translated into public engagement activities. Bella Eacott, who is Research and Curriculum Manager for Clod Ensemble, participated in the Dartington symposium. One of Clod Ensemble's primary aims is to develop capabilities in clinicians that are core to the performing arts, such as collaboration, expression, invention, non-verbal awareness, observation, vocal clarity, narrative insight, critical reflexivity, tolerance of ambiguity, appreciation and celebration of diversity and difference, inclusive judgement and self-care. These are essential for excellent clinical teamwork and patient care. Running throughout these educational activities are key questions such as 'What is health and what is illness?', 'How are health and illness performed?', 'What is the "body" that performs health and illness across differing historical and cultural contexts?' and 'What are the guiding metaphors that shape performance involving the "healthy" and "ill" body?'

The latter question, central to our symposium, is poorly researched in terms of embodied metaphors as these appear through 'scripted' public performances in the profession of medicine. What anthropologists, ethnographers (including auto-ethnography by clinicians) and sociologists of medicine show us are the direct consequences for dramatic performance of medicine that flow from the two didactic or master metaphors of the body as machine and medicine as war or conflict.

First, if the body is treated as a machine, then doctors assume a role of engineer, and performance is geared towards facilitating the smooth running of the machine. The performance is one of maintenance. Just as the plumber is not expected to necessarily engage in anything but surface conversation with a customer, so the doctor is positioned, performatively, as one who diagnoses faults and proceeds to fix them. Indeed, oiling the body does not even require oiling the conversation with the patient about the body. The fact that the machine that is being fixed is a flesh-and-blood human with experience and feelings is secondary to the performance of instrumentality. Second, if the disease is to be eradicated or fought, then, in order to separate the 'enemy' of the infection or organ failure from the person who carries that infection or failure, the person, performatively, must be disembodied. The performance then follows the metaphor.

'Machine' has the same root as 'machinate' – to plot, scheme or contrive behaviour. This returns us to the dramaturgical model of medicine, in which the doctor plays a role according to a script. Medicine as machination is, however, both cold and hollow; it is necessary to objectify the patient in order to stay in character. This is a tired and outdated form of clinical encounter. This model, of course, raises many contradictions – the central one of which is that the doctor's performance in the bald terms set out above is inhumane, unethical and an-aesthetic. It is literally nonsensical, avoiding the issue that humans are sentient beings whose common sense is that of self-perception (including pain and pleasure) that must be made sense of socially or collaboratively.

Self-perception (Heller-Roazen 2007) makes meaning of symptoms, but such meaning is opaque until it is made transparent through sharing and generating meanings with others. Therefore, doctors' performances cannot be dictated solely by the scripts generated under the guidance of the master metaphors of the body as machine (by implication, devoid of self-perception) and medicine as conflict (by implication, devoid of a meaningful conversation with the 'enemy' of infection or organ failure, for example).

Aristotle noted that humans cannot be 'untouchables', where touch is 'the most acute' of the senses – the soft human flesh calls out for contact and for mutual understanding of its inner messages. Performance in the arts ritualizes and codes such sensations to critically examine their meanings. But performance in medicine is merely coded without this critical insight, so that medicine is acted out according to a regime that requires a supplement of 'medicine watch-ers' (I borrow this term, introduced earlier, from Allan Peterkin, a psychiatrist and medical educator from Toronto) – sociologists, anthropologists, psycholo-gists, artists and so forth who engage with medicine – to perform critical reflec-tion on medicine. This has become formalized as the medical humanities (Bleakley 2014b, 2015).

Medicine, then, continues to perform the body under the guidance of the twin dominant metaphors of body as machine and medicine as war. Here, doctors' bodies are socialized and educated as instruments of diagnosis of machine failure and interventionists in machine maintenance, and as interventionist warriors now drawing on a variety of sophisticated armaments, primarily diagnostic imaging technologies, gene therapies and pharmacological weaponry.

I am, of course, deliberately stripping back medicine's performance to its bare bones for rhetorical purposes. All of the doctors I know are concerned about this historical guiding metaphor legacy and are deliberately engaged, through medical education and the medical humanities, in some level of active resistance to these metaphor hegemonies, eager to promote new metaphors that will shape a future landscape of authentic interprofessional team care and patient-centred practice (Bleakley 2014a).

However, many of those doctors will baulk at the next stage of the argument against the hegemony of the medical model, a view elaborated at the symposium through the performance work and theory of Martin O'Brien. Martin's work moves us into an important area of debate concerning the right of the person as patient to perform his or her symptoms in a way that he or she sees fit – especially as this goes against the grain of orthodox medical and clinical practice and opinion – as reclamation of an identity otherwise colonized by medicine.

The emergence of the zombie metaphor

The embodied metaphor can get sick and symptomize – tired out, played out, dull, listless. But what if the sick body acts as a platform for the creative, as the Romantic Movement and Nietzsche in particular insisted? A key modern figure here is Georges Bataille (1897–1962), born three years before Nietzsche's death, whose work on transgression and limit experiences provides a frame of reference for understanding the beauty and potential of the sick body. Further, what if the sick body – by being adopted as the site of art through performance – is metaphorized?

Gianna Bouchard (also a participant in the Dartington symposium) and Martin O'Brien co-edited a special issue of the journal *Performance Research* (2014, Vol. 19, No. 4) – 'On Medicine'. This collected some of the latest thinking on the turbulent relationship between the discourses of medicine and performance art. Within medical education, recognition of 'performance' is characteristically limited to rather tepid discussions about the roles and uses of actor-patients within simulation and assessment scenarios, such as medical students practising, or being assessed on, consultations and physical examinations. Typically, students find the psychiatric consultation to be the most challenging. While performance art has an intense and well-developed relationship with medical tropes (for example, in the work of Bob Flanagan and Sheree Rose, Orlan, Ron Athey, Stelarc, Ive Tabar and Peggy Shaw), medicine has not reciprocated by, for example, introducing insights from, or collaborating with, performance artists to bring an extra dimension to medicine and surgery curricula. Performance is probably the most neglected area in the medical/health humanities (Bates *et al.* 2014), or is diluted from the radical performance art end of the spectrum, where 'performance' acquired through medical education is, for example, compared to string music education (Wooliscroft and Phillips 2003).

In the summer of 2015, at an international medical humanities conference that I organized at Dartington Hall, Martin O'Brien performed a new version of an ongoing piece called 'Mucus Factory' – the new piece was entitled 'It's Good to Breathe In (This Devon Air)' (Bleakley *et al.* 2017). Martin is a graduate of Dartington College from its heyday as the most progressive performing arts institution in the UK (and is now a lecturer at Queen Mary University, London). 'Mucus Factory', in Martin's own words, is 'a mixture of a durational physiotherapy session, a technique designed to clear the airways, and an artificial attempt to use mucus as a substance for vanity and pleasure' (http://martin obrienperformance.weebly.com/performance.html). In his Dartington performance, after cutting the shape of his lungs on his chest with a scalpel, through vigorous chest self-physiotherapy he brings up and collects mucus in specimen jars and then uses this as hair gel, carrying this out in several ritualistic cycles to purposefully create monotony.

Martin appropriates physiotherapy – claimed as a professional allied-medical technique – as a performance, in self-treatment. In his own description (paraphrased): as a person living with cystic fibrosis (CF), Martin uses physical endurance, disgust, long durations and pain-based practices to address a politics of the sick queer body and examine what it means to be born with a life-threatening disease, politically and philosophically. In my words, his work is an act of resistance, not to illness per se but to the medical appropriation of his body in the service of normative models of health. Through such work, he reclaims agency and celebrates his given body and being. At the Dartington symposium, Martin showed a clip of a film of a new development of 'Mucus Factory', in which he begins by cutting the shape of lungs onto (and into) his chest with a scalpel, as he did at the previous Dartington performance a year earlier.

In this work, Martin purposefully multiplies metaphors, through pun and double plays, such as 'fluidity' and 'inscription'. The tangible fluid is coughed-up mucus, abject matter used as hair gel or dangled into his mouth so that disgust and attraction are mischievously conjoined. The physiotherapy is less massage and more a paradoxical beating up, a self-imposed violence; but it is also an animal chest pounding, an act of agency and ownership of identity, a simultaneous boundary making and undoing, a territorial deterritorializing. The cutting of the shape of the lungs is another disguised act – as reclamation of the interior body, inscribing of identity, and a positive appropriation of the surgeon's rights and rites.

As somebody who lives with CF, where overproduction of mucus is literally drowning the lungs and impacting and obstructing the intestines, Martin draws on Lauren Berlant's (2011) notion of 'slow death' to describe how his own endurance performances are inevitable and not contrived (O'Brien 2014). Endurance in art and endurance in life coincide. 'Slow death' seems to be the major metaphor that shapes his work. Medicine's interest in impulse and heroism necessarily rejects the metaphor of 'slow death'. The hero either keeps death at bay at all costs, or dies suddenly in battle.

Subsequently, Martin's interest in the zombie, discussed below, might be seen as a shift in interest from the leading metaphor of 'slow death' to 'suspended death'. The zombie, says Jacques Derrida, poisons systems of order. It is the symbol par excellence for breaking down oppositional categories (life/death). As an enfleshed ghost, the zombie is Derrida's favourite metaphor for deconstruction (Casciato 2009).

Again, neither of the zombie metaphors of 'slow death' or 'suspended death' interests modern medicine, and this is what makes the work of artists like Martin so important in the context of discussing medical metaphors. Such work celebrates what medicine denies, even as medicine and its allies, such as physiotherapy, work in good faith and wholeheartedly on behalf of the patient. Martin says: 'I submit to medicine in order to survive – in order to endure longer', but his endurance art is surely subverting medicine at the same time; perhaps not inverting, but multiplying up, the medical gaze (O'Brien 2014, p. 63). While the chronically ill body necessarily demands submission to regimes of regulation and maintenance, these can be subverted in acts of empowerment. Ironically, medicine's master metaphors of the body as machine and medicine as war can themselves be seen as 'zombie metaphors' or the walking dead. 'Dead' metaphors, as discussed in Chapter 2, are metaphors that have moved beyond status even as idioms, to become clichéd. 'Medicine as war' is still used by Macmillan Cancer Support, reminding people that they need support to 'fight' against cancer ('Cancer is the toughest fight most of us will have to face').

As heart disease and cancer have just been overtaken by dementia as the leading cause of death in England and Wales, due to an ageing population, the UK Alzheimer's Society (www.alzheimers.org.uk) continues to employ as its banner 'Leading the fight against dementia'. Alzheimer's Research UK talks of 'defeating dementia', and examples are given of individuals' 'battles' against dementia (www.bbc.co.uk/news/health-37972141). Individuals like Martin, suffering from CF, can afford a wry smile in the face of this dementia epidemic, because CF sufferers will live a relatively short life. Martin has embraced life's insult to create intensity, and in the process rejects the war metaphors by which medicine operates, replacing them with the sensual, in which life is treated as a suspended sentence. This is also a pun for an unfinished act of language. Martin's risky durational performances, then, consistently move him to the brink, to the edge of the sentence, embracing the unknown.

To return to the value of performance art, Gianna Bouchard (Bouchard and O'Brien 2014, p. 94) suggests: 'Live Art can erode and undermine the perceived creeping loss of agency over our bodies, reclaiming them from the dominant discourses of medicine and science.' Petra Kuppers (2006, p. 203) calls this the 'reembodying of medically derived body knowledge'. This can be seen as a replacement of medicine's dominant metaphors by those of artists; in Martin's case, when he writes that 'performance functions as a metaphor for illness experience', this can readily be reversed, whereby illness experience is a metaphor for performing death in life. As Martin's latest work claims, this is the worldview of the zombie, who lives just at that point where the sentence is running out.

Martin's second film excerpt at the symposium presentation introduced a positively disturbing metaphor – of the sick body and medical patient as zombie. This metaphorical frame inverts and subverts dominant metaphors for medical work and upholds the tradition of the artist as diagnostician of culture, whose main work is to challenge habitual perceptions and frames of reference. In zombie guise, Martin performs an identity of resistance to medical norms through celebration of the body under duress and at its limits.

'Zombie' appears as a metaphor in language as the common similes 'transfixed like a zombie' and 'wide-eyed like a zombie'. 'Zombie' is an anglicized version of the Haitian French *zombi*, which, in turn, is a version of the Haitian Creole *zonbi*. In Haitian folklore, now a syncretic union of West African vodou and Catholicism, the zombie is a reanimated human corpse, the living dead or 'undead' roaming the earth. The reanimation is the work of vodou. In popular culture, the zombie is the work of mad science. The poet Robert Southey, in a history of Brazil, first introduced 'zombie' into the English language in 1819. Mary Shelley's *Frankenstein* drew on a well-established European folklore tradition referring to the undead amongst us. The zombie film tradition was initiated in Victor Halperin's 'White Zombie' from 1932, starring Bela Lugosi, and it was in modern film that the zombie was re-created through George Romero's *Night of the Living Dead*, although the term 'zombie' was never used in the film. Here, the zombie feeds on human flesh and savours brains. This notion of the zombie gave rise to the current 'zombie apocalypse', in which civilization is threatened by a zombie infestation.

This returns us to Martin's 'slow death' and the dialogue with a disorder that threatens to drown his body in overproduction of mucus, which can be reimagined as 'suspended death'. This metaphor challenges the dominant medical frame of body as machine, but invites comparison with Deleuze and Guattari's (1988b) version of 'machine' as deterritorialized assemblages, liquid machines that are nomadic and spontaneously morph into new shapes and expressions. The zombie, then, is both a metaphor for a medical condition and an emblem of resistance against the medical normalizing of bodies. 'Zombie' can be claimed as a metaphor, as it transfers death across from the really dead to the living dead or the dead renewed, thus transfiguring the living, or elevating their status from normal to pathologically enervating.

Serendipitously, one of Martin's performance father-figures, Bob Flanagan, met one of Martin's artistic mentors, Sheree Rose, at a Halloween party, at which Bob was made up as a zombie. Martin's 2015 zombie film 'The Unwell' offers a dystopic and liminal future in the image of an acceptable, even welcome, plague that rids us of material desire:

> This used to be the most optimistic city in the world. Now it's full of darkness illuminated by the fading street lamps. Out of this darkness stumbles life quite different from us. The unwell negotiate this landscape in a way we could not.

This city has no crime, no poverty and no war – 'nothing to fear. There is only sickness and this sickness is itself a form of existence, a way of seeing and being, a way of breathing and moving' (quotes used with permission of the author).

Martin sums up his zombie existence as 'survival of the sickest' (http://martin obrienperformance.weebly.com) – a replacement of both the Darwinian trope (survival of the fittest) and the 'medicine as war' master metaphor – in which those who suffer 'illness' are in healthy competition for the best restatement of 'quality of life' indicators. This thoroughly subverts the direction of travel of all 'health' agencies, such as the World Health Organization, whose stated aim is to 'reduce risks' to health and wellbeing. For example, the 2002 WHO Report is full of the rhetoric of combat against ill health and the creeping dangers of 'risk', seen as a 'threat' to humankind globally: 'These are dangerous times for the wellbeing of the world.' This is described as a 'drama' in which the key players are no longer the impoverished but the well-off, gradually – in zombie terms – 'eating their own flesh' through excessive consumption of fatty foods, alcohol and frenetic lifestyles. A new order of governmental control is needed to bring some shape and order to this wild trajectory of self-imposed symptoms. Desire must be curbed.

This scenario is heaven-sent for students of Michel Foucault, whose life's work was the exposure of forms of 'governmentality', from the macro-level of big metaphors and big ideas such as the classification of knowledge, through to the micro-levels of self-imposed governance that we blindly call 'conscience'. Martin's work illustrates Foucault's notion of aesthetic self-forming through resistance to normative discourse and associated metaphors.

We can also make sense of Martin's ontological positioning as 'endurance zombie' within a tradition stemming from Friedrich Nietzsche and reworked by Foucault, valuing the transvaluation of all values. Nietzsche famously questions taken-for-granted moralities and asks whether we can adopt a position of tolerance when faced with alien values. The zombie, of course, represents such values for most of us, and this is why the literalizing of the metaphor in living, breathing endurance performance is challenging for the WHO 'wellness' mentality and mainstream medicine, as well as for the person on the street who accepts medicine without any critical interrogation or active sensibility.

Foucault's body of work systematically maps out the historical conditions of possibility under which once-included citizens are now excluded through regimes that afford identities of 'the mad', 'the prisoner', 'the sick (clinical patient)' and the 'sexually perverse'. Control of citizenry operates at gross (sovereign power) and fine (capillary power) levels. The state or government includes and excludes through contested definitions and imposition of penalties, while 'governmentality' seeps down to the self as a capillary mechanism, reaching into the finest aspects of life, such as exercise, moral choice and sexual identity, even into 'conscience'.

Foucault surprises at every turn: classification is not a values-free expression of scientific logic but a political act of judgement and control over knowledge. The empty lazar houses once used by lepers afford convenient housing for moral irritants as towns and cities are cleansed of their village idiots, prostitutes, single mothers and beggars, who, in turn, are 'treated', or 'reformed' by quasi-scientific reclassification. Institutions are built to scrutinize and 're-form' the wayward in a drive to normalize and discipline. Irritated by seeing persons at home under the family's terms, doctors invent a space and a set of techniques in which the patient can be reduced to symptoms, managed and medicalized (the 'clinic'). Finally, sex was never repressed during the Victorian era and is not 'liberated' now, but is represented and managed in differing ways – such as the emergence of a 'liberated' confessional normative sexuality in modern times that still continues to marginalize many sexual practices and choices as perverse.

Martin O'Brien (2014) notes how biomedical science – seen through a Foucauldian lens – is a major instrument of disciplining and normalizing the body, or 'administering life' in Foucault's term. The production of 'docile bodies' through such bio-power again depends on the application of the major metaphors of the body as machine (inspection and regulation are passed off as regular maintenance) and medicine as war (the person must be suspended in order to clear a space for the battle with the toxic invader or mutant gene). In terms of chronic illness, as Martin notes, the 'patient' must be subjugated as a long-term regime of 'care' is introduced with regular inspections and moral censures ('How many units of alcohol have you drunk this week?', 'Have you taken your medication?').

Here, the default body is the healthy body that is well oiled, maintained, regularly inspected and always ready for battle, and works within set limits of what is tolerated as normal sexual behaviour. This neatly bypasses the individual, unique, idiosyncratic and sensuous materiality of the body with its inner sense-impressions or acute sensibility. The individual's sensibility is rendered insensible as sensibility capital fails to be distributed between doctor and patient, but is instead lodged with the doctor and the medical establishment sandwiched between its twin moralizing metaphors of war and machine.

It is through idiosyncratic performance practices, currently shaped by the guiding metaphor of the zombie, that Martin challenges the dominant medical discourse and reclaims inner-directed bodily sensibility. In his performance, he is controlled yet retains control; his genitals are pinned, yet he is fully eroticized; he is force fed liquids yet retains bladder control; and he suffocates by choice – not at the hands of authoritarian political strangulation. Again, these are suspended sentences, and acts of proper moral impudence and political defiance or resistance. It is metaphorical work made flesh, but the flesh is that of the flesh-eating zombie, a flesh that is at once both pushed to its limits and demedicalized. In its direct engagement with the abject, it is work that necessarily places an audience to be figuratively eaten up from within. Within the zombie metaphor, for the performer, this is necessary work – a vocation, a calling, a placement, and never an avocation.

Metaphor, our symposium disclosed, is a many-headed beast that provides both succour and stigma. Reflecting everyday dilemmas, art, such as performance art, is in a unique position to reflect back to us, through metaphor, how our lives are shaped by metaphor, and how unconscious we are of such shaping. Thirty years ago, Charles Krauthammer (1986) wrote an article in the *Los Angeles Times* asking: 'What are we hiding under the bandages of metaphor?', a powerful metaphorical image in its own right. He noted that medical metaphors, themselves often militaristic and stigmatizing, had been purloined by the military, so that enemies become 'cancers' to be eradicated, and military air- and ground-strikes should be 'surgical', with no 'collateral damage' or civilian harm.

Summary

An apology

Like a dragonfly, I have sometimes alighted on a topic briefly, only to nervously flit to something else. There are good reasons for this. For example, I have not concentrated on metaphors of pain because this area is so well served by other literature (Fuller and Hughes 2003; Padfield *et al.* 2003; Semino 2010; Frank 2011; Buchbinder 2015; Neilson 2015; Stewart 2016). Similarly, I have not focused on summary metaphors for the doctor–patient relationship, although that is where I alighted at the close of the previous chapter in a radical rethink of medicine as 'patient-directed', beyond paternalism and even patient-centred medicine, and driven by the surprising creativity of sickness (O'Brien 2014). The doctor–patient relationship is also an area that has been well documented: from the well-known 'paternalism' and 'consumerism' metaphors (Childress and Siegler 1984; Beisecker and Beisecker 1993) to the newly minted dance metaphor of 'tango', emphasizing democracy in the medical encounter (Balcu 2013). Situating himself in the zeitgeist of the noughties, Stewart (2016) suggests that metaphors of the future shaping healthcare practices will be 'dialogically co-constructed' between providers and patients – perhaps a form of 'tango'? Does the sick body 'tango', or is that a conceit?

In terms of specialties, I have concentrated on the visual specialties of pathology, radiology and dermatology in Chapters 5 and 6, because it is here that resemblances are most used in clinical judgement and appreciation. Why write a chapter (7) on psychiatry and not one on, say, paediatrics? My defence is that psychiatry is an area that I know something about; similarly with medical education (Chapter 8) and the use of poetry in the medical humanities (Chapter 9).

So, although this book can claim to be the first comprehensive and systematic account of metaphors in medicine, it necessarily has its limits. Where its strength rests, I think, is in developing arguments made in previous books for democratizing medicine (Bleakley *et al.* 2011; Bleakley 2014a), primarily through the medical humanities as core and integrated provision in medical education (Bleakley 2014b, 2015). I now suggest that the primary medium for democratizing medicine is what arts and humanities share in common: the reflexive employment of metaphor as metaphor on the up, and not metaphor that shuts down thinking. Medicine as an institution and culture is shaped historically by meta-metaphor, and this, in turn, shapes the work and identities of doctors. We must be able to grapple with these historical effects with an eye to the future shape of medical practice.

I hope that I have demonstrated throughout this book just how such historical shaping occurs. A reflexive awareness of the work of metaphor in medicine by doctors and medical educators can, I believe, shift the work of metaphor: from structuring the everyday conceptual system of medical culture to transforming that culture. The aims of such a transformation are: first, improvement of patient care and safety; second, deeper public engagement with medicine; and third, transforming medical culture from instrumental expression to critical reflexivity, whereby practitioners are able to gain critical distance from their practices and review them for their guiding values and impact. This is a poetic, as well as a scientific, enterprise.

A recap

What is a metaphor?

Metaphors are historically and culturally contingent tropes that can turn language and communication from the mundane and instrumental into the expressive and aesthetic in uplifting ways, but can also close down imagination and thinking in discomfiting ways. Metaphors are like bees – they generally work hard to maintain the overall hive of language as a productive organism, but they also carry a sting. Some go on solo flights for reconnaissance, and some (meta-metaphors) are queen bees around which swarms of admiring workers gather; while others, again, like to sting. Metaphors do work – through thinking, feeling and performing socially. But they also like to just hang around, to be admired, to irritate, to be discussed and analysed, to be mobilized, and just to preen themselves and show off their plumage. Metaphors can be killers – suffocating with pillows while disguised as lovers.

The way metaphors perform can be mapped as a spectrum (see Table 12.1).

Table 12.1 Spectrum of metaphors

Sinister	Neutral	Dexter
Malign	Benign	Transformative
Stain	Linguistic padding	Turning the ordinary into the extraordinary
Wrack	May provide initial traction for innovation	
Ruin		
Close down thinking		Thinking otherwise
Stink	Bland	Perfumed

Metaphors in medicine

Metaphors can be used in medicine:

1   to think with, as:

- differential diagnosis/treatment options/prognosis;
- reflective and critical approach towards own practice and positioning in medical culture and institution;
- reflective about epistemological underpinning to practice;
- engaging in values clarification and relativization;
- using language in exploratory as well as explanatory ways;
- innovation (thinking 'otherwise');

2   to communicate with, as:

- challenging the assumption that language communicates truth and fact in a value-free manner – rather, language can be representational, rhetorical, expressive and ideological;
- as a means for articulating ontological positions such as identities;
- discursive (arguing points of view within a certain frame);
- dialogical;
- displaying power (both claiming authority and reframing authority as resistance and forming of democratic habits).

Ten things discussed in this book that medical educators should know

1   Medicine is soaked in metaphors.
2   As a culture and institution, medicine has historically been shaped by the leading or didactic metaphors of 'medicine as war' and 'the body as a machine', permeating to the level of regulation of individual doctors as identity construction. Such meta-metaphors may once have been transformative but now can be unhelpful, even stigmatizing. These dominant metaphors are complex and have numerous faces and expressions, including context specificity (see the following section).
3   Medicine characteristically refuses metaphor for the plain, literal and descriptive.
4   Perhaps as a result of such refusal (point 3 above), metaphor returns in a distorted form as 'backstage' derogatory medical slang. It is regularly argued that medical slang may offer a safety valve for the emotional pressures that clinical practice brings, but this view can be challenged. The use of derogatory medical slang is unethical, is avoidable and brings medicine into disrepute.
5   Doctors use metaphor as a rhetorical (persuasive) device, primarily as a pretence of certainty under conditions of uncertainty and ambiguity. Metaphor, then, offers a rhetorical device to grapple with causal ambiguities. This

maintains authority over patients, junior doctors and non-medical healthcare colleagues, for example through portraying them in morally favourable (gaining favour) or unfavourable (demonstrating authority) ways. *That* metaphors persuade may be self-evident; *how* and *why* they persuade is the subject of this book.

6   Doctors' and patients' uses of metaphors may clash, misalign and generate mutual misunderstanding.

7   In contrast to point 6 above, doctors and patients may use metaphors positively, as transformative devices for opening up communication.

8   Doctors think with metaphors for diagnostic purposes, fundamentally at the level of analogy, resemblance or aphorism in pattern recognition. Whereas medicine is largely pragmatic, metaphors can concretize concepts productively ('illness scripts') or unproductively ('hard wired').

9   Once a 'no go' area for medicine, metaphors are now used politically by doctors as rhetorical devices – for example, 'patient safety' is employed as a metaphor to prick the conscience of political masters and managers, when introducing longer shifts and expectations for working at night and on weekends puts patients at risk because of overstretching resources, and disadvantages young women doctors with children, who find it difficult to arrange 'unsociable hours' childcare (Boseley 2016).

10   Doctors self-display through use of metaphors and resemblances as part of expressive style and aesthetic.

Same metaphor/different genres or contexts

Elena Semino (2011) shows how the same metaphor may be adopted and then utilized differently across differing 'genres', or discourses of practice. She illustrates this with the metaphor of 'gate' as this is adopted in theories of pain control. As previously discussed, Mara Buchbinder (2015) shows how the metaphor of 'stickiness' is adopted in differing ways according to context in the arena of pain management in paediatric medicine, particularly as this involves multidisciplinary teams. In this book, I have shown how a variety of metaphors are imported into, and refracted through, medicine as opposed to other professions, cultures, institutions, discourse practices or genres. Metaphors also grow within medicine – crystallizing, deposited, iatrogenic, self-serving and as forms of resistance. An 'in progress' example of this is the metaphor of 'risk' (see point 9 above), which has outgrown its literal nature to be utilized rhetorically.

At the time of writing, English junior doctors are in dispute with the UK government over a new contract that demands a 'seven-day NHS', based on a misreading by the government of research supposedly showing a 'weekend effect' (another interesting metaphor), whereby more patients die at the weekends than on weekdays. The government claims that there is inadequate medical cover on weekends. Closer analysis shows that the 'weekend effect' is not a consistent phenomenon and that patients admitted at weekends tend to be sicker (Boseley 2016). Junior doctors, who already work weekend shifts, say that this project cannot be achieved with the current level of resourcing (not just in medicine but across health and social care as a network). More consultants, nurses and support staff would need to be called in to meet the government's demands. The medical and nursing workforce employs the human metaphors of 'stretched' resources at 'breaking point', while the government employs managerial metaphors of 'rationalization' of resources and better 'strategic planning'.

Junior doctors (the term 'junior' is a mis-metaphor; it covers all doctors below consultant grade, and so includes many experienced doctors at registrar grade) have already engaged in industrial strikes under the threat of the government imposing a contract. This radical politicizing of doctors is new in UK medicine. At the core of the debate is the metaphor of 'risk' and that metaphor's relative rhetorical strength.

Baldly, 'risk' for the government is putting patients who are hospitalized at weekends at risk because of lack of a full workforce (GP practices are mainly closed at weekends as well) – this is based on strongly contested evidence, as noted above. The metaphor of 'risk' is then outwardly patient focused but actually construed as one of 'efficiency' – efficient management of available resources. Junior doctors' metaphor of 'risk' is different. Here, patients are at 'risk' if they are exposed to potentially poorer care from clinical teams because of lack of resources, such as enough doctors and nurses working night rotas within any one ward. In this case, 'risk' equates with a deficit in 'quality of care' in clinical-psychological terms related to doctors' stress, and is not set within an economic model (Peterkin and Bleakley 2017). 'Risk' is then outwardly focused on doctors at risk through overwork, but this overlays a primary concern to offer patients safe practice. Thus, the same metaphor ('risk') has different meanings across the genres of healthcare management and healthcare clinical practice. Another way of looking at the ongoing junior doctors' dispute is, then, as a clash of metaphors.

Conclusion

Ways in which metaphors in medicine 'work'

I have argued that analogies (metaphors and resemblances) in medicine serve at a minimum the following functions.

1 Giving meaning to life swinging between pleasure and pain

Metaphors are classically described as transforming the ordinary into the extra-ordinary through transposition, gaining deeper meanings or more effective traction ('he's milking the audience', 'I couldn't fathom her questions'). However, metaphors can symptomize (turn hollow, sour, bad but harmless, or at worst become dangerous), acting as symptoms ('she's gone off the rails', 'he takes so many pills that he rattles', 'she's a vegetable now', 'the cancer's winning the battle'). Metaphors may describe suffering, but they suffer themselves, as symptoms of cultural shrinkage and atrophy. The life history of 'big' metaphors – from celebrity status to incognito and possible erasure – can be traced as an inverted U curve from potent, through hollow, to 'dead' metaphors. Metaphors are regularly revived on cycles of fashion, reinventing themselves (for example, 'cut and paste' CRISPR gene technologies, discussed in point 3 below), but they, too, ultimately 'circle the drain', suffering the same fate as flesh. Perhaps death can be reconfigured as the exhaustion of metaphor for the terminal embrace of the literal – as when Ariel, in Shakespeare's *The Tempest*, sings to Ferdinand (lost on the island) that 'Full fathom five thy father lies.' This is no metaphor but literal truth – Ferdinand's father has supposedly drowned. (Alonso, Ferdinand's father and King of Naples, is not, in fact, dead, so Shakespeare, through Ariel, puns on 'lies'.)

2 Reconfiguring ambiguities

Metaphors such as 'sticky neurons' and 'sticky brains' (Chapter 1) offer a handle, or tangibility, for an otherwise difficult to grasp, or intangible, object or process – paradoxically, even where the metaphor itself may be ambiguous, such as 'sticky brain' (the brain is not sticky; it is the perseverative behaviour of the child with unexplained symptoms of chronic pain that is 'sticky') and the notion that symptoms may be 'all in the mind', or stuck to a psychological impulse that per-sistently drips like a leaky tap. The metaphor offers something to work with, to converse with – a sensory image, even if a ghost anatomy. The brain is not figured out (certainty) but con-figured (held as uncertainty and ambiguity) through the metaphor. Teaching medical students how to think metaphorically and how to appreciate metaphors in medicine may, then, be a way of educating for tolerance of ambiguity, a central value for doctors, as discussed throughout this book.

Metaphors bring syncopation to what would otherwise be a militaristic marching music of medical practice, potentially one of arrogant certainty. Medi-cine should be performed just off the beat, where improvisation is allowed – essential as we move from the formulaic approach of evidence-based (population-based) medicine to a tailored medicine for each individual patient. This is even more essential as we see an increase in the numbers of patients pre-senting with mental health issues, or with medically unexplained symptoms. Doctors must learn to inhabit the 'swampy lowlands' of clinical practice rather than crave the 'high ground' of certainty (see Chapter 8). Education in a meta-phorical imagination may help.

3 Acting ideologically

Metaphors shape a culture (its values, practices and consequent identity con-structions), both maintaining, and breaking with, tradition. At the level of the general culture, metaphors can act as 'medicine', treating symptoms. This medicinal activity is culturally sanctioned and organized as 'art'. Artists can be 'diagnosticians of culture', challenging unproductive habits and tired ways of seeing. Metaphors constitute the artists' collective pharmacopoeia.

At the level of medical culture, metaphors are adopted and shaped historically as leading, dominant or didactic (Chapter 4). These metaphors shape the culture and are hard to shift, even as they may stigmatize. They become resistant to change through subtle transformations – for example, the 'medicine as war' metaphor adapts from epidemiological application to 'targets' in personalized medicine. Also, the 'body as machine' metaphor is hardy, and it, too, has adapted to the world of personalized medicine, particularly within the sphere of genetic engineering.

CRISPR (Clustered Regularly Interspaced Short Palindromic Repeats) is an industry-based 'genome editing tool'. The acronym itself is a metaphor – the tech-nology is 'crisper', quicker and leaner, with 'robust cutting activity' (www.sigma aldrich.com/catalog/product/sigma/crispr?lang=en&region=GB). The acronym spelt out also bears an uncanny resemblance to the sticky brains/ perseverative behaviour syndrome. The technology is regularly depicted as acting like a scalpel or scissor blade. DNA sequences can be snipped, edited and rewritten through 'cutting and pasting' nucleotides from the genes of one organism and into the genes of another to 'engineer' desired traits, drawing on, and reinvigor-ating, familiar (and potentially tired) information technology tropes (Specter 2016). Who does not want a 'crisp' science? Nobody craves medicine that is like floppy lettuce, dry and curly white bread sandwiches, or out of date yoghurt with prominent mould – yet medicine deals on a daily basis with the unrefrigerated, and the hospital is an incubator for moulds. (Nosocomial and iatrogenic infections are largely avoidable through handwashing – not a metaphor, unless you are Lady Macbeth or a handwringing healthcare manager).

If a dominant metaphor shapes medical culture's mindset and practices ('the body as machine' and the production of impersonalism), can the culture be changed through changing the dominant metaphor? How would this happen – as a slow historical process, as a sharp educational intervention, as a policy decision, or because of a demographic sea change, such as more women than men now entering medicine? In the current climate, as discussed in Chapter 4, it is more likely that a spray of 'local', context-specific metaphors will emerge to replace current, inappropriate and potentially destructive, monolithic metaphors such as 'the war on cancer'. Certainly, medicine should cultivate metaphors of 'embrace' and 'holding' as alternatives to martial and violence metaphors; and we should remind ourselves that 'hospital' has the same root as 'hospitality', so that metaphors of welcoming, sheltering and feeding are already in the DNA of medicine and healthcare and could be foregrounded.

4 Keeping us close to the body at its limits

Metaphors both shape and generate insight into relative 'health' and 'suffering' where metaphors are embodied and grounded in activity. Metaphors are 'good to sense with' as well as good to think with. As medicine starts with the body and its afflictions, or in public health the body of the population, so everyday metaphors are often bodily based ('he made my blood boil', 'you must be taking the piss'), and bodily processes are territorialized by metaphors – such as 'sick societies' and 'that's a lame excuse' (Fleischman 2001).

5 Keeping us close to the mind at its limits

Mental illness has been described as a metaphor (Chapter 7). This is not a sceptical view, but rather, recognition that in some ways the world of metaphor and the world of the mind at its limits collide. This includes 'mindsets' that underpin symptoms such as addictions, and patterns of behaviour such as regular noncompliance with prescriptions. Perhaps points 4 and 5 here should be combined as 'bodymind' within the spirit of 'embodied metaphors'.

6 Affording diagnostic potential

Analogies are 'good to think with', or better, 'good to sense with'. Medical metaphors and similes are 'good to think medicine with'. Doctors think with metaphors. Resemblances in particular (prominent in the visual specialties – radiology, pathology and dermatology) are central to Type 1 clinical reasoning (pattern recognition) and associated diagnostic acumen (education of the senses).

7 Promising relational potential: conversations with colleagues and consultations with patients

Doctors employ the metaphor of 'knowledge translation' to encompass, for example, how they draw on and utilize biomedical research knowledge, statistical information, and knowledge from studies carried out in the social sciences (such as communication skills and patient satisfaction studies). In a review of the literature on knowledge translation, Greenhalgh and Wieringa (2011) ask: 'Is it time to drop the "knowledge translation" metaphor?' They note that a number of metaphors commonly employed in the social sciences – such as knowledge as 'socially constructed', 'embodied', 'performed', and owned and distributed as 'capital' according to prevailing power structures – do not readily translate back to medicine, where scientific modes, 'evidence-based' knowledge, and pragmatic 'know-do' mindsets dominate the discourse.

Something will, then, be lost in translation between disciplines – perhaps nuances, but more importantly, whole epistemological stances and meanings. Prior to knowledge 'translation', it is important to articulate the metaphors that shape differing kinds of knowledge such as 'tacit' and 'performative'. General practitioners observed by Gabbay and Le May (2010) drew on what the authors call 'mindlines' to make clinical decisions. These are tacit, embodied metaphors rather than evidence-based directives expressing expertise – fundamentally Type 1 reasoning, drawing on pattern recognition or resemblances ('I've seen this many times before, I can recall particular patients with these symptoms and this is how they presented and later responded to treatment'). Such mindlines are not static but are adapted through discussions with colleagues, reading new research and case studies, attending conferences, and so forth.

This shaping is a process of sharing stories and distilling key metaphors from those stories. But the stories themselves are shaped by big metaphors held by the culture, such as the body as machine, or patient as compliant customer (paternalism + economics). 'Mindlines' is, perhaps, an unhelpful metaphor, more so than 'sticky brains'. Does tacit knowledge follow 'lines', such as 'lines of thought' or 'lines of flight'? Better metaphors for the way that tacit knowing is organized, summoned and expressed are surely to be drawn from complexity theory, such as 'systems', 'attractors' and 'emergence'. 'Tangles' may be more appropriate than 'lines'. Perhaps 'mindline' resonates with the notion of an Australian Aboriginal 'songline', as described by Bruce Chatwin (1986), which is a compressed story or mythology.

Patients themselves use different metaphorical expressions and constructs from their doctors to make sense of symptoms. This gap must be bridged for optimal patient care. Patient communities who are experts in their own conditions (for example, unexplained chronic pain, rare blood cancers, voice hearers) should be studied early in medical education so that medical students can become familiar with the metaphorical vocabulary of these groups and develop 'otherness'. Patients' voices must not be 'lost in translation' across to the world of medical metaphors or its reductive scientific specialist languages (see Chapter 10; Marshall and Bleakley 2013).

8 *Offering a form of defence against the pressures of the work*

Doctors are taught to endure hardship by stripping away unnecessary labour (for example, deeper emotional interaction or entanglement with patients), but paradoxically, the constant grind of literalism and reductionism in itself takes its toll. I describe this below through the metaphor of 'driving with the brakes on'. Metaphors can be invited into medicine (or, as they are already there, can be acknowledged and employed for good effect) to refresh imagination for clinical work. Paradoxically, 'lean' medicine can be harder work emotionally and psychologically, since what is held at bay or is repressed can return in a distorted form. This is readily advertised in the continuing use of 'dark' medical slang (Chapter 3), for example, or in the typical passive aggressive profiles of layers of healthcare organizations from clinical teams to overarching, politically shaped health services.

9 *Promising an identity construction*

Metaphors are used to position doctors and then to create identities: doctors or surgeons; medical and surgical specialties; in relation to other healthcare professionals; through expanding roles (for example, doctor as teacher and manager); and in relation to organizational contexts (clinical team, department, hospital, general practice, hospital trust, National Health Service, private sector). Elkind (1998), referring to doctors' perceptions of the UK National Health Service (NHS), notes how practitioners' metaphorizing can follow didactic models such as the body as a machine, whereby the NHS is reduced to a perceived machine and the doctor becomes a cog within it. Other metaphors used to describe the NHS are organic (organism), paralleling a religion (the organization has founding principles and a vision), and economic (NHS as marketplace, patients as customers). Whichever metaphor is adopted then shapes the identity of the doctor (for example, as heart or brain in an organism, as priest in a religion, or as vendor in a marketplace).

Rodriguez and Bélanger (2014, p. 41) asked Canadian practitioners within the Quebec primary healthcare system to characterize that system through narrative accounts. A core metaphor of the 'journey' reappeared across accounts, in which the development of a multidisciplinary collaborative practice included: 'an uneasy departure, uncertainty about the destination, conflict amongst members who jump ship or stay on board, negotiations about the itinerary, and, finally, enduring challenges in leading the way and being pioneers of change'. Here, organizational identities such as 'leadership' or 'key participant' are shaped according to the 'journey' metaphor with its submetaphors such as 'jumping ship'.

Metaphors that medical students, and then doctors, entertain, embody and perform can shape conflicting identities. Korkmaz and Senol (2014) asked 178 first year medical students in Turkey to complete the prompt: 'A physician is like _____ because _____ ', thus inviting a simile. The responses were coded for similarity and frequency, resulting in six distinct metaphor groups. What is interesting is how new medical students already embody strong metaphorical frames that are contradictory. Thus, the doctor was seen as 'a figure of kindness and help' and as a 'healthcare provider' at the same time as 'a knowledge provider', a 'superior figure' and a 'symbol of prestige'. Metaphors of power and authority mix with those of care and largesse, summarized in the potentially mixed metaphor of the doctor 'as a cooperative leader'.

Is medicine's refusal of metaphor akin to driving with the brakes on?

Hard-nosed philosophers of language argue that language conceals reality and, therefore, we have to strip away language's veils – especially metaphors – to get at nature (Shibles 1971). Science works with this assumption and medicine follows science. Hence, metaphors should be excluded from medicine. However, as this book demonstrates, medicine is replete with metaphors, and medical practices such as diagnosis cannot proceed without metaphors. Indeed, metaphor itself is medicine – in the wider culture generally prescribed by artists, performers and writers.

In previous work (Bleakley *et al.* 2011; Bleakley 2014a, 2014b, 2015), while broadcasting great admiration for the work that most doctors do, I have argued that systemic faults in medical education shape cultures of medicine that operate like a car that is driven at one and the same time with the accelerator to the floor and the brakes on. It has not escaped my attention that this analogy is 'mechanical' – an alternative would be two people running a 'three-legged' race when there is an opportunity for both to run free and for one to be available to help the other. This metaphor also invites reflection on collaboration, such as the patient–doctor relationship and clinical teamwork. Such collaboration is often accepted grudgingly, such that two people enact a three-legged race, hampered by a self-inflicted binding.

Paradoxes such as driving with the brake on and collaborating as a three-legged race are grounded in largely unexamined, big, values-referenced fault lines that are historical effects of medical culture. Previously, I have argued that medicine may be at worst failed, and at best hampered, by its subscription to heroic individualism in an age of collaborative teamwork; by doctor-centredness in an age of patient-centredness and the expert patient; by masculinism in an age in which more women than men practice medicine; by instrumentalism, impersonalism and refusal of the aesthetic in an age in which we need humanistic professionals who exude style rather than impersonality; and, finally, by elitism or subscription to unproductive authority structures and an apolitical stance in an age in which we need principled, democratic medicine celebrating difference and social justice.

In this book, I bring this critique to a head, suggesting that medical education's refusal to address the value of metaphor in medicine has led to a one-dimensional approach: objective, literal, instrumental and flat. Driving metaphor out of medicine also drives out an interest in the aesthetics of practice. Such flatness numbs, educating for impersonalizing patients ('cases' rather than persons; facts and charts rather than stories; norm-referenced to populations rather than seen as idiosyncratic). More, the repression of metaphor has historically led to its distorted appearance as 'gallows humour' (Piemonte 2015) or potentially insulting backstage banter about patients, historically institutionalized in unsavoury medical slang.

To realize the power of metaphor in medicine – for both good and bad – is to recognize the central place of the imagination in medicine. As most cognitive psychologists, brain scientists, linguists and anthropologists will tell you (Fauconnier and Turner 2002), making metaphor is what drives imagination, and imagination, in turn, is the engine of innovation. However, as discussed throughout this book, tired and dead metaphors, or metaphors gone off and gone bad, can work against productive imagination. In an era in which we are trying to establish authentic collaborative teamwork and patient-centredness against the grain of the tradition of heroic medicine, continued use of the didactic metaphors of medicine as combat and the body as machine adds to medicine's overall refusal of, and resistance to, metaphorical thinking. This is, again, to restate the metaphors, like driving with the brakes on, or running a race three-legged when the runners could be free. Medical education has developed a habit of self-hampering, even self-harming.

While doctors, properly and justifiably, claim that they are underresourced, overworked and generally fatigued (Peterkin and Bleakley 2017), and the outcome of this fatigue may be to put patients at risk and also to put themselves at risk (showing in symptoms such as high rates of suicide, suicide ideation, and drug and alcohol abuse), an historical culture lingers in which doctors (and surgeons in particular) also perversely relish driving themselves into the ground in this way. Instead of complaining about chronic underresourcing of health services, atrocious lighting and heating conditions and poor food in hospitals, and structural problems in the culture, such as endemic bullying and oppressive and unproductive hierarchy, putting up with these has, historically, become a kind of badge of honour and a rite of passage. Many, however, are now calling for a sea change in medical culture, in which tired and unproductive authority structures will be replaced with working democracies, and where whistleblowing on bad practice will no longer be stigmatized and avoided (see Rodulson *et al.* 2015, where we discuss that there has to be a better metaphor than 'whistleblowing' for ethically and professionally correct intervention). This is reflected in new forms of medical education (Cooke *et al.* 2010; Bleakley *et al.* 2011; Bleakley 2014a) and in a growing political awareness and activism amongst doctors celebrating social justice (Bleakley 2016; Peterkin and Bleakley 2017).

Where doctors continue to put up with medical traditions that are patently inappropriate – such as denial of ambiguity in diagnostic work, denial that poor communication with patients and colleagues in team settings is a risk to both patients' and practitioners' health and safety, and the rationalization of medically unexplained symptoms – the brakes must come off, and the accelerator must be used more sensitively; the three-legged collaboration must become four-legged. Embrace the metaphor! You have nothing to lose but your metaphorical chains!

Metaphors are naturally occurring phenomena in the big habitat of language ('metaphor spotting' is detailed in Appendix 1). Medical metaphors offer a specific niche in that bigger habitat. Where metaphors appear – or 'self-display' – we might first respond to them aesthetically rather than instrumentally, appreciating them before we explain them away. Metaphor spotting is often just the prelude to explaining their functions, but let us give metaphors time to breathe and enjoy exposure as they sing, display their plumage, engage in their dances, and colour our world as our thinking refracts through the medium of metaphor. Metaphors do substantial work in medicine, and most of this book is devoted to an exposition of what that work means and where it has value, but let us linger on the fact that many metaphors display beauty, grace and impact (lingering as symptom presentations). Let us celebrate their distinctive presences.

Appendix 1

Twenty-two ways of looking at a metaphor

Linguists distinguish between differing kinds of metaphors, but often the distinctions are arbitrary and the overlaps more significant than the distinctions. Richard Nordquist (2015) describes 22 kinds of metaphor:

1 Absolute

Here, the tenor, or source, cannot be easily distinguished from the vehicle, or target. This is sometimes called a blended or paralogical metaphor. It is a kind of anti-metaphor. An example is 'Death is a journey' – how could we possibly know, as we are not yet dead?

2 Burlesque

Here, the comparison is hugely exaggerated, extraordinarily comic or grotesque. Nordquist's example is from the novelist Ford Maddox Ford's *The Good Soldier* (1915): 'It was a very black night and the girl was dressed in cream-coloured muslin, and must have glimmered under the tall trees of the dark park like a phosphorescent fish in a cupboard.'

3 Catachrestic

This is a figuratively effective but strained metaphor that is logically misused, such as 'decimate' for 'devastate'. It is common in medical metaphors – for example, where blood vessels are described as 'rivers', we also find tributaries, bridges and so forth, as if these were natural extensions.

4 Complex

Also known as a compound or telescoped metaphor; here, the literal meaning is expressed through a combination of primary metaphors. The target becomes the source for the next metaphor, as with Nordquist's example: 'This man was hair-trigger angry, and boiling over with the venom inside of him' (Howard Fast, *Power*, 1962).

5 *Conceptual*

Here, one idea is understood in terms of another, such as 'time is money'.

6 *Conduit*

This is a specific type of conceptual metaphor referring to processes of communication, such as 'getting your point across', 'she gave away her best ideas', 'your real feelings are finally coming across'. Michael Reddy estimates that 70 per cent of expressions used to talk about language and communication are conduit metaphors, arguing that metaphor use is everyday and neither ornamental nor special. Lakoff and Johnson (1980) describe Reddy's work as an inspiration for *Metaphors We Live By* and describe conduit metaphors as central to the architecture of cognition. Joe Grady (1998) critiques both models, suggesting that 'conduit' is a much more diffuse and complex category than the 'parcel' (container and communication) example offered by Reddy and elaborated by Lakoff and Johnson. The logic of the 'conduit' is fragmented, suggesting that it is a surface manifestation of a number of more general organizing metaphors.

7 *Conventional*

Better known as an idiom, this is a wholly familiar comparison that has perhaps become hackneyed, such as 'all the world's a stage', but is not yet a 'dead' metaphor (see type 9 below).

8 *Creative*

An original comparison that is poetic, literary, novel or unconventional. Richard Rorty (1991) calls a metaphor 'a voice from outside logical space'. A creative metaphor calls one 'to change one's language and one's life', rather than offering 'a proposal about how to systematize them'. An example is from W.B. Yeats' poem 'Byzantium', where Yeats refers to 'That dolphin-torn, that gong-tormented sea.' One would not expect dolphins leaping to be described as 'tearing' the sea, as Yeats does ('dolphin-torn'). This is a savage yet apt metaphor for such large-bodied creatures. More, why is the sea 'gong-tormented'? This suggests that there is some sinister sound emanating from the sea in its throes, even a spiritual torment. Yeats thus makes us look at the sea again as wracked and even in pain, rather than as energized.

9 *Dead*

Here, the metaphor has lost its presence and force through overuse. Both I.A. Richards and Lakoff and Turner challenge the notion of dead metaphors, suggesting that they may now simply be unconscious or tacit. The most deeply entrenched metaphors may even be the most powerful, as they work effortlessly. Examples of dead metaphors are the 'arms' of the chair and the 'foot' of the bed.

10 Extended

Also known as a conceit or a megametaphor, here the metaphor (as comparison) runs on through a series of sentences, the end point of which may be an allegory. The novelist Michael Chabon (2007) writes about family gatherings:

> It never takes longer than a few minutes, when they get together, for everyone to revert to the state of nature, like a party marooned by a shipwreck.... Also the storm at sea, the ship, and the unknown shore. And the hats and the whiskey stills that you make out of bamboo and coconuts. And the fire that you light to keep away the beasts.

11 Grammatical

One grammatical structure is substituted for another, resulting in a more compressed expression. Nordquist gives an example: 'the fifth day saw them at the summit'. Here, the fifth day unexpectedly becomes the subject of the sentence, rather than the climbers.

12 Kenning

A hangover from Old English and Norse poetry, a kenning is a highly compressed object-referenced figurative expression used in place of a noun or name, such as 'bone-house' for body, 'word-hoard' for lexicon, 'whale-road' for sea, 'sea-horse' for boat and 'iron-shower' for the rain of spears during a battle.

13 Mixed

Mixed metaphors are often already dead, or clichés (dead on their feet), such as this journalistic excerpt from the *Detroit News*, quoted in the *New Yorker*, 26 November 2012:

> I don't think we should wait until the other shoe drops. History has already shown what is likely to happen. The ball has been down this court before and I can see already the light at the end of the tunnel.

The journalist must surely have had his or her tongue firmly in his or her mouth.

14 Ontological

Here, something concrete is projected onto something abstract, such as boxing or battle applied to economics: 'fighting inflation', 'another round of cuts', 'the economy is taking a beating'. Medicine draws heavily on such metaphors: 'the hospital is a battleground'.

15 *Organizational*

An organization's key values or practices are captured in a pithy comparison: 'workers are cogs in the machine'.

16 *Personification*

An inanimate object or an abstraction is given human characteristics, as with this example from Nordquist: 'The fog had crept into the taxi where it crouched panting in a traffic jam. It oozed in ungenially, to smear sooty fingers over the two elegant young people who sat inside' (Margery Allingham, 1952, *The Tiger in the Smoke*).

17 *Primary*

Here, the metaphor is intuitively understood: 'to know is to see'.

18 *Root*

This is a master or basic metaphor, even a myth, capturing a worldview, such as an origin myth. It builds on primary metaphors (type 17 above): 'life is a journey', 'the universe is a machine', 'the universe is a complex system', 'social interaction is a game', 'life is a drama' ('do you like the part you're playing?').

19 *Structural*

Similar to an ontological metaphor (type 14 above), a complex concept or abstraction is presented in terms of a concrete 'big' notion, such as 'argument is war', or 'medicine is war (on disease)'.

20 *Submerged*

One of the terms – either source or target – is implied rather than stated explicitly: 'he mended her feelings' for 'he tried to make her feel better'. Harvey Birenbaum (1988) suggests that submerged metaphors 'lend the force of their associations in a subliminal way but are likely to be disruptive if they are realized too explicitly'.

21 *Therapeutic*

This is a figurative comparison used by a therapist to help a client or patient – commonly discussed in psychoanalysis, for example 'unblocking a memory'. Therapeutic storytelling draws heavily upon the supposed healing power of metaphor, whereby the metaphor allows a circumstance to be seen in a new light.

Much of the basic technical vocabulary of psychoanalysis is already metaphorical: defence mechanism, projection, displacement, rationalization, slip of the tongue, repression, and so forth.

22 Visual

Particularly used in television advertising – a visual image is used instead of a word or phrase. Cars become animals stalking the streets.

Appendix 2

How is metaphor use researched empirically, and how do we decide on what constitutes a metaphor in text, talk, action or image?

Research into the use of metaphors in medicine is almost certain to be driven by the pragmatic needs of the clinical community, which centres on continuous quality improvement of patient care and safety. This community champions evidence-based practice and will crave evidence based on empirical research in the field of metaphor and clinical practice. Primary questions will be:

1   What didactic metaphors shape the medical and medical education landscapes, and how might these didactic metaphors shift, be replaced, or be tailored according to the needs of individuals and discrete discourse communities across differing genres such as specialty clinical talk, interprofessional care discussions, patient consultations, patient online forums, public healthcare education, arts and humanities interventions, clinical texts, and so forth? Best-fit methods to research these questions:

   - analysing 'real world' clinical talk and activity;
   - analysing online communities such as patient forums and blogs;
   - historical archives such as clinical texts that can be explored through (a) linguistic corpus analysis and (b) Foucauldian discourse analysis to determine (potentially multiple and competing) historical conditions of possibility for the emergence of a dominant or didactic metaphor.

   This spectrum of research is already established with the Lancaster University Metaphor in End-of-Life Care (MELC) project (http://ucrel.lancs.ac.uk/melc/) (Demmen *et al.* 2015; Semino *et al.* 2015; Potts and Semino 2017), creating a first-class model for other research groups.

2   How and why are metaphors currently employed in varieties of clinical practice, such as diagnostic methods, communication with patients and colleagues in team settings, and organizational structures?

3   How is metaphor use distributed across practitioners, specialties and organizational structures?

4   How and why are metaphors employed in clinical texts?
     This is best done through linguistic corpus analysis (Deignan 2005).
5   How should historically sensitive metaphors be archived?

Included in such research is establishing that a lexical item (a word, a fragment or a sentence), the atmosphere of a text (e.g. rhetorical, ironic, cynical, descriptive or instrumental, aesthetic, ethical, political), and/or an activity (e.g. non-verbal proxemics captured on video) is indeed, *according to context*, being employed as a metaphor. A standard way of doing this is to employ 'Pragglejaz in practice', or to find 'metaphorically used words in natural discourse' (Steen *et al.*, in Low *et al.* 2010, pp. 165–84). The 'Pragglejaz' Metaphor Identification Procedure (MIP) refers to a systematic method originally devised by a group of 10 researchers, the first letters of whose Christian names spell Pragglejaz (www.lancaster.ac.uk/staff/eiaes/Pragglejaz_Group_2007.pdf).

The validity of research depends upon prior relative visibility and stability of the phenomenon under investigation. If a researcher decides in advance that surgery can be researched as performative 'theatre' because an operating room is called a 'theatre', he or she will be disappointed to find that surgical theatre teams do not see 'theatre' as metaphorical in this sense. Of course, their activities can be read as performative theatre, but when they say the word 'theatre', this cannot be read as a metaphor. In context, it is a literal description of a surgical site or space. Similarly, 'at the bedside' is literal description for a hospital team visiting a patient and perhaps teaching around that patient, but it does not, in that team's eyes, offer a 'device for seeing something in terms of something else' (Burke's 1945 definition of a metaphor). 'Bedside' for a medical anthropologist or sociologist, however, may signify a host of metaphorical possibilities.

A 'round' for a doctor is literally going around the ward to visit patients with a clinical team and junior doctors plus medical students who learn on the job. A 'grand round' is not some spectacular improvement on a 'round' but is the literal translation of a patient's diagnosis, treatment and prognosis – the patient having been visited on the ward round – to a lecture theatre for teaching purposes. To a medical educator, anthropologist or sociologist, again, the 'grand' round may act as a metaphor signifying the medical hierarchy at work. 'Pimping' in a North American medical education context means to make the student appear small or insignificant – teaching by ritual humiliation. In a European medical context, where it is commonly associated with procuring money through controlling prostitution and its monetary profit, the metaphor is meaningless.

Thus, it is vital to identify metaphors in context as 'metaphors for whom?' Instead of relying on intuitive judgements about what constitutes metaphor process or product (outcome), Pragglejaz offers protocol. (A reminder: Donald Schön differentiates between a metaphoric product as a 'frame' or 'perspective' – 'we're into a new ball game' – and a process by which new ways of looking at the world come into being – the government threatens UK doctors with an imposed, much-contested and disliked employment contract, leading to junior doctors becoming 'political animals').

Here, in a simplified form, are the steps of 'contextually sensitive' MIP:

1 Familiarization: read the entire text discourse or watch videotape of practice to establish a sense of what is going on.
2 Determine the lexical units to be analysed (words, phrases, activities).
3 For each lexical unit, determine its contextual meaning. For example, when a surgeon says to his or her assistant 'close up', there is no metaphor or rhetoric at work – the surgeon is asking the assistant (usually a registrar) to suture the patient's wound. If the registrar says to the scrub nurse after the surgeon has left 'he's really stitched me up, this is a ragged wound to close', he or she is employing a metaphor ('stitched me up'; 'ragged wound' is a literal description). When a urologist says to a male patient 'we've got your waterworks under control', he is using this mechanical metaphor for the benefit of the patient (even if the patient resents his body being objectified), and not for the benefit of himself and the clinical team, because he (and the urology nurse) are not thinking 'waterworks' but 'bladder', 'urethra' and 'catheterization'.
4 For each lexical unit, determine whether it has a more basic meaning than the one used in the given context: that is, more concrete, more precise, historically older.
5 Decide whether the lexical unit in context contrasts with the basic meaning but can be understood or is illuminated by it.
6 If the answer to point 5 is 'yes', then the lexical unit can be marked as metaphorical.

Here is an example: a patient is admitted to Accident and Emergency with a severe abdominal pain. The Year 2 Foundation doctor on duty says 'I'll get you something to make you feel more comfortable and then we'll have a look at you.' Ten minutes later, a nurse appears in the cubicle with a glass of water and one paracetamol tablet. For the patient, the doctor was using 'comfortable' relatively, even metaphorically. The patient is expecting heavier-duty dosage or different sedation. The lexical unit – in this case, a word – 'sedation' is used metaphorically from the patient's perspective.

A retired heart surgeon is talking to a cardiologist about what is being found during his own angiogram. They disagree about potential treatment. The heart surgeon says: 'Stick a stent in; it's just a mechanical problem, like pipecleaning.' The cardiologist disagrees: 'I don't think the artery is constricted enough to warrant a stent and it's distal; let's manage it through lifestyle and a drug regime: low dose aspirin, statin, alpha-blocker, and ACE inhibitor.' 'Pipecleaning' is used metaphorically and is an historically contingent metaphor. Few people smoke pipes, and smoking can be a cause of arterial blockage. The lexical unit has a more basic and concrete meaning and is historically older than 'pipecleaning' used as a metaphor. The cardiologist does not use a single metaphor, bar (arguably) 'alpha blocker' and 'ACE inhibitor'. While these are common medical descriptors and thus dead metaphors to the medical community, 'blocking' and 'inhibiting' – it can be argued – are used metaphorically in the descriptors. There is no rhetorical outcome for this, however, whereas 'pipecleaning' embodies rhetorical capital.

Appendix 3

A note on aphorisms

Aphorisms or maxims are cousins to metaphors. 'Aphorism' comes from the Greek *aphorismos*, meaning to have limits. They are pithy or terse sayings – often humorous – expressing a principle or an insight and boxed up to be memorable: 'when you hear hoofbeats, don't think zebras' (stick to the obvious and the expected, don't expect or cultivate the obscure); or, one of William Osler's notable pithy sayings: 'The good physician treats the disease; the great physician treats the patient who has the disease.'

Whereas a metaphor is an already collapsed, tight expression that opens up a wealth of associations, working in terms of an expansion or 'big bang', aphorisms are all about collapse. Multiple and complex issues and meanings are focused in memorable phrases or sayings. Doctors like aphorisms because they work in the same way as traditional case histories and presentations – tight, collapsed, lean, to the point and functional. This book is about metaphors and not aphorisms, although they have elements in common. For a review of the history and purposes of aphorisms in medicine, see Levine and Bleakley (2012).

Bibliography

About Gwinyai Masukume. (Undated). Improbable research. Available at: www.improbable.com/about/people/GwinyaiMasukume.html. Last accessed: 26 March 2017.

Agamben G. (1998). *Homo Sacer: Sovereign Power and Bare Life*. Palo Alto, CA: Stanford University Press.

Ahmed H, Ogala WN, Ibrahim M. Culinary metaphors in Western medicine: a dilemma of medical students in Africa. *Medical Education*. 1992; 26: 423–4.

Alford H. (1739). *The Works of John Donne, D.D., Dean of St Paul's 1621–1631, With a Memoir of His Life. Vol. II*. London: John W. Parker.

Allum VJ. (undated). What does English for Medical Purposes cover? AuthorsDen. Available at: www.authorsden.com/visit/viewarticle.asp?id=66339. Last accessed: 30 August 2016.

Almendraia A. The whimsical way medical students learn about the body. *The Huffington Post*. 10 July 2014. Available at: www.huffingtonpost.com/2014/07/10/food-metaphors-in-medicine_n_5572347.html. Last accessed: 11 August 2016.

Altoona Family Physicians Residency. The Altoona list of medical analogies (undated). Available at: www.altoonafp.org/analogies.htm. Last accessed: 30 August 2016.

Alzheimer's Society. (Undated). Available at: www.alzheimers.org.uk. Last accessed: 26 March 2017.

Amini B. Honeycombing (lungs). Radiopaedia. Available at: http://radiopaedia.org/articles/honeycombing. Last accessed: 26 March 2017.

Andrade-Filho Jde S. Analogies in medicine: intruder noodles. *Revista do Instituto de Medicina Tropical de São Paulo*. 2011a; 53: 345.

Andrade-Filho Jde S. Analogies in medicine: the American killer. *Revista do Instituto de Medicina Tropical de São Paulo*. 2011b; 53: 339.

Andrade-Filho Jde S. Analogies in medicine: marine pilot's wheel. *Revista do Instituto de Medicina Tropical de São Paulo*. 2012a; 54: 330.

Andrade-Filho Jde S. Analogies in medicine: picture frame and tapir's nose. *Revista do Instituto de Medicina Tropical de São Paulo*. 2012b; 54: 298.

Andrade-Filho Jde S. Analogies in medicine: anchovy paste in the liver. *Revista do Instituto de Medicina Tropical de São Paulo*. 2012c; 54: 234.

Andrade-Filho Jde S. Analogies in medicine: little thief in the skin. *Revista do Instituto de Medicina Tropical de São Paulo*. 2012d; 54: 118.

Andrade-Filho Jde S. Analogies in medicine: violin strings adhesions. *Revista do Instituto de Medicina Tropical de São Paulo*. 2013a; 55: 435–6.

Andrade-Filho Jde S. Analogies in medicine: spaghetti and meatballs. *Revista do Instituto de Medicina Tropical de São Paulo*. 2013b; 55.

Andrade-Filho Jde S. Analogies in medicine: gimlet in Chagas disease. *Revista do Instituto de Medicina Tropical de São Paulo.* 2013c; 55: 68.

Andrade-Filho Jde S. Analogies in medicine: starry-sky appearance. *Revista do Instituto de Medicina Tropical de São Paulo.* 2014a; 56: 541–2.

Andrade-Filho Jde S. Analogies in medicine: slapped cheek appearance. *Revista do Instituto de Medicina Tropical de São Paulo.* 2014b; 56: 458.

Andrade-Filho Jde S. Analogies in medicine: white clay-pipe stem 'cirrhosis'. *Revista do Instituto de Medicina Tropical de São Paulo.* 2014c; 56: 92.

Andrade-Filho Jde S, Pena GP. Analogies in medicine. *International Journal of Surgical Pathology.* 2001; 9: 345–6.

Andrade-Filho Jde S, Pena GP. Analogies in medicine: fungus and liturgy. *Revista do Instituto de Medicina Tropical de São Paulo.* 2010; 52: 288.

Annas GJ. Reframing the debate on health care reform by replacing our metaphors. *New England Journal of Medicine.* 1995; 332: 744–7.

Annas GJ. Toward an ecology of health. Beyond the military and market metaphors. *Healthcare Forum.* 1996; 39: 30–4.

Anon. Doctors' slang, medical slang and medical acronyms and veterinary acronyms & vet slang. Available at: http://messybeast.com/dragonqueen/medical-acronyms.htm. Last accessed: 26 March 2017.

Aristotle. (1996). *Poetics.* Harmondsworth: Penguin Classics.

Arrigo BA. Martial metaphors and medical justice: implications for law, crime, and deviance. *Journal of Political and Military Sociology.* 1999; 27: 307–22.

Arroliga AC, Newman S, Longworth DL, Stoller JK. Metaphorical medicine: using metaphors to enhance communication with patients who have pulmonary disease. *Annals of Internal Medicine.* 2002; 137: 376–9.

Austin JL. (1975, 2nd edn). *How to Do Things with Words.* Cambridge, MA: Harvard University Press.

Bachelard G. (1977). *The Psychoanalysis of Fire.* Boston, MA: Beacon Press.

Bachelard G. (1988). *Air and Dreams: An Essay on the Imagination of Movement.* Dallas, TX: Dallas Institute.

Bachelard G. (1989). *The Flame of a Candle.* Dallas, TX: Dallas Institute.

Bachelard G. (1992). *The Poetics of Space.* Boston, MA: Beacon Press.

Bachelard G. (1994). *Water and Dreams: An Essay on the Imagination of Matter.* Dallas, TX: Dallas Institute.

Bachelard G. (2002). *Earth and Reveries of Will: An Essay on the Imagination of Matter.* Dallas, TX: Dallas Institute.

Baker SR, Noorelahi YM, Ghosh S, Yang LC, Kasper DJ. History of metaphoric signs in radiology. *European Journal of Radiology.* 2013; 82: 1584–7.

Baker SR, Partyka L. Relative importance of metaphor in radiology versus other medical specialties. *Radiographics.* 2012; 32: 235–40.

Bakhtin M. (1982). *The Dialogic Imagination: Four Essays.* Austin, TX: University of Texas Press.

Balcu I. Tango as metaphor for doctor/patient relations: Patients 2.0 – Kathy Kastner. 9 October 2013. Available at: http://e-patients.net/archives/2013/10/tango-as-metaphor-for-doctorpatient-relations-patients-2-0-kathy-kastner.html. Last accessed: 3 September 2016.

Bamforth I. (2015). *A Doctor's Dictionary: Writings on Culture and Medicine.* London: Carcanet.

Barfield O. (1928/2010). *Poetic Diction: A Study in Meaning*. London: Barfield Press.

Bates V, Bleakley A, Goodman S. (eds) (2014). *Medicine, Health and the Arts: Approaches to the Medical Humanities*. London: Routledge.

Battistatou A, Zolota V, Scopa C. The gourmet 'pathologist'. *International Journal of Surgical Pathology*. 2000; 8: 341–2.

Bauman Z. (2000). *Liquid Modernity*. London: Polity Press.

BBC News Channel. (2003). Doctor slang is a dying art. Available at: http://news.bbc.co.uk/1/hi/3159813.stm. Last accessed: 18 August 2016.

BBC News Channel. (2014). The seven best metaphors for the economy. Available at: www.bbc.co.uk/news/business-30208476. Last accessed: 26 March 2017.

BBC News Channel. (2016). Junior doctors' row: the basics of the dispute. Available at: www.bbc.co.uk/news/health-36672762. Last accessed: 1 October 2016.

Beauchamp TL, Childress JF. (2013, 7th ed.). *Principles of Biomedical Ethics*. Oxford: OUP.

Beisecker AE, Beisecker TD. Using metaphors to characterize doctor–patient relationships: paternalism versus consumerism. *Health Communication*. 1993; 5: 41–58.

Bell C. War and the allegory of medical intervention: why metaphors matter. *International Political Sociology*. 2012; 6: 325–8.

Benedek M, Beaty R, Jauk E, Koschutnig K, Fink A, Silvia PJ, Dunst B, Neubauer AC. Creating metaphors: the neural basis of figurative language production. *NeuroImage*. 2014; 90: 99–106.

Berlant L. (2011). *Cruel Optimism*. Durham, NC: Duke University Press.

Bhabha H. (2004, 2nd edn). *The Location of Culture*. London: Routledge.

Birenbaum H. (1988). *Myth and Mind*. Lanham, MD: University Press of America.

Bjørkløf GH, Kirkevold M, Engedal K, Selbaek G, Helvik AS. Being stuck in a vice: the process of coping with severe depression in late life. *International Journal of Qualitative Studies on Health and Well-being*. 2015; 10: 271–87.

Bleakley A. (Undated). Thinking with metaphors in medicine: re-shaping clinical work. Available at: www.medicalmetaphors.com. Last accessed: 26 March 2017.

Bleakley A. Greens and greenbacks. *Spring*. 1992; 52: 68–71.

Bleakley A. From reflective practice to holistic reflexivity. *Studies in Higher Education*. 1999; 24: 315–30.

Bleakley A. (2004). Doctors as connoisseurs of informational images: aesthetic and ethical self-forming through medical practice. In: J Satterthwaite, E Atkinson, W Martin (eds) *Educational Counter-Cultures: Confrontations, Images, Vision*. London: Trentham.

Bleakley A. (2006). Towards an aesthetics of healthcare practice: learning the art of clinical judgement. In: *Theory and Practice in Nursing Education*. University of Aarhus, Denmark.

Bleakley A. (2014a). *Patient-centred Medicine in Transition: The Heart of the Matter*. Dordrecht: Springer.

Bleakley A. (2014b). The medical humanities in medical education: toward a medical aesthetics of resistance. In: T Jones, D Wear, L Friedman (eds) *Health Humanities Reader*. New York, NY: Rutgers University Press.

Bleakley A. (2015). *Medical Humanities and Medical Education: How the Medical Humanities Can Shape Better Doctors*. London: Routledge.

Bleakley A. The perils and rewards of critical consciousness raising in medical education. *Academic Medicine*. 2016; 91: 289–91.

Bleakley A, Bligh J. Distributing menus to hungry learners: can learning by simulation become simulation of learning? *Medical Teacher*. 2006; 28: 606–13.

Bleakley A, Jolly M. Writing out prescriptions: hyperrealism and the chemical regulation of mood. *Advances in Health Sciences Education: Theory and Practice*. 2012; 17: 779–90.

Bleakley A, Bligh J, Browne J. (2011). *Medical Education for the Future: Identity, Power and Location*. Dordrecht: Springer.

Bleakley A, Farrow, R, Gould D, Marshall R. Learning how to see: doctors making judgements in the visual domain. *Journal of Workplace Learning*. 2003a; 15: 301–6.

Bleakley A, Farrow, R, Gould D, Marshall R. Making sense of clinical reasoning: judgement and the evidence of the senses. *Medical Education*. 2003b; 37: 544–52.

Bleakley A, Lynch L, Whelan G (eds) (2017). *Dangerous Currents: Risk and Regulation at the Interface of Medicine and the Arts*. Newcastle: Cambridge Scholars Publishing.

BNF Publications. (Undated). Available at: www.bnf.org/about/. Last accessed: 26 March 2017.

Borges JL. 'Slow nightfall' and blindness. Available at: www.brainyquote.com/quotes/quotes/j/jorgeluisb125297.html. Last accessed: 18 August 2016.

Boseley S. Fewer people die in hospital at weekends, study finds. *Guardian*. Friday 6 May 2016. Available at www.theguardian.com/society/2016/may/06/fewer-die-in-hospital-weekends-study-jeremy-hunt-doctors-contract. Last accessed: 3 September 2016.

Bouchard G, O'Brien M. (eds) Editorial: on medicine. *Performance Research Medicine*. 2014; 19, No. 4.

Bradley J. From the sweet taste of urine to MRI: how doctors lost their senses. The Conversation. 10 July 2014. Available at https://theconversation.com/from-the-sweet-taste-of-urine-to-mri-how-doctors-lost-their-senses-28905. Last accessed: 29 August 2016.

Brockway L. Tell us: What's your medical metaphor? TEDMED. 8 April 2015. Available at http://blog.tedmed.com/tell-us-whats-your-medical-metaphor/. Last accessed: 29 August 2016.

Brown D. Judge backs dying child's bid to have body frozen. *The Times*. 18 November 2016, front page.

Broyard A. Good books about being sick. 1 April 1990. Available at www.nytimes.com/1990/04/01/books/good-books-abut-being-sick.html?pagewanted=all. Last accessed: 20 August 2016.

Buchbinder M. 'Sticky' brains and sticky encounters in an American pediatric pain clinic. *Culture, Medicine and Psychiatry*. 2012; 36: 102–23.

Buchbinder M. (2015). *All in Your Head: Making Sense of Pediatric Pain*. Oakland, CA: University of California Press.

Burke K. (1945). *A Grammar of Motives*. Berkeley, CA: University of California Press.

Burke K. Review: democracy of the sick. *The Kenyon Review*. 1959; 21: 639–43.

Burnside JW. Medicine and war: a metaphor. *Journal of the American Medical Association*. 1983; 249: 2091.

Callahan JF. (2004). *Ralph Ellison's Invisible Man: A Casebook*. Oxford: OUP.

Cameron L. (2003). *Metaphor in Educational Discourse*. London: Continuum.

Cameron L, Low G. (eds) (1999). *Researching and Applying Metaphor*. Cambridge: CUP.

Campo R. Poetry Foundation: Rafael Campo. Undated. Available at www.poetry foundation.org/poems-and-poets/poets/detail/rafael-campo. Last accessed: 29 Augus 2016.

Cardiovascular basics. Picmonic. Available at: www.picmonic.com/pathways/medicine/courses/standard/physiology-184/cardiovascular-basics-287. Last accessed: 26 March 2017.

Carter AH. Metaphors in the physician-patient relationship. *Soundings*. 1989; 72: 153–64.

Casciato C. (2009). Jacques Derrida on Zombies. The Inevitable Zombie Apocalypse. Available at www.inevitablezombieapocalypse.com/2009/04/jacques-derrida-on-zombies/. Last accessed: 5 September 2016.

Cassels C. Stimulant use exceptionally high among medical students. Medscape News and Perspectives. 6 February 2013. Available at www.medscape.com/viewarticle/778843. Last accessed: 18 August 2016.

Chabon M. (2007). *The Yiddish Policeman's Union*. New York, NY: HarperCollins.

Chamber TS. (1999). *The Fiction of Bioethics: Cases as Literary Texts*. London: Routledge.

Chatwin B. (1986). *The Songlines*. Harmondsworth: Penguin Books.

Cheng C. Food analogies can help teach medicine. Counsel & Heal News. 10 July 2014. Available at www.counselheal.com/articles/10421/20140710/food-analogies-can-help-teach-medicine.htm#ixzz3m70yYxvO. Last accessed: 29 August 2016.

Childress JF, Siegler M. Metaphors and models of doctor-patient relationships: their implications for autonomy. *Theoretical Medicine*. 1984; 5: 17–30.

Cichminska M, Topolewska M. Conceptual metaphors in *House MD*. *Prace Jezykoznawcze* UWM Olsztyn 2010; 65–76. Available at www.academia.edu/11455453/Conceptual_metaphors_in_House_M.D. Last accessed: 18 August 2016.

Cixous H. (1991). *Coming to Writing and Other Essays*. Cambridge, MA: Harvard University Press.

Clark A. (2008). *Supersizing the Mind*. Oxford: OUP.

Clark A. (2016). *Surfing Uncertainty*. Oxford: OUP.

Clark A, Chalmers DJ. The extended mind. *Analysis*. 1998; 58: 10–23.

Clod Ensemble. Performing medicine. Available at: performingmedicine.com. Last accessed: 26 March 2017.

Clow B. Who's afraid of Susan Sontag? or, the myths and metaphors of cancer reconsidered. *Social History of Medicine*. 2001; 14: 293–312.

Cone J. (2013). Tolerating ambiguity in four simple steps. Interaction Associates. Undated. Available at http://interactionassociates.com/insights/blog/tolerating-ambiguity-four-simple-steps#.Vymv1l6TOTM. Last accessed: 29 August 2016.

Cooke M, Irby DM, O'Brien BC. (2010). *Educating Physicians: A Call for Reform of Medical School and Residency*. San Francisco, CA: Jossey-Bass.

Coombs RH, Chopra S, Schenk DR, Yutan E. Medical slang and its functions. *Social Science & Medicine*. 1993; 36: 987–98.

Cooper C. Ethnic doctors far less likely to reach senior posts in NHS. *Independent*. 26 September 2013. Available at www.independent.co.uk/life-style/health-and-families/health-news/ethnic-doctors-far-less-likely-to-reach-senior-posts-in-nhs-8842397.html. Last accessed: 29 August 2016.

Cooper C. Mind your language: 'Battling' cancer metaphors can make terminally ill patients worse. *Independent*. 3 November 2014. Available at www.independent.co.uk/life-style/health-and-families/health-news/mind-your-language-battling-cancer-metaphors-can-make-terminally-ill-patients-worse-9836322.html. Last accessed: 15 August 2016.

Cooper D. (1967). *Psychiatry and Anti-Psychiatry*. London: Paladin.

Couser G. Thomas. Disability as metaphor. *Prose Studies: History, Theory, Criticism.* 2005; 27: 141–54.

Cussins A. Content, embodiment, and objectivity: the theory of cognitive trails. *Mind.* 1992; 101: 651–88.

Custers EJFM. Thirty years of illness scripts: theoretical origins and practical applications. *Medical Teacher.* 2015; 37: 457–62.

Davies K. The body and doing gender: the relations between doctors and nurses in hospital work. *Sociology of Health & Illness.* 2003; 25: 720–42.

De Leonardis F. War as medicine: the medical metaphor in contemporary Italian political language. *Social Semiotics.* 2008; 18: 33–45.

Deignan AH. (2005). *Metaphor and Corpus Linguistics.* Amsterdam: John Benjamins.

Deleuze G. (1998). *Essays Critical and Clinical.* London: Verso.

Deleuze G, Guattari F. (1988a/2004). *Anti-Oedipus: Capitalism and Schizophrenia.* London: Continuum.

Deleuze G, Guattari F. (1988b/2004). *A Thousand Plateaus.* London: Continuum.

DeLillo, D. (1997). *Underworld.* New York, NY: Charles Scribner's Sons.

DeLillo, D. (2016). *Zero K.* New York, NY: Scribner Book Company.

Demjen Z, Semino E, Koller V. Metaphors for 'good' and 'bad' deaths: a health professional view. *Metaphor and the Social World.* 2016; 6: 1–19.

Demmen J, Semino E, Demjen Z, Koller V, Hardie A, Rayson P, Payne SA. Computer-assisted study of the use of violence metaphors for cancer and end of life by patients, family carers and health professionals. *International Journal of Corpus Linguistics.* 2015; 20: 205–31.

Derrida J. (1998). *Archive Fever: A Freudian Impression.* Chicago: University of Chicago Press.

Dewey J. (2013). *Democracy and Education: An Introduction to the Philosophy of Education by John Dewey.* Charleston, NC: CreateSpace Independent Publishing Platform.

Diekema DS, Fost N. Ashley revisited: a response to the critics. *The American Journal of Bioethics.* 2010; 10: 30–44.

Docherty J. Four reasons to use the war metaphor with caution. The Center for Justice and Peacebuilding. 16 September 2001. Available at www.emu.edu/cjp/publications/beyond-september-11th/2001/use-the-war-metaphor-with-caution/. Last accessed: 29 August 2016.

Donaldson J. (2015). *Missing Link: The Evolution of Metaphor and the Metaphor of Evolution.* Montreal: McGill-Queen's University Press.

Donoghue D. (2014). *Metaphor.* Cambridge, MA: Harvard University Press.

Dubiel H. (2009). *Deep within the Brain: Living with Parkinson's Disease.* New York: Europa editions.

Dubiel H. What is 'Narrative Bioethics'? *Frontiers in Integrative Neuroscience.* 2011; 5: 10.

Dunbar K, Blanchette I. The in vivo/in vitro approach to cognition: the case of analogy. *Trends in Cognitive Sciences.* 2001; 5: 334–9.

Dutton K. (2012). *The Wisdom of Psychopaths: What Saints, Spies, and Serial Killers Can Teach Us about Success.* London: Arrow.

Earp BD, Everett JAC, Madva EN, Hamlin JK. Out, damned spot: can the 'Macbeth Effect' be replicated? *Basic and Applied Social Psychology.* 2014; 36: 91–8.

Ehrenreich B. (2001). Welcome to cancerland. *Harper's Magazine.* November 2001. Available at http://harpers.org/archive/2001/11/welcome-to-cancerland/. Last accessed: 29 August 2016.

Eisner EW. (1998). *The Enlightened Eye: Qualitative Inquiry and the Enhancement of Educational Practice*. Upper Saddle River, NJ: Merrill.

Elkind A. Using metaphor to read the organisation of the NHS. National Health Service. *Social Science & Medicine*. 1998; 47: 1715–27.

Empson W. (1930). *Seven Types of Ambiguity*. London: The Hogarth Press.

Engeström Y. (2008). *From Teams to Knots*. Cambridge: CUP.

Engeström Y. (2009). The Future of Activity Theory: A Rough Draft. Keynote lecture given at ISCAR conference, San Diego, 2008. Available at: http://lchc.ucsd.edu/mca/Paper/ISCARkeyEngestrom.pdf. Last accessed: 13 November 2016.

Engeström Y. (2010). Activity theory and learning at work. Available at www.helsinki.fi/cradle/documents/Engestrom%20Publ/Chapter%20for%20Malloch%20book.pdf. Last accessed: 3 September 2016.

Eviatar Z, Just MA. Brain correlates of discourse processing: an fMRI investigation of irony and conventional metaphor comprehension. *Neuropsychologia*. 2006; 44: 2348–59.

Faber P, Linares CM. (2004). The role of imagery in specialized communication. In: B Lewandowska-Tomaszczyk, A Kwiatkowska (eds) *Imagery and Language*. Frankfurt: Peter Lang, 585–602.

Farquhar F, Fitzsimons P. Lost in translation: the power of language. *Educational Philosophy and Theory*. 2011; 43: 652–62.

Fauconnier G, Turner M. (2002). *The way we think: Conceptual blending and the mind's hidden complexities*. New York, NY: Basic Books.

Fenster M. Seeing the State: transparency as metaphor. *Administrative Law Review*. 2010; 62: 617–72. University of Florida Levin College of Law Research Paper No. 2010–07. Available at: http://ssrn.com/abstract=1562762. Last accessed: 2 November 2016.

Finatto MJB. Metaphors in scientific and technical languages: challenges and perspective. *Documentação de Estudos em Lingüística Teórica e Aplicada*. 2010; 26 especial: 645–56.

Fleischman S. (2001). Language and medicine. In: D Schiffrin, D Tannen, H Hamilton (eds.) *The Handbook of Discourse Analysis*. Oxford: Blackwell, 470–502.

Fleming A, Cutrer W, Reimschisel T, Gigante J. You too can teach clinical reasoning! *Pediatrics*. 2012; 130: 795–7.

Flexner A. (1910). *Medical Education in the United States and Canada*. New York, NY: Carnegie Foundation for the Advancement of Teaching. (Revised 1973: New York, NY: Heritage Press).

Fludernik M. (ed.) (2011). *Beyond Cognitive Metaphor Theory: Perspectives on Literary Metaphor*. London: Routledge.

Foley P. 'Black Dog' as metaphor for depression: a brief history. 2005. Available at www.blackdoginstitute.org/au/media/eventscal/index.cfm. Last accessed: 15 August 2016.

Food related medical terms. (Undated). Available at: http://foodmedicaleponyms.blogspot.co.uk. Last accessed: 26 March 2017.

Foucault, M. (1964). *Madness and Civilization*. London: Routledge.

Foucault M. (1970). *The Order of Things*. New York, NY: Pantheon Books.

Foucault M. (1976/1989) *The Birth of the Clinic: An Archaeology of Medical Perception*. London: Routledge.

Foucault M. (1988). *Technologies of the Self*. Amherst, MA: University of Massachusetts Press.

Fox AT, Fertleman M, Cahill P, Palmer RD. Medical slang in British hospitals. *Ethics & Behavior*. 2003; 13: 173–89.

Francis M. (2013). *Muscovy*. London: Faber & Faber.

Frank A. Project MUSE – metaphors of pain. *Literature and Medicine*. 2011; 29: 182–96.

Frank A. (2013). *The Wounded Storyteller*. Chicago, IL: University of Chicago Press.

Freire P. (1973). *Education for Critical Consciousness*. New York, NY: Crossroad Publishing Company.

Frieden HJ, Dolev JC. Medical analogies: their role in teaching dermatology to medical professionals and patients. *Journal of the American Academy of Dermatology.* 2005; 53: 863–6.

Frueh J. (1996). *Erotic Faculties*. Berkeley, CA: University of California Press.

Fuks A. The military metaphors in modern medicine. Freeland: Oxfordshire Inter-disciplinary net. 2009. Available at www.inter-disciplinary.net/wp-content/uploads/2009/06/hid_fuks.pdf. Last accessed: 19 August 2016.

Fuller G, Hughes T. Metaphors and analogies in neurology: from Kerplunk to dripping taps. *Practical Neurology.* 2003; 3: 142–9.

Furlan J. (2014). 5 Poems from 'Prelude To Bruise' Read By Saeed Jones. Buzzfeed. Available at: www.buzzfeed.com/juliafurlan/5-poems-from-prelude-to-bruise-read-by-saeed-jones?utm_term=.kuyXZz4yn#.ppMajmw92. Last accessed: 26 March 2017.

Furnham A, Marks J. Tolerance of ambiguity: a review of the recent literature. *Psychology.* 2013; 4: 717–28.

Furnham A, Ribchester T. Tolerance of ambiguity: a review of the concept, its measurement and applications. *Current Psychology.* 1995; 14: 179–99.

Gabbay J, Le May A. (2010). *Practice-based Evidence for Healthcare: Clinical Mindlines*. London: Routledge.

Galewski M. May I take your metaphor? – how we talk about cancer. 28 September 2015. Available at http://scienceblog.cancerresearchuk.org/2015/09/28/may-i-take-your-metaphor-how-we-talk-about-cancer/. Last accessed: 15 August 2016.

Geary J. (2011). *I Is an Other: The Secret Life of Metaphor and How It Shapes the Way We See the World*. New York, NY: HarperPerennial.

Gentner D, Markman A. Structure mapping in analogy and similarity. *American Psychologist.* 1997; 52: 45–56.

George DR. Overcoming the social death of dementia through language. *Lancet.* 2010; 376: 586–7.

George DR, Whitehouse PJ. The War (on Terror) on Alzheimer's. *Dementia (London).* 2014; 13: 120–30.

Gholipour B. Strawberry cervix? Doc reviews food words used in medicine. Live Science. 9 July 2014. Available at www.livescience.com/46732-food-references-in-medical-terms.html. Last accessed: 4 September 2016.

Gibson JJ. (1979). *The Ecological Approach to Visual Perception*. Boston, MA: Houghton Mifflin.

Ginn S. Metaphors in medicine. The *BMJ* blogs 23 August 2011. Available at http://blogs.bmj.com/bmj/2011/08/23/stephen-ginn-metaphors-in-medicine/. Last accessed: 4 September 2016.

Gladwell M. (2009). *Outliers*. London: Penguin.

Gleyse J. The machine body metaphor: from science and technology to physical education and sport, in France (1825–1935). *Scandinavian Journal of Medicine & Science in Sports.* 2013; 23: 758–65.

Goffman E. (1959). *The Presentation of Self in Everyday Life*. New York, NY: Random House.

Gollwitzer M, Meltzer A. Macbeth and the joystick: Evidence for moral cleansing after playing a violent video game. *Journal of Experimental Social Psychology.* 2012; 48: 1356–60.

Grady J. (1998). The 'conduit' metaphor revisited: a reassessment of metaphors for communication. In: J-P Koenig (ed.) *Discourse and Cognition: Bridging the Gap*. Stanford, CA: Center for the Study of Language and Information (CSLI) Publications, 205–18.

Greenberg L. (2009). *The Body Broken: A Memoir*. New York, NY: Random House.

Greenblatt, Stephen (1980). *Renaissance Self-Fashioning: From More to Shakespeare*. Chicago: University of Chicago Press.

Greenhalgh T, Wieringa S. Is it time to drop the 'knowledge translation' metaphor? A critical literature review. *Journal of the Royal Society of Medicine*. 2011; 104: 501–9.

Guiot C, Delsanto PP, Deisboeck TS. Morphological instability and cancer invasion: a 'splashing water drop' analogy. *Theoretical Biology & Medical Modelling*. 2007; 4: 4.

Gwyn R. (1999) 'Captain of my own ship': metaphor and the discourse of chronic illness. In: L Cameron and G Low (eds) *Researching and Applying Metaphor*. Cambridge: CUP.

Haidet P. Jazz and the 'art' of medicine: improvisation in the clinical encounter. *Annals of Family Medicine*. 2007; 5: 164–9.

Hall J. (2013). *Essays on Performance Writing etc Vol 1*. Exeter: Shearsman Books.

Harden H. (2013). Understanding leadership as decision making in a healthcare context: exploring skillful relating, institutional talk and the emergence of multi-ontology sense-making in cancer care networks in Australia. PhD thesis. Griffith University.

Hardy JN. Metaphor may fill the space created by uncertainty. *BMJ*. 2012; 345: e5468.

Hatala AR. The status of the 'biopsychosocial' model in health psychology: towards an integrated approach and a critique of cultural conceptions. *Open Journal of Medical Psychology*. 2012; 1: 51–62.

Heller-Roazen D. (2007). *The Inner Touch: Archaeology of a Sensation*. New York, NY: Zone Books.

Hilligoss B. Selling patients and other metaphors: a discourse analysis of the interpretive frames that shape emergency department admission handoffs. *Social Science & Medicine*. 2014; 102: 119–28.

Hilligoss B, Mansfield JA, Patterson SE, Moffatt-Bruce SD. Collaborating or 'selling' patients? A conceptual framework for emergency department-to-inpatient handoff negotiations. *Joint Commission Journal on Quality and Patient Safety*. 2015; 41: 134–43.

Hillman J. (1977). *Re-visioning Psychology*. London: HarperCollins.

Hillman J, Roscher W. (2000). *Pan and the Nightmare*. Dallas, TX: Spring Books.

Hoda RS, Hoda SA. (2004). *Fundamentals of Pap Test Cytology*. Totowa: NJ: Humana Press.

Hodges B. The many and conflicting histories of medical education in Canada and the USA: an introduction to the paradigm wars. *Medical Education*. 2005; 39: 613–21.

Hodgkin P. Medicine is war: and other medical metaphors. *BMJ (Clinical research ed.)*. 1985; 291: 1820–1.

Hofstadter D, Sander E. (2013). *Surfaces and Essences: Analogy as the Fuel and Fire of Thinking*. New York: Basic Books.

Homer. *The Iliad*. Trans. R Fagles (1998). New York, NY: Penguin Books, lines 415–19.

Hoybye MT, Johansen C, Tjornhoj-Thomsen T. Online interaction. Effects of storytelling in an internet breast cancer support group. *Psychooncology*. 2005; 14: 211–20.

Hudak PL, McKeever P, Wright JG. The metaphor of patients as customers: implications for measuring satisfaction. *Journal of Clinical Epidemiology*. 2003; 56: 103–8.

Hunter KM. (1993). *Doctors' Stories: The Narrative Structure of Medical Knowledge*. Princeton, NJ: Princeton University Press.

Hunter KM. Eating the curriculum. *Academic Medicine: Journal of the Association of American Medical Colleges.* 1997; 72: 167–72.

Hutchings D. Communicating with metaphor: a dance with many veils. *The American Journal of Hospice & Palliative Care.* 1998; 15: 282–4.

Irigaray L. (2004). *An Ethics of Sexual Difference.* London: Continuum.

Ishiguro K. (2005). *Never Let Me Go.* London: Faber & Faber.

Jones AH. Narrative in medical ethics. *BMJ.* 1999; 318: 253–6.

Jones S. (2014). *Prelude to a Bruise.* Minneapolis, MI: Coffee House Press.

Kamps H. The patient as a text – metaphors in medicine. *Tidsskrift for den Norske læge-forening: tidsskrift for praktisk medicin, ny række.* 1999; 119: 2677–80.

Kanthan R, Mills S. Using metaphors, analogies and similes as aids in teaching pathology to medical students. *The Journal of the International Association of Medical Science Educators.* 2006; 16: 19–26.

Kipersztok L, Masukume G. Food for thought: palatable eponyms from pediatrics. *Malta Medical Journal.* 2014; 26: 51–5.

Kirklin D. Metaphors for medicine: revealing reflections or just popular parodies? *Journal of Medical Ethics: Medical Humanities.* 2001; 27: 89.

Kirklin, D. Truth telling, autonomy and the role of metaphor. *Journal of Medical Ethics* 2007; 33: 11–14.

Kistner U. Illness as metaphor? The role of linguistic categories in the history of medicine. *Studies in 20th Century Literature.* 1998; 22: Iss.1, Article 3.

Knorr-Cetina K. From pipes to scopes: the flow architecture of financial markets. *Distinktion: Journal of Social Theory.* 2003; 4: 7–23.

Kolko J. (2010). Sensemaking and framing: a theoretical reflection on perspective in design synthesis. In: the 2010 Design Research Society conference proceedings. Available at www.jonkolko.com/writingSensemaking.php. Last accessed: 16 August 2016.

Korkmaz H, Senol YY. Exploring first grade medical students' professional identity using metaphors: implications for medical curricula. *Medical Education Online.* 2014; 19: 20876.

Kost A, Chen FM. Socrates was not a pimp: changing the paradigm of questioning in medical education. *Academic Medicine.* 2015; 90: 20–4.

Krauthammer C. What are we hiding under the bandages of metaphor? *Los Angeles Times.* 18 May 1986. Available at http://articles.latimes.com/1986-05-18/opinion/op-21115_1_metaphor. Last accessed: 6 September 2016.

Kuppers P. (2006). *The Scar of Visibility: Medical Performances and Contemporary Art.* Minneapolis, MN: University of Minnesota Press.

Lakhtakia R. Twist of taste: gastronomic allusions in medicine. *Medical Humanities.* 2014; 40: 117–18.

Lakoff G, Johnson M. (1980). *Metaphors We Live By.* Chicago: University of Chicago Press.

Lakoff G, Johnson M. (1999). *Philosophy in the Flesh: The Embodied Mind and Its Challenge to Western Thought.* Ney York, NY: Basic Books.

Lakoff G, Turner M. (1989). *More than Cool Reason: A Field Guide to Poetic Metaphor.* Chicago, IL: University of Chicago Press.

Lam V. (2012). *The Headmaster's Wager.* London: HarperCollins UK.

Lammers T, Aime S, Hennink WE, Storm G, Kiessling F. Theranostic nanomedicine. *Accounts of Chemical Research.* 2011; 44: 1029–38.

Lane HP, McLachlan S, Philip J. The war against dementia: are we battle weary yet? *Age and Ageing.* 2013; 42: 281–3.

Langum V. (2013). Metaphor as medicine in medieval surgical manuals. UGPS Working Paper Series. Umea University. Available at www.academia.edu/19502646/Metaphor_as_Medicine_in_Medieval_Surigcal_Manuals [sic]. Last accessed: 18 August 2016.

Lapsley P, Groves T. The patient's journey: travelling through life with a chronic illness. *BMJ.* 2004; 329: 582.

Latour B. (2002). *Iconoclash: Beyond the Image Wars in Science, Religion, and Art.* Karlsruhe: Zentrum für Kunst und Medientechnologie (ZKM).

Latour B. (2010). *Reassembling the Social: An Introduction to Actor-Network-Theory.* Oxford: OUP.

Lauveng A. (2012). *A Road Back from Schizophrenia: a Memoir.* New York, NY: Skyhorse Publishing.

Leaf C. Why we're losing the war on cancer (and how to win it). *Fortune.* 2004; 149: 76–82.

Levine D, Bleakley A. Maximising medicine through aphorisms. *Medical Education.* 2012; 46: 153–62.

Lévi-Strauss C. (1969). *The Raw and the Cooked: Introduction to a Science of Mythology.* Vol. 1. New York, NY: Harper & Row.

LexiCon Research Group, University of Granada. (Undated). Available at: http://lexicon.ugr.es. Last accessed: 26 March 2017.

Low G, Todd Z, Deignan A, Cameron L (eds) (2010). *Researching and Applying Metaphor in the Real World.* Amsterdam: John Benjamins.

Lynn M. (2012). Pipes, reins, & the cerebral winepress: mechanical metaphor in Vesalius' *Fabrica.* Wonders & Marvels. Available at www.wondersandmarvels.com/2012/07/metaphor-vesalius-fabrica.html. Last accessed: 10 August 2016.

Lyotard J-F. (1979). *The Postmodern Condition: A Report on Knowledge.* Manchester: Manchester University Press.

Macbeck CE, Olesen F. Metaphorically transmitted diseases. How do patients embody medical explanations? *Family Practice.* 1997; 14: 271–8.

McCartney M. The fight is on: military metaphors for cancer may harm patients. *BMJ.* 2014; 349: g5155.

MacGill M. Food analogies work well for smell and look of disease, says pathologist. Medical News Today. 10 July 2014. Available at www.medicalnewstoday.com/articles/279339.php. Last accessed: 4 September 2016.

Mack P. (2011). *A History of Renaissance Rhetoric 1380–1620.* Oxford: OUP.

McLeary P. (2015). *The Cable.* Available at: http://foreignpolicy.com/2015/11/18/russia-insults-u-s-war-strategy-with-weird-cat-metaphor/. Last accessed: 26 March 2017.

MacNeill D. So you think gestures are nonverbal? *Psychological Review.* 1985; 92: 350–71.

Maglie R. (2009). *Understanding the Language of Medicine.* Rome: ARACNE editrice.

Maier B, Shibles WA. (2011). *The Philosophy and Practice of Medicine and Bioethics: A Naturalistic-Humanistic Approach.* Dordrecht: Springer.

Malone P. Why can't you talk to your radiologist? (and why sometimes you should). DC MedicalMalpractice & Patient Safety Blog. 7 December 2014. Available at www.protectpatientsblog.com/2014/12/why_cant_you_talk_to_your_radi.html. Last accessed: 6 September 2016.

Mangione S. The stethoscope as metaphor. *Cleveland Clinic Journal of Medicine* 2012; 79: 545–6.

Marshall R, Bleakley A. The death of Hector: pity in Homer, empathy in medical education. *Medical Humanities.* 2009; 35: 10–12.

Marshall R, Bleakley A. Lost in translation: Homer in English; the patient's story in medicine. *Medical Humanities.* 2013; 39: 47–52.

Martin E. (1994). *Flexible Bodies: Tracking Immunity in American Culture from the Days of Polio to the Age of AIDS.* Boston, MA: Beacon Press.

Martinez-Hernaez A. Biomedical psychiatry and its concealed metaphors: an anthropological perspective. *Collegium antropologicum.* 2013; 37: 1019–25.

Masukume G. Food for thought. *Croatian Medical Journal.* 2012; 53: 77–9.

Masukume G, Zumla A. Analogies and metaphors in clinical medicine. *Clinical Medicine (London).* 2012; 12: 55–6.

Mather C. The pipeline and the porcupine: alternate metaphors of the physician-industry relationship. *Social Science & Medicine.* 2005; 60: 1323–34.

Mattingly C. The machine-body as contested metaphor in clinical care. *Genre.* 2011; 44: 363–80.

Medicine pathways. Picmonic. Available at: www.picmonic.com/pathways/medicine. Last accessed: 26 March 2017.

Meisenberg BR, Meisenberg SW. The political use of the cancer metaphor: negative consequences for the public and the cancer community. *Journal of Cancer Education.* 2015; 30: 389–9.

Menary R. (ed.) (2010). *The Extended Mind.* London: MIT Press.

Menéndez-Viso A. Black and white transparency: contradictions of a moral metaphor. *Ethics and Information Technology.* 2009; 11: 155–62.

Merckelbach H, Devilly GJ, Rassin E. Alters in dissociative identity disorder. Metaphors or genuine entities? *Clinical Psychology Review.* 2002; 22: 481–97.

Metamia. (Undated). Available at: www.metamia.com. Last accessed: 26 March 2017.

Metaphor in End-of-Life Care (MELC) group. Available at www.research.lancs.ac.uk/portal/en/projects/metaphor-in-end-of-life-care(669c6aff-0494-4422-a341-2a8a039367a7).html; http://ucrel.lancs.ac.uk/melc/. Last accessed: 26 March 2017.

Milam EC, Mu EW, Orlow SJ. Culinary metaphors in dermatology: eating our words. *Journal of the American Medical Association Dermatology.* 2015; 151: 912. Available at: http://archderm.jamanetwork.com/article.aspx?articleid=2168932. Last accessed: 26 March 2017.

Miller L. Doctor at war, doctors washing feet. *Narrative Inquiry in Bioethics.* 2014; 4: 202–4.

Mitchell G, Ferguson-Pare M, Richards J. Exploring an alternative metaphor for nursing: relinquishing military images and language. *Canadian Journal of Nursing Leadership.* 2003; 16: 48–58.

Montgomery K. (2006). *How Doctors Think: Clinical Judgment and the Practice of Medicine.* Oxford: OUP.

Montgomery SL. (1996). Illness and image: on the contents of biomedical discourse. In: SL Montgomery (ed.) *The Scientific Voice.* New York, NY: The Guilford Press, 134–95.

Mossaheb N, Aschauer HN, Stoettner S, Schmoeger M, Pils N, Raab M, Willinger U. Comprehension of metaphors in patients with schizophrenia-spectrum disorders. *Comprehensive Psychiatry.* 2014; 55: 928–37.

Mullins S, Spence SA. Re-examining thought insertion: semi-structured literature review and conceptual analysis. *The British Journal of Psychiatry.* 2003; 182: 293–8.

Mustacchi P, Krevans JR. Metaphorically speaking: the metaphor of health care provision as a factory. *Western Journal of Medicine.* 2001; 175: 14–6.

Neilson S. Pain as metaphor: metaphor and medicine. *Medical Humanities.* 2015; 42: 3–10.

Neuroscience for Kids. The synapse. 4 September 2016. Available at: https://faculty. washington.edu/chudler/synapse.html. Last accessed: 6 September 2016.

Nevins M. (2010). *Abraham Flexner: A Flawed American Icon.* Bloomington, IN: iUniverse.

Nicholas G. Metaphors and malignancy: making sense of cancer. *Current Oncology.* 2013; 20: e608–9.

Nietzsche F. (2015 reprint). *On Truth and Lies in a Nonmoral Sense.* Charleston: CreateSpace.

Nimnuan C, Hotopf M, Wessely S. Medically unexplained symptoms: an epidemiological study in seven specialities. *Journal of Psychosomatic Research.* 2001; 51: 361–7.

Nordquist R. Metaphor (figure of speech and thought). 3 December 2015. Available at: http://grammar.about.com/od/mo/g/metaphorterm.htm. Last accessed: 18 August 2016.

Not to Be Reproduced. (Undated). Wikipedia. Available at: https://en.wikipedia.org/wiki/ Not_to_be_Reproduced. Last accessed: 26 March 2017.

Nowotny H. (2015). *The Cunning of Uncertainty.* Cambridge: Polity.

O'Brien M. (Undated). Martin O'Brien: performance artist. Available at: http://martin obrienperformance.weebly.com/performance.html. Last accessed: 26 March 2017.

O'Brien M. Performing chronic: chronic illness and endurance art. *Performance Research.* 2014: 19: 54–63.

Ofri D. Poetry in medicine. (Undated). Available at http://danielleofri.com/poetry-in-medicine/. Last accessed: 17 August 2016.

Olsman E, Duggleby W, Nekolaichuk C, Willems D, Gagnon J, Kruizinga R. Leget C. Improving communication on hope in palliative care. A qualitative study of palliative care professionals' metaphors of hope: grip, source, tune, and vision. *Journal of Pain and Symptom Management.* 2014; 48: 831–8.

Osherson S, AmaraSingham L. (1981). The machine metaphor in medicine. In: E Mishler, G Mishler, L AmaraSingham (eds) *Social Contexts of Health, Illness and Patient Care.* New York, NY: Cambridge University Press, 218–49. Out of print chapter. Available at http://n.ereserve.fiu.edu/010007672-1.pdf. Last accessed: 2 September 2016.

Ott PW. Medicine as metaphor: John Wesley on therapy of the soul. *Methodist History.* 1995; 33: 178–91.

Padel R. (1992). *In and out of the Mind: Greek Images of the Tragic Self.* Princeton, NJ: Princeton University Press.

Padfield D. 'Representing' the pain of others. *Health.* 2011; 15: 241–57.

Padfield D, Hurwitz B, Pither C. (2003). *Perceptions of Pain.* Stockport: Dewi Lewis Publishing.

Padfield D, Janmohamed F, Zakrzewska JM, Hurwitz B. A slippery surface ... can photo-graphic images of pain improve communication in pain consultations? *International Journal of Surgery.* 2010; 8: 144–50.

Parsons GN, Kinsman SB, Bosk CL, Sankar P, Ubel PA. Between two worlds medical student perceptions of humor and slang in the hospital setting. *Journal of General Internal Medicine.* 2001; 16: 544–9.

Patten SB. Medical models and metaphors for depression. *Epidemiology and Psychiatric Sciences.* 2015; 24: 303–8.

Pauli HG, White KL, McWhinney IR. Medical education, research, and scientific think-ing in the 21st century. *Education for Health.* 2000; 13: 15–25, 165–72, 173–86.

Pena E. Lost in translation: methodological considerations in cross-cultural research. *Child Development.* 2007; 78: 1255–64.

Pena GP, Andrade-Filho Jde S. Analogies in medicine: valuable for learning, reasoning, remembering and naming. *Advances in Health Sciences Education: Theory and Practice*. 2010; 15: 609–19.

Penson RT, Schapira L, Daniels KJ, Chabner BA, Lynch TJ. Cancer as metaphor. *The Oncologist*. 2004; 9: 708–16.

Performing Medicine. (Undated). Available at: http://performingmedicine.com/category/performance/. Last accessed: 26 March 2017.

Peterkin A, Bleakley A. (2017). *Staying Human during the Foundation Programme: How to Thrive after Medical School*. London: Taylor & Francis.

Phillips A. (1994). *On kissing, tickling, and being bored*. Cambridge, MA: Harvard University Press.

Pickering N. (2006). *The metaphor of mental illness*. Oxford: OUP.

Piemonte N. Last laughs: gallows humor and medical education. *The Journal of Medical Humanities*. 2015; 36: 375–90.

Pies R. Mind-language in the age of the brain: is 'mental illness' a useful term? *Journal of Psychiatric Practice*. 2015; 21: 79–83.

Pilkington E. The Ashley treatment: 'Her life is as good as we can possibly make it.' *Guardian*. 15 March 2012. Available at: www.theguardian.com/society/2012/mar/15/ashley-treatment-email-exchange. Last accessed: 31 August 2016.

Pinar WF. (1975). The method of 'Currere'. Paper presented at the Annual Meeting of the American Research Association, Washington DC, April 1975. Available at: http://files.eric.ed.gov/fulltext/ED104766.pdf. Last accessed: 13 November 2016.

Plath S. (1960). *The Colossus and Other Poems*. London: William Heinemann.

Plath S. (1960). Metaphors. Genius. Available at: http://genius.com/Sylvia-plath-metaphors-annotated. Last accessed: 26 March 2017.

Polanyi M. (1983). *The Tacit Dimension*. Gloucester: Smith.

Polanyi M, Prosch H. (1975). *Meaning*. Chicago: University of Chicago Press.

Potts A, Semino E. (forthcoming 2017). Healthcare professionals' online use of violence metaphors for care at the end of life in the US: a corpus-based comparison with the UK. *Corpora*.

Pragglejaz Group. MIP: a method for identifying metaphorically used words in discourse. *Metaphor and Symbol* 2007; 22: 1–39. Available at: www.lancaster.ac.uk/staff/eiaes/Pragglejaz_Group_2007.pdf. Last accessed: 26 March 2017.

Radiology Quality Institute. (2012). Radisphere: diagnostic accuracy in radiology: defining a literature-based benchmark. Available at: www.radisphereradiology.com/wp-content/uploads/Diagnostic-Accuracy-in-Radiology. Last accessed: 3 October 2016.

Radiopaedia. (Undated). Available at: https://radiopaedia.org. Last accessed: 26 March 2017

Reber AS. (1996). *Implicit Learning and Tacit Knowledge: An Essay on the Cognitive Unconscious*. Oxford: OUP.

Reddy M. The conduit metaphor: a case of frame conflict in our language about language. In: A Ortony (ed.) (1993, 2nd edn) *Metaphor and Thought*. Cambridge: CUP, 164–201.

Regehr G. It's NOT rocket science: rethinking our metaphors for research in health professions education. *Medical Education*. 2010; 44: 31–9.

Reisfield GM, Wilson GR. Use of metaphor in the discourse on cancer. *Journal of Clinical Oncology*. 2004; 22: 4024–7.

Rhodes LA. 'This will clear your mind': the use of metaphors for medication in psychiatric settings. *Culture, Medicine and Psychiatry* 1984; 8: 49–70.

Richards IA. (1965). *The Philosophy of Rhetoric.* Oxford: OUP.

Ricoeur P. (2003). *The Rule of Metaphor: The Creation of Meaning in Language.* London: Routledge.

Risen C. The Lady Macbeth effect. *New York Times Magazine.* 10 December 2006. Available at: www.nytimes.com/2006/12/10/magazine/10Section2a.t-9.html?_r=0. Last accessed: 6 September 2016.

Ritchie D. 'Argument is war' – or is it a game of chess? Multiple meanings in the analysis of implicit metaphors. *Metaphor and Symbol.* 2003; 18: 125–46.

Rodriguez C, Bélanger E. Stories and metaphors in the sensemaking of multiple primary health care organizational identities. *BMC Family Practice.* 2014; 15: 41.

Rodulson V, Marshall R, Bleakley A. Whistleblowing in medicine and in Homer's *Iliad. Medical Humanities.* 2015; 41: 95–101.

Rorty R. (1991). *Essays on Heidegger and Others.* New York, NY: Cambridge University Press, 12–13.

Rosai J. (2004). *Rosai and Ackerman's Surgical Pathology.* St Louis, MO: Mosby, 721.

Rosen M. Performance poetry: the word of the moment. *Guardian.* Friday 9 May 2014. Available at: www.theguardian.com/commentisfree/2014/may/09/performance-poetry-turner-prize-judges-spoken-word. Last accessed: 6 September 2016.

Rosenman S. Metaphor in clinical practice. *Australian Family Physician.* 2008a; 37: 865–6.

Rosenman S. Metaphor, meaning and psychiatry. *Australasian Psychiatry: Bulletin of Royal Australian and New Zealand College of Psychiatrists.* 2008b; 16: 391–6.

Salager-Meyer, F. Metaphors in medical English prose: a comparative study with French and Spanish. *English for Specific Purposes.* 1990; 9: 145–59.

Santarpia A, Venturini A, Blanchet A, Cavallo M. Metaphorical conceptualizations of the body in psychopathology and poetry. *Documentação de Estudos em Lingüística Teórica e Aplicada.* 2010; 26 especial: 435–51.

Scarry E. (1985). *The Body in Pain: The Making and Unmaking of the World.* Oxford: OUP.

Schaefer M, Rotte M, Heinze H-J, Denke C. Dirty deeds and dirty bodies: embodiment of the Macbeth effect is mapped topographically onto the somatosensory cortex. *Scientific Reports.* 2015; 5: Article number 18051.

Schleifer R, Vannatta JB. (2013). *The Chief Concern of Medicine: The Integration of the Medical Humanities and Narrative Knowledge into Medical Practices.* Ann Arbor, MI: University of Michigan Press.

Schön D. (1983). *The Reflective Practitioner.* New York, NY: Basic.

Schön D. (1990). *Educating the Reflective Practitioner: Towards a New Design for Teaching and Learning in the Professions.* Oxford: Jossey-Bass.

Schwartz A. (2016). *ADHD Nation: The Disorder. The Drugs. The Inside Story.* London: Little, Brown.

Schwartz ES. Metaphors and medically unexplained symptoms. *The Lancet.* 2015; 386: 734–5.

Selzer R. (1996) *Mortal Lessons: Notes on the Art of Surgery.* San Diego: Harvest.

Semino E. Descriptions of pain, metaphor and embodied simulation. *Metaphor and Symbol.* 2010; 25: 205–26.

Semino, E. The adaptation of metaphors across genres. *Review of Cognitive Linguistics.* 2011; 9: 130–52.

Semino E, Demjen Z, Demmen J, Koller V, Payne S, Hardie A, Rayson P. The online use of Violence and Journey metaphors by patients with cancer, as compared with health professionals: a mixed methods study. *BMJ Supportive & Palliative Care.* 2017; 7: 60–6.

Sfard A. On two metaphors for learning and the danger of choosing just one. *Educational Researcher.* 1998; 27: 4–13.

Shen, W. (2014). Is the quest to build a kinder, gentler surgeon misguided? Available at: https://psmag.com/is-the-quest-to-build-a-kinder-gentler-surgeon-misguided-3950dee829fa#.azxd62ipp. Last accessed: 29 September 2016.

Shenoi J. The art of analogies in the clinic. 7 March 2011. Available at: www.onclive.com/publications/oncology-fellows/2010/August-2010/The-Art-of-Analogies-in-the-Clinic#sthash.FFnKeKUz.dpuf. Last accessed: 21 August 2016.

Shibles W. (1971). *Metaphor: An Annotated Bibliography and History.* Whitewater, WI: The Language Press.

Sigma-Aldrich. (Undated). Custom CRISPR products. Available at: www.sigmaaldrich.com/catalog/product/sigma/crispr?lang=en&region=GB. Last accessed: 26 March 2017.

Sinha P. Medicine at the mercy of a metaphor: why we need to speak differently about death and disease. *The Huffington Post.* 25 February 2015. Available at: www.huffingtonpost.com/pranay-sinha/medicine-at-the-mercy-of-_b_6746176.html. Last accessed: 18 August 2016.

Skelton JR, Wearn AM, Hobbs FDR. A concordance-based study of metaphoric expressions used by general practitioners and patients in consultation. *British Journal of General Practice* 2002; 52: 114–18.

Skelton JR, Whetstone J. English for Medical Purposes and Academic Medicine: looking for the common ground. *Ibérica* 2012; 24: 87–102.

Skott C. Expressive metaphors in cancer narratives. *Cancer Nursing.* 2002; 25: 230–5.

Slobod D, Fuks A. Military metaphors and friendly fire. *Canadian Medical Association Journal.* 2012; 184: 144.

Smith DW. (2005). Critical, clinical. In: CJ Stivale (ed.) *Gilles Deleuze: Key Concepts.* Stocksfield: Acumen.

Smith JN, Gunderman RB. Should we inform patients of radiology results? *Radiology.* 2010; 255: 317–21.

Sontag S. (1978). *Illness as Metaphor.* New York, NY: Farrar, Straus & Giroux.

Sontag S. (1989). *AIDS and Its Metaphors.* New York, NY: Farrar, Straus & Giroux.

Specter M. How the DNA revolution is changing us. *National Geographic.* August 2016. Available at: www.nationalgeographic.com/magazine/2016/08/dna-crispr-gene-editing-science-ethics/. Last accessed: 4 November 2016.

Steslow K. Metaphors in our mouths: the silencing of the psychiatric patient. *The Hastings Center Report.* 2010; 40: 30–3.

Stevens W. (1954). *Collected Poems.* New York, NY: Knopf.

Stewart M. (2016) The road to pain reconceptualisation: do metaphors help or hinder the journey? Pre-publication. Available at http://knowpain.co.uk/the-road-to-pain-reconceptualisation-do-metaphors-help-or-hinder-the-journey/. Last accessed: 1 September 2016.

Stineman MG, Streim JE. The biopsycho-ecological paradigm: a foundational theory for medicine. *PM & R: the Journal of Injury, Function, and Rehabilitation.* 2010; 2: 1035–45.

Stolberg M. Metaphors and images of cancer in early modern Europe. *Bulletin of the History of Medicine.* 2014; 88: 48–74.

Stroud JH, Sardello R. (2015). *Gaston Bachelard: An Elemental Reverie of the World's Stuff.* Dallas, TX: Dallas Institute Publications.

Study group discussion: Food analogies in Medicine. (2015). Medicowesome. Available at: http://medicowesome.blogspot.co.uk/2015/02/study-group-discussion-food-analogies. html. Last accessed: 26 March 2017.

Styron W. (1992). *Darkness Visible.* London: Vintage.

Szasz T. (1974). *The Myth of Mental Illness.* New York, NY: Harper.

Taussig M. (2001). *The Nervous System.* London: Routledge.

Temmerman R. (2000). *Towards New Ways of Terminology Description: The Sociocognitive Approach.* Amsterdam: John Benjamins.

Terry SI, Hanchard B. Gastrology: the use of culinary terms in medicine. *BMJ* 1979; 2: 1636–9.

Thagard P. (1997). Medical analogies: why and how? In: P Langley, M Shafto (eds) *Proceedings of the Nineteenth Annual Conference of the Cognitive Science Society.* Mahwah: Erlbaum.

The Treachery of Images. (Undated). Wikipedia. Available at: https://en.wikipedia.org/ wiki/The_Treachery_of_Images. Last accessed: 26 March 2017.

Thomas SP. Anger: the mismanaged emotion. *Dermatology Nursing.* 2003; 15: 351–7.

University of Ottawa. (Undated). Two rival medical models of disease. Available at: www.med.uottawa.ca/sim/data/Models/Osler_Garrod.htm. Last accessed: 26 March 2017.

Urbanski M, Bréchemier ML, Garcin B, Bendetowicz D, Thiebaut de Schotten M, Foulon C, Rosso C, Clarençon F, Dupont S, Pradat-Diehl P, Labeyrie MA, Levy R, Volle E. Reasoning by analogy requires the left frontal pole: lesion-deficit mapping and clinical implications. *Brain.* 2016; 139(Pt 6): 1783–99.

Vaihinger H. (1924). *The Philosophy of 'As If'.* London: Routledge.

Vaisrub S. (1977). *Medicine's Metaphors: Messages & Menaces.* New Jersey, NJ: Medical Economics Co.

Valle RS, von Eckartsberg R (eds) (1981). *The Metaphors of Consciousness.* New York: Plenum Press.

Vallely SR, Mills JO. Should radiologists talk to patients? *BMJ.* 1990; 300: 305–6.

Van Nes F, Abma T, Jonsson H, Deeg D. Language differences in qualitative research: is meaning lost in translation? *European Journal of Ageing.* 2010; 7: 313–16.

Van Rijn-van Tongeren GW. (1997). *Metaphors in medical texts.* Amsterdam: Rodopi.

Verghese A. (Undated). Q/A with Abraham Verghese. Available at: http://abraham verghese.com/home/faq/. Last accessed: 26 Mar 2017.

Verghese A. 'Soundings'. *Granta.* 1992; 31: 81–90.

Verghese A. (1994). *My Own Country: A Doctor's Story of a Town and Its People in the Age of AIDS.* New York, NY: Simon & Schuster.

Verghese A. (2009). *Cutting for Stone.* London: Chatto & Windus.

Verghese A. A doctor's touch. TED talk. 2011. Available at www.ted.com/talks/ abraham_verghese_a_doctor_s_touch; www.youtube.com/watch?v=sxnlvwprf_c. Last accessed: 6 September 2016.

Verghese A. Rituals, metaphors and medicine in a tech age. 2014a. Available at: www. youtube.com/watch?v=iQ7rnWyAbZo. Last accessed: 29 August 2016.

Verghese A. 2014b. TEDMED. A linguistic prescription for ailing communication. Available at: www.tedmed.com/talks/show?id=292979. Last accessed: 29 August 2016.

Verghese A. Dying patients benefit from doctors' honest communication, compassion. Life Matters Media. 25 April 2015. Available at: www.lifemattersmedia.org/2015/04/ abraham-verghese-dying-patients-benefit-from-doctors-honest-communication- compassion/. Last accessed: 6 September 2016.

Vogt P, Mach F. The war is over – let us learn to work together. *Revue médicale suisse.* 2015; 11: 1163–4.

Volk P. On language; medical edibles. 19 August 1990. *New York Times Magazine.* Available at: www.nytimes.com/1990/08/19/magazine/on-language-medical-edibles. html. Last accessed: 20 August 2016.

Warren VL. The 'medicine is war' metaphor. *HEC Forum.* 1991; 3: 39–50.

Way EC. (1994). *Knowledge Representation and Metaphor.* Oxford: Intellect.

Webb JR, Valasek MA, North CS. Prevalence of stimulant use in a sample of US medical students. *Annals of Clinical Psychiatry.* 2013; 25: 27–32.

Wieringa S, Greenhalgh T. 10 years of mindlines: a systematic review and commentary. *Implementation Science.* 2015; 10: 45. Available at: http://implementationscience. biomedcentral.com/articles/10.1186/s13012-015-0229-x. Last accessed: 18 August 2016.

Wiggins NM. Stop using military metaphors for disease. *BMJ.* 2012; 345: e4706.

Williams WC. (1923/2015). *Spring and All.* Eastford, CT: Martino Fine Books.

Wiltshire J. (1991). *Samuel Johnson in the Medical World.* Cambridge: CUP.

Wirtztum E, van der Hart O, Friedman B. The use of metaphors in psychotherapy. *Journal of Contemporary Psychotherapy.* 1988; unpaginated. Available at www. onnovdhart.nl/articles/metaphors.pdf. Last accessed: 6 September 2016.

Wohlmann A. (Undated). Available at: www.grk.lifesciences-lifewriting.uni-mainz.de/ research-projects/dr-anita-wohlmann-medical-metaphors/. Last accessed: 26 March 2017.

Wohlmann A. (2015). Medical metaphors. Life Sciences Writing. 2015. Available at www.grk.lifesciences-lifewriting.uni-mainz.de/research-projects/dr-anita-wohlmann-medical-metaphors/. Last accessed: 16 August 2016.

Woods C. 'Everything is medicine': Burke's master metaphor? *KB Journal.* 2009; 5: not paginated. Available at: http://digitalcommons.unl.edu/cgi/viewcontent.cgi?article=103 0&context=commstudiespapers. Last accessed: 18 August 2016.

Wooliscroft JO, Phillips R. Medicine as a performing art: a worthy metaphor. *Medical Education.* 2003; 37: 934–9.

Xie J, Lee S, Chen X. Nanoparticle-based theranostic agents. *Advanced Drug Delivery Reviews.* 2010; 62: 1064–79.

Yates F. (1966). The *Art of Memory.* London: Bodley Head.

Zeev-Wolf M, Faust M, Levkovitz Y, Harpaz Y, Goldstein A. Magnetoencephalographic evidence of early right hemisphere overactivation during metaphor comprehension in schizophrenia. *Psychophysiology.* 2015; 52: 770–81.

Zhong CB, Liljenquist K. Washing away your sins: threatened morality and physical cleansing. *Science.* 2006; 313: 1451–2.

Index

Page numbers in **bold** denote figures, those in *italics* denote tables.

CPSIA information can be obtained
at www.ICGtesting.com
Printed in the USA
BVHW041334260821
615312BV00014B/397